Evaluating Novel Biomarkers for Personalized Medicine

Evaluating Novel Biomarkers for Personalized Medicine

Editors

Tudor Drugan
Daniel Leucuta

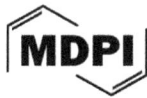

Basel • Beijing • Wuhan • Barcelona • Belgrade • Novi Sad • Cluj • Manchester

Editors
Tudor Drugan
Medical Informatics and
Biostatistics
Iuliu Hatieganu University of
Medicine and Pharmacy
Cluj-Napoca
Romania

Daniel Leucuta
Medical Informatics and
Biostatistics
Iuliu Hatieganu University of
Medicine and Pharmacy
Cluj-Napoca
Romania

Editorial Office
MDPI
St. Alban-Anlage 66
4052 Basel, Switzerland

This is a reprint of articles from the Special Issue published online in the open access journal *Diagnostics* (ISSN 2075-4418) (available at: www.mdpi.com/journal/diagnostics/special_issues/7YI40QN1E4).

For citation purposes, cite each article independently as indicated on the article page online and as indicated below:

Lastname, A.A.; Lastname, B.B. Article Title. *Journal Name* **Year**, *Volume Number*, Page Range.

ISBN 978-3-7258-0692-8 (Hbk)
ISBN 978-3-7258-0691-1 (PDF)
doi.org/10.3390/books978-3-7258-0691-1

© 2024 by the authors. Articles in this book are Open Access and distributed under the Creative Commons Attribution (CC BY) license. The book as a whole is distributed by MDPI under the terms and conditions of the Creative Commons Attribution-NonCommercial-NoDerivs (CC BY-NC-ND) license.

Contents

About the Editors vii

Preface ix

Tudor Drugan and Daniel Leucuța
Evaluating Novel Biomarkers for Personalized Medicine
Reprinted from: *Diagnostics* **2024**, *14*, 587, doi:10.3390/diagnostics14060587 1

Efsun Somay, Erkan Topkan, Busra Yilmaz, Ali Ayberk Besen, Hüseyin Mertsoylu and Ugur Selek
Predicting Teeth Extraction after Concurrent Chemoradiotherapy in Locally Advanced Nasopharyngeal Cancer Patients Using the Novel GLUCAR Index
Reprinted from: *Diagnostics* **2023**, *13*, 3594, doi:10.3390/diagnostics13233594 5

Alexandru Stan, Paul-Adrian Călburean, Reka-Katalin Drinkal, Marius Harpa, Ayman Elkahlout, Viorel Constantin Nicolae, et al.
Inflammatory Status Assessment by Machine Learning Techniques to Predict Outcomes in Patients with Symptomatic Aortic Stenosis Treated by Transcatheter Aortic Valve Replacement
Reprinted from: *Diagnostics* **2023**, *13*, 2907, doi:10.3390/diagnostics13182907 18

Josipa Radić, Sanja Lovrić Kojundžić, Andrea Gelemanović, Marijana Vučković, Danijela Budimir Mršić, Daniela Šupe Domić, et al.
Serum Adropin Levels and Body Mass Composition in Kidney Transplant Recipients—Are There Sex Differences?
Reprinted from: *Diagnostics* **2023**, *13*, 2768, doi:10.3390/diagnostics13172768 29

Nicoleta Ștefania Motoc, Iulia Făgărășan, Andrada Elena Urda-Cîmpean and Doina Adina Todea
Prognosis Predictive Markers in Patients with Chronic Obstructive Pulmonary Disease and COVID-19
Reprinted from: *Diagnostics* **2023**, *13*, 2597, doi:10.3390/diagnostics13152597 42

Crina Claudia Rusu, Ina Kacso, Diana Moldovan, Alina Potra, Dacian Tirinescu, Maria Ticala, et al.
Triiodothyronine and Protein Malnutrition Could Influence Pulse Wave Velocity in Pre-Dialysis Chronic Kidney Disease Patients
Reprinted from: *Diagnostics* **2023**, *13*, 2462, doi:10.3390/diagnostics13142462 59

Larisa Cujba, Cristina Stan, Ovidiu Samoila, Tudor Drugan, Ancuta Benedec (Cutas) and Cristina Nicula
Identifying Optical Coherence Tomography Markers for Multiple Sclerosis Diagnosis and Management
Reprinted from: *Diagnostics* **2023**, *13*, 2077, doi:10.3390/diagnostics13122077 70

Ioana-Andreea Gheban-Roșca, Bogdan-Alexandru Gheban, Bogdan Pop, Daniela-Cristina Mironescu, Vasile Costel Siserman, Elena Mihaela Jianu, et al.
Identification of Histopathological Biomarkers in Fatal Cases of Coronavirus Disease: A Study on Lung Tissue
Reprinted from: *Diagnostics* **2023**, *13*, 2039, doi:10.3390/diagnostics13122039 85

**Ioana-Andreea Chiș, Vlad Andrei, Alexandrina Muntean, Marioara Moldovan,
Anca Ștefania Mesaroș, Mircea Cristian Dudescu and Aranka Ilea**
Salivary Biomarkers of Anti-Epileptic Drugs: A Narrative Review
Reprinted from: *Diagnostics* **2023**, *13*, 1962, doi:10.3390/diagnostics13111962 . . . . **99**

**Lavinia Patricia Mocan, Ioana Rusu, Carmen Stanca Melincovici, Bianca Adina Boșca,
Tudor Mocan, Rareș Crăciun, et al.**
The Role of Immunohistochemistry in the Differential Diagnosis between Intrahepatic Cholangiocarcinoma, Hepatocellular Carcinoma and Liver Metastasis, as Well as Its Prognostic Value
Reprinted from: *Diagnostics* **2023**, *13*, 1542, doi:10.3390/diagnostics13091542 . . . . **122**

**Vlad-Ionuț Nechita, Nadim Al Hajjar, Cristina Drugan, Cristina-Sorina Cătană, Emil Moiș,
Mihaela-Ancuța Nechita and Florin Graur**
Chitotriosidase and Neopterin as Two Novel Potential Biomarkers for Advanced Stage and Survival Prediction in Gastric Cancer—A Pilot Study
Reprinted from: *Diagnostics* **2023**, *13*, 1362, doi:10.3390/diagnostics13071362 . . . . **135**

Sonya Youngju Park, Deog-Gon Cho, Byoung-Yong Shim and Uiju Cho
Relationship between Systemic Inflammatory Markers, GLUT1 Expression, and Maximum 18F-Fluorodeoxyglucose Uptake in Non-Small Cell Lung Carcinoma and Their Prognostic Significance
Reprinted from: *Diagnostics* **2023**, *13*, 1013, doi:10.3390/diagnostics13061013 . . . . **145**

About the Editors

Tudor Drugan

Professor Tudor Drugan has been working at the Medical Informatics Discipline since 1995, covering cycle I (Bachelor's Degree, Faculty of Medicine: Biostatistics and Medical Informatics, Scientific Research Methodology, Critical Appraisal of Medical Scientific Literature), cycle II (Scientific Research Methodology and Bioinformatics courses for UMF master's degrees), and cycle III (Scientific Research Methodology for the Doctoral School of UMF).

His areas of interest include medical scientific research methodologies, biostatistics, bioinformatics, computer-assisted medical education, and artificial intelligence applications in medical research.

Daniel Leucuta

As a senior lecturer, Daniel Leucuța has been working at the Department of Medical Informatics and Biostatistics from 2005, where he teaches Biostatistics and Medical Informatics, Critical Appraisal of Medical Scientific Literature, and Scientific Research Methodology (for students, masters, and PhD students).

His main topics of interest include systematic reviews and meta-analyses, quality assessment of articles, and statistical analyses (multivariate methods).

Preface

Standard and cutting-edge biomarkers used for the diagnosis and evaluation of different illnesses will be covered in this Special Issue. Emphasis will be placed on personalized medicine, since this innovative strategy enables healthcare professionals to identify the most effective therapies for each patient using diagnostic tests and biomarkers.

Evidence-based findings indicate that many medications are unsuccessful for some individuals; as such, this method is crucial. Healthcare professionals can create individual preventative plans and treatment plans by considering the patient's medical history, as well as biomarkers throughout the diagnosis process. This strategy benefits patients and the healthcare system, according to several cost-effective studies.

Treatments that are customized for each patient offer both medical and financial benefits, making them not only essential for patients and physicians, but also welcomed by regulatory agencies as well as insurance providers.

Tudor Drugan and Daniel Leucuta
Editors

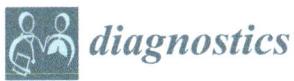 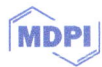

Editorial

Evaluating Novel Biomarkers for Personalized Medicine

Tudor Drugan * and Daniel Leucuța

Department of Medical Informatics and Biostatistics, Faculty of Medicine, Iuliu Hațieganu University of Medicine and Pharmacy, 400349 Cluj-Napoca, Romania
* Correspondence: tdrugan@umfcluj.ro

1. Introduction

Personalized medicine, sometimes referred to as precision medicine, is a paradigm shift in healthcare. This model is based on the concept of customizing prevention and treatment approaches to particular cohorts of individuals, drawing on the genetic predispositions, lifestyle choices, and distinctive personal circumstances of individuals. Therefore, uniform therapeutic modalities are not implemented across patient populations as they are with conventional therapies; rather, individual patient characterization and comprehensive pre-testing are emphasized to discern the optimal treatment avenue. Remarkably, traditional one-size-fits-all therapeutic concepts often ignore critical individual variables such as genetic makeup, health status, age, and gender, hence resulting in variable treatment outcomes, from remarkable efficacy to complete inefficiency.

Modern medical research has been increasingly devoted to pioneering individualized diagnostic methodologies and pharmacotherapies personalized to the distinct needs of each patient. Within this context, biomarkers specific to disease provide useful information about the type, molecular etiology, and stage of a disease, leading the way for personalized therapeutic intervention [1,2]. A biomarker can be measured quantitatively and is indicated according to objective evidence representing a biological process, the stage of a disease, or the response of an organism to a given therapeutic intervention.

These biomarkers include a wide array of biological substances or characteristics, such as molecules, nucleic acids (DNA—Deoxyribonucleic Acid, mRNA—Messenger Ribonucleic Acid), microRNA, small interfering RNA, proteins, proteoglycans, lipids, sphingolipids, cells, and imaging features that are detectable and quantifiable in biological samples such as blood, urine, tissues, or imaging scans [3,4].

In assessing patients' health, biomarkers play a crucial role in several aspects:

- Disease Diagnosis: Biomarkers can assist in the early recognition and diagnosis of disease, mainly in targeting molecular signatures or definite abnormalities that are linked to a condition. For example, high levels of certain proteins in the blood could signify cancer is present in the body.
- Prognosis of Disease: Biomarkers may also become useful information tools for prognosis, that is, predicting how a disease is likely to develop or run its course. This is able to help physicians estimate how the disease will progress over time, the risk of it recurring, and overall survival rates, which all help to manage patients and aid in the prescription of treatments.
- Choice of Treatment: Biomarkers can help to decide who may best be treated using a particular therapy. Biomarker-guided therapy can hence select the right treatment for the right patients based on individual characteristics so as to optimize the treatment efficacy and minimize any adverse effects.
- Biomarker assessment can be used to monitor the response to treatment to longitudinally capture its course and any deviations that occur in biological markers associated with disease progression or the therapeutic response from baseline to the final round. In general, the use of biomarkers is increasing across the board and within

Citation: Drugan, T.; Leucuța, D. Evaluating Novel Biomarkers for Personalized Medicine. *Diagnostics* **2024**, *14*, 587. https://doi.org/10.3390/diagnostics14060587

Received: 20 February 2024
Accepted: 6 March 2024
Published: 11 March 2024

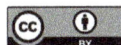

Copyright: © 2024 by the authors. Licensee MDPI, Basel, Switzerland. This article is an open access article distributed under the terms and conditions of the Creative Commons Attribution (CC BY) license (https://creativecommons.org/licenses/by/4.0/).

different medical disciplines to further develop personalized medicine and deliver precision healthcare.

The assessment of biomarkers in medical studies is systematically undertaken to estimate validity, reliability, and clinical utility in light of providing an appropriate diagnosis, prognosis, or prediction or following diagnosis progress. In terms of the process, biomarker assessment generally includes some essential steps:

- Biomarker identification and selection: Relevant biomarker candidates are identified based on preclinical studies, exploratory analyses, and literature reviews and should be related to the indication of these studies, if relevant. A biomarker is a molecular, cellular, or imaging-based characteristic that facilitates distinguishing between the different stages of a disease and predicting the impact of therapeutic interventions.
- Analytical validation: This is how the technical performance characteristics of an assay measuring biomarkers or of the method of measurement itself are examined. Here, the parameters evaluated are the sensitivity, specificity, accuracy, precision, reproducibility, and robustness of biomarker measurement to ensure its reliability across laboratories and platforms.
- Validation of clinical utility: In addition to defining diagnostic or prognostic accuracy, validation of a biomarker includes evaluation of its clinical utility, where clinical utility means the impact of using a biomarker on patient management decisions, therapeutic outcomes, and healthcare resource utilization.
- Long-term monitoring and further research: Following regulatory approval and adoption into practice, monitoring and further research will have to continue with a view to realizing in real-life settings what can be achieved using biomarker-guided interventions, including their long-term safety and effectiveness. Finally, the execution of follow-up post-marketing surveillance, longitudinal observational studies, and comparative effective research aimed at refining clinical algorithms and optimizing the patient outcomes may be required.

In summary, assessing biomarkers in medical research involves a complex procedure demanding rigorous scientific examination, clinical verification, and regulatory supervision to guarantee their dependable and purposeful utilization in healthcare environments. Proficient biomarker assessment has the potential to expedite the advancement of personalized medicine methodologies, enhance clinical decision-making, and ultimately elevate the quality of patient care.

2. Brief Overview and List of Contributions

The Special Issue of the MDPI scientific journal *Diagnostics*, entitled "Evaluating Novel Biomarkers for Personalized Medicine", will focus on this exact topic. Indeed, the eleven articles in this issue cover a wide array of medical subfields, with a scope intended to be widely applicable and demonstrative of the great importance of the research on biomarkers in personalized healthcare. From predicting the treatment outcomes in cancer to assessing inflammatory status in cardiovascular disease, important insights into how biomarkers may transform clinical practice are provided.

For instance, the use of the newly developed GLUCAR Index is assessed for the prediction of the risk of teeth extraction among nasopharyngeal cancer patients receiving chemoradiotherapy and of the inflammatory status of patients who have undergone transcatheter aortic valve replacement due to symptomatic aortic stenosis using machine learning techniques.

Further, the action of serum adropin levels in kidney transplant recipients; the prognostic markers in patients suffering from chronic obstructive pulmonary disease and COVID-19; and the effect of triiodothyronine and protein malnutrition on pulse wave velocity in pre-dialysis patients with chronic kidney disease are all analyzed.

Furthermore, it includes pioneering research on the detection of optical coherence tomography markers for multiple sclerosis diagnosis and management, histopathological biomarkers in coronavirus disease fatalities, and the value of immuno-histochemistry in determining the prognosis for different liver cancers.

Lastly, discussed as newly developed biomarkers are chitotriosidase and neopterin for the prognosis in gastric cancer; systemic inflammatory markers and their interaction with glucose transporter expression in non-small-cell lung carcinoma; and salivary biomarkers of anti-epileptic drugs.

These articles therefore indicate the evolving status of the research on biomarkers and its vital involvement in driving personalized medicine, ultimately leading to much more focused and effective patient care strategies.

3. Conclusions

In conclusion, biomarkers greatly contribute to correctly assessing a patient's status in personalized medicine, as they provide invaluable insight into individual biological characteristics and the process of disease. Thus, according to the careful estimation of biomarkers in individuals, healthcare providers are able to design treatment strategies, optimize the therapeutical outcomes, and eventually provide improved patient care within a new era of personalized medicine.

Funding: This research received no external funding.

Conflicts of Interest: The authors declare no conflict of interest.

List of Contributions

1. Somay E, Topkan E, Yilmaz B, Besen AA, Mertsoylu H, Selek U. Predicting Teeth Extraction after Concurrent Chemoradiotherapy in Locally Advanced Nasopharyngeal Cancer Patients Using the Novel GLUCAR Index. Diagnostics (Basel). 2023 Dec 4;13(23):3594. doi: 10.3390/diagnostics13233594.
2. Stan A, Călburean PA, Drinkal RK, Harpa M, Elkahlout A, Nicolae VC, Tomșa F, Hadadi L, Brînzaniuc K, Suciu H, Măruşteri M. Inflammatory Status Assessment by Machine Learning Techniques to Predict Outcomes in Patients with Symptomatic Aortic Stenosis Treated by Transcatheter Aortic Valve Replacement. Diagnostics (Basel). 2023 Sep 11;13(18):2907. doi: 10.3390/diagnostics13182907.
3. Radić J, Lovrić Kojundžić S, Gelemanović A, Vučković M, Budimir Mršić D, Šupe Domić D, Novaković MD, Radić M. Serum Adropin Levels and Body Mass Composition in Kidney Transplant Recipients-Are There Sex Differences? Diagnostics (Basel). 2023 Aug 26;13(17):2768. doi: 10.3390/diagnostics13172768.
4. Motoc NȘ, Făgărășan I, Urda-Cîmpean AE, Todea DA. Prognosis Predictive Markers in Patients with Chronic Obstructive Pulmonary Disease and COVID-19. Diagnostics (Basel). 2023 Aug 4;13(15):2597. doi: 10.3390/diagnostics13152597.
5. Rusu CC, Kacso I, Moldovan D, Potra A, Tirinescu D, Ticala M, Rotar AM, Orasan R, Budurea C, Barar A, Anton F, Valea A, Bondor CI, Ticolea M. Triiodothyronine and Protein Malnutrition Could Influence Pulse Wave Velocity in Pre-Dialysis Chronic Kidney Disease Patients. Diagnostics (Basel). 2023 Jul 24;13(14):2462. doi: 10.3390/diagnostics13142462.
6. Cujba L, Stan C, Samoila O, Drugan T, Benedec Cutas A, Nicula C. Identifying Optical Coherence Tomography Markers for Multiple Sclerosis Diagnosis and Management. Diagnostics (Basel). 2023 Jun 15;13(12):2077. doi: 10.3390/diagnostics13122077.
7. Gheban-Roșca IA, Gheban BA, Pop B, Mironescu DC, Siserman VC, Jianu EM, Drugan T, Bolboacă SD. Identification of Histopathological Biomarkers in Fatal Cases of Coronavirus Disease: A Study on Lung Tissue. Diagnostics (Basel). 2023 Jun 12;13(12):2039. doi: 10.3390/diagnostics13122039.
8. Mocan LP, Rusu I, Melincovici CS, Boșca BA, Mocan T, Crăciun R, Spârchez Z, Iacobescu M, Mihu CM. The Role of Immunohistochemistry in the Differential Diagnosis between Intrahepatic Cholangiocarcinoma, Hepatocellular Carcinoma and Liver

Metastasis, as Well as Its Prognostic Value. Diagnostics (Basel). 2023 Apr 25;13(9):1542. doi: 10.3390/diagnostics13091542.
9. Nechita VI, Hajjar NA, Drugan C, Cătană CS, Moiş E, Nechita MA, Graur F. Chitotriosidase and Neopterin as Two Novel Potential Biomarkers for Advanced Stage and Survival Prediction in Gastric Cancer-A Pilot Study. Diagnostics (Basel). 2023 Apr 6;13(7):1362. doi: 10.3390/diagnostics13071362.
10. Park SY, Cho DG, Shim BY, Cho U. Relationship between Systemic Inflammatory Markers, GLUT1 Expression, and Maximum 18F-Fluorodeoxyglucose Uptake in Non-Small Cell Lung Carcinoma and Their Prognostic Significance. Diagnostics (Basel). 2023 Mar 7;13(6):1013. doi: 10.3390/diagnostics13061013.
11. Chiș IA, Andrei V, Muntean A, Moldovan M, Mesaroș AȘ, Dudescu MC, Ilea A. Salivary Biomarkers of Anti-Epileptic Drugs: A Narrative Review. Diagnostics (Basel). 2023 Jun 4;13(11):1962. doi: 10.3390/diagnostics13111962.

References

1. Curry, T.B.; Matteson, E.L.; Stewart, A.K. Introduction to the Symposium on Precision Medicine. *Mayo Clin. Proc.* **2017**, *92*, 4–6. [CrossRef] [PubMed]
2. Sigman, M. Introduction: Personalized medicine: What is it and what are the challenges? *Fertil. Steril.* **2018**, *109*, 944–945. [CrossRef] [PubMed]
3. Bartlett, M.G.; Chen, B. Editor-in-Chief editorial and introduction to 'Metabolomics and biomarkers' special issue. *Biomed. Chromatogr.* **2016**, *30*, 5–6. [CrossRef] [PubMed]
4. Kerioui, M.; Bertrand, J.; Bruno, R.; Mercier, F.; Guedj, J.; Desmée, S. Modelling the association between biomarkers and clinical outcome: An introduction to nonlinear joint models. *Br. J. Clin. Pharmacol.* **2022**, *88*, 1452–1463. [CrossRef] [PubMed]

Disclaimer/Publisher's Note: The statements, opinions and data contained in all publications are solely those of the individual author(s) and contributor(s) and not of MDPI and/or the editor(s). MDPI and/or the editor(s) disclaim responsibility for any injury to people or property resulting from any ideas, methods, instructions or products referred to in the content.

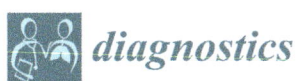

Article

Predicting Teeth Extraction after Concurrent Chemoradiotherapy in Locally Advanced Nasopharyngeal Cancer Patients Using the Novel GLUCAR Index

Efsun Somay [1], Erkan Topkan [2,*], Busra Yilmaz [3], Ali Ayberk Besen [4], Hüseyin Mertsoylu [5] and Ugur Selek [6]

[1] Department of Oral and Maxillofacial Surgery, Faculty of Dentistry, Baskent University, Ankara 06490, Turkey; efsuner@gmail.com
[2] Department of Radiation Oncology, Faculty of Medicine, Baskent University, Adana 01120, Turkey
[3] Department of Oral and Maxillofacial Radiology, School of Dental Medicine, Bahcesehir University, Istanbul 34349, Turkey; busra.yilmaz1@bau.edu.tr
[4] Clinics of Medical Oncology, Adana Seyhan Medical Park Hospital, Adana 01120, Turkey; besenay@gmail.com
[5] Clinics of Medical Oncology, Istinye University, Adana Medical Park Hospital, Adana 01120, Turkey; mertsoylu@hotmail.com
[6] Department of Radiation Oncology, School of Medicine, Koc University, Istanbul 34450, Turkey; ugurselek@yahoo.com
* Correspondence: docdretopkan@gmail.com

Abstract: To evaluate the value of the newly created GLUCAR index in predicting tooth extraction rates after concurrent chemoradiotherapy (C-CRT) in locally advanced nasopharyngeal carcinomas (LA-NPCs). **Methods:** A total of 187 LA-NPC patients who received C-CRT were retrospectively analyzed. The GLUCAR index was defined as 'GLUCAR = (Fasting **Glu**cose × **C**RP/**A**lbumin **R**atio) by utilizing measures of glucose, C-reactive protein (CRP), and albumin obtained on the first day of C-CRT. **Results:** The optimal GLUCAR cutoff was 31.8 (area under the curve: 78.1%; sensitivity: 70.5%; specificity: 70.7%, Youden: 0.412), dividing the study cohort into two groups: GLUCAR < 1.8 (N = 78) and GLUCAR ≥ 31.8 (N = 109) groups. A comparison between the two groups found that the tooth extraction rate was significantly higher in the group with a GLUCAR ≥ 31.8 (84.4% vs. 47.4% for GLUCAR < 31.8; odds ratio (OR):1.82; $p < 0.001$). In the univariate analysis, the mean mandibular dose ≥ 38.5 Gy group (76.5% vs. 54.9% for <38.5 Gy; OR: 1.45; $p = 0.008$), mandibular V55.2 Gy group ≥ 40.5% (80.3 vs. 63.5 for <40.5%, $p = 0.004$, OR; 1.30), and being diabetic (71.8% vs. 57.9% for nondiabetics; OR: 1.23; $p = 0.007$) appeared as the additional factors significantly associated with higher tooth extraction rates. All four characteristics remained independent predictors of higher tooth extraction rates after C-CRT in the multivariate analysis ($p < 0.05$ for each). **Conclusions:** The GLUCAR index, first introduced here, may serve as a robust new biomarker for predicting post-C-CRT tooth extraction rates and stratifying patients according to their tooth loss risk after treatment.

Keywords: nasopharyngeal cancer; tooth extraction; glucose; C-reactive protein; albumin

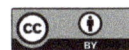

1. Introduction

Nasopharyngeal cancers (NPCs) rank as the 23rd most prevalent form of cancer globally, with an approximate total of almost 130,000 new cases reported annually [1]. They are highly aggressive malignant tumors that originate from the nasopharyngeal epithelium and significantly contribute to the morbidity and mortality associated with head and neck cancers. Despite significant progress in the field of diagnostic imaging and mass screening techniques, the majority of NPC patients (70–75%) present with locally advanced disease

(LA-NPCs) due to the peculiar location of the malignancy [2,3]. Definitive platinum-based concurrent chemoradiotherapy (C-CRT) with intensity-modulated radiotherapy (IMRT) has superseded radiation alone or sequential chemoradiotherapy regimens in the treatment of medically fit LA-NPCs, as it has demonstrated a substantial improvement in locoregional disease control and survival rates, as well as a notable reduction in most severe toxicities [4,5].

In addition to its antitumor actions, high doses of ionizing radiation in the head and neck region may also harm healthy tissues within or near the radiation field. These tissues usually include the skin, muscles, oral mucosa, salivary glands, teeth, and upper and lower jaw bones, some of which are unavoidably encompassed by the planning target volume [6]. As a result, high doses of radiotherapy (RT) can cause a number of oral toxicities, including radiation caries, osteoradionecrosis, hyposalivation, dysgeusia, dysphagia, trismus, and tooth loss [7]. RT and C-CRT have been known to cause significant damage to teeth, vascularization, and supporting tissues, inevitably leading to tooth extractions and a decline in oral functions and related quality of life (QoL) measures [8]. Additionally, pre-C-CRT tooth extractions have been recently shown to be associated with weight loss > 5% during the C-CRT course in oropharyngeal cancer patients [9], a well-recognized predictor of poorer survival outcomes in almost all solid cancers [10]. Therefore, tooth loss before, during, or after oncological therapy may not only impair oral functioning but also contribute to malnutrition and a poor disease prognosis. From this perspective, it is essential to ascertain new biological indicators to precisely predict the likelihood of tooth loss at any point throughout cancer treatment, which might facilitate the timely implementation of preventative or therapeutic interventions for those at high risk.

Historically, little research has been conducted to investigate the impact of various biomarkers on the occurrence of tooth loss after C-CRT and RT. In a study conducted by Yilmaz et al. [11], it was demonstrated that among 263 patients with LA-NPC, those with low pretreatment hemoglobin (Hb) levels (Hb ≤ 10.6 g/dL) had a higher incidence of tooth extraction following C-CRT compared to those with high Hb levels (83.9% vs. 78.1% for Hb > 10.6 g/dL; $p < 0.001$). A separate investigation, including a cohort of 246 patients diagnosed with locally advanced squamous cell head and neck cancer, indicated a significant correlation between the need for tooth extraction after C-CRT and higher values of the systemic immune inflammation index (SII) measured before treatment initiation ($p = 0.001$). This inflammatory biomarker reflects the congruence between the patient's inflammatory and immune status, regardless of the underlying cause, and was more common in the group with the determined SII cutoff value (cutoff: 558) compared to the group with lower values [12]. These studies have clarified that hypoxia-, immune-, and inflammation-related biomarkers can predict tooth loss after C-CRT for people with head and neck cancer, including LA-NPCs. Hence, further research in this field is now more promising than ever before.

Periodontal disease and dental caries are the most common causes of tooth loss, and inflammation plays a crucial role in both. Some inflammatory markers, such as high glucose levels in the blood, can cause microvascular and macrovascular changes that lead to periodontal disease and compulsory tooth extractions [13]. In a study conducted by Suzuki et al., using the National Database of Health Insurance Claims and Specific Health Checkups of Japan, it was shown that individuals belonging to the diabetes mellitus (DM) group had a greater prevalence of tooth loss compared to those in the control group, irrespective of gender [14]. Patients diagnosed with DM tended to lose their posterior teeth at earlier ages than those in the control group. Additionally, individuals within the DM cohort had a higher prevalence of tooth loss, irrespective of the presence or absence of periodontal disease treatment. Similarly, elevated levels of C-reactive protein (CRP), an established marker of acute and chronic inflammation, strongly indicate the presence of destructive periodontal disease and inevitable tooth loss [15–18]. Another acute-phase reactant protein that may be associated with tooth loss rates is albumin. Yoshihara et al. found a significant correlation between the number of missing teeth in 5 or 10 years and decreased serum albumin levels in patients with low serum albumin levels [19]. Likewise, the results of another study revealed that patients with hypoalbuminemia were at high risk for root caries and related tooth loss [20].

Based on the robust findings of the studies mentioned above, it can be confidently stated that elevated levels of glucose and CRP, along with reduced levels of albumin, serve as highly accurate predictors of tooth loss rates following hyperinflammatory conditions, including the LA-NPC patients undergoing definitive C-CRT. Therefore, motivated by the compelling evidence, we hypothesized that the integration of pretreatment glucose (GLU) and CRP-to-albumin ratio (CAR) measurements, namely, the GLUCAR index, should provide improved predictive capabilities for the unavoidable tooth extractions in patients with LA-NPC undergoing definitive C-CRT. Consequently, this retrospective research was conducted to examine the significance of the newly proposed GLUCAR index in predicting tooth loss rates after C-CRT in these patient groups.

2. Patients and Methods

2.1. Ethics, Consent, and Permission

The institutional review board of the Baskent University Medical Faculty approved the retrospective study design before compiling any data (project no: DKA:19/39). Eligible patients provided informed consent before undergoing oral and dental evaluations and C-CRT, allowing for collecting and analyzing blood samples, sociodemographic and medical data, dental X-rays, and academic presentations. This retrospective study was conducted in collaboration between the Department of Radiation Oncology and the Dentistry Clinics of the Baskent University Medical Faculty, and was approved by the institutional review board.

2.2. Patient Population

The Dentistry Clinics at Baskent University's Adana Research and Treatment Center analyzed the records of LA-NPC patients who received C-CRT and had pre- and post-C-CRT oral and dental examinations between February 2010 and January 2023. To be included in this study, patients had to meet the following criteria: age of 18 years, histopathologic evidence of squamous cell carcinoma, locally advanced disease as per the 8th edition of the American Joint Cancer Committee (AJCC) cancer staging criteria, no previous history of other cancers, no history of systemic chemotherapy or head and neck RT, and accessible complete blood count and biochemistry test results before C-CRT. Access to pre- and post-C-CRT dental and panoramic radiography examination records was an absolute requirement for eligibility. Patients with tumor or lymph node invasion in the mandible, a previous diagnosis of osteoradionecrosis of jaws or a history of jaw surgery, and the use of steroids or other immune modifiers, as well as blood transfusions within 30 days before the start of C-CRT were all ineligible for the study. Patients with active systemic inflammatory diseases, such as rheumatological, nephritic, respiratory disorders, viral hepatitis, immune suppressive, collagen vascular, chronic inflammatory, and glucose storage diseases, were excluded from the study. These restrictions were deliberately implemented to reduce the possibility of biased effects resulting from pre-existing inflammatory and immunological diseases and medication usage. Furthermore, to mitigate the influence of their partiality on the results, individuals with periodontitis, cardiovascular diseases, vascular disorders, stroke, metabolic syndrome, and diabetes, which are among the variables that make individuals more susceptible to tooth loss, were also eliminated from this research.

2.3. Baseline Oral Examination

All patients received a comprehensive dental evaluation from a skilled oral and maxillofacial surgeon (ES) before C-CRT, following the guidelines of the American Dental Association (ADA) and the US Food and Drug Administration (FDA) [21]. Radiographic examinations were performed using panoramic scans as part of standard dental care for every head and neck cancer patient following the instructions provided by the manufacturer

(J Morita, Veraviewepocs 2D, Kyoto, Japan). All teeth were examined for dental caries using World Health Organization criteria with illuminated and explorer mirrors [22]. Teeth that had no periodontal support, were too decayed to be restored, and had apical lesions that were too large to be treated with root canal treatment were extracted. Shallow tooth decay lesions were treated with the use of dental fillings. The patients received instruction on oral hygiene practices, and dental scaling procedures were conducted to promote the ongoing maintenance and enhancement of oral hygiene.

2.4. GLUCAR Index Calculation and Measurement

We developed the novel GLUCAR index as '*GLUCAR = [Fasting glucose (mg/dL) × CRP (mg/dL)/albumin (g/dL)]*' by using pretreatment glucose, CRP, and albumin measures obtained from the standard complete blood count tests performed on the first day of the C-CRT. The Abbott Architect c8000 Biochemistry Autoanalyzer (Abbott Architect c8000 Biochemistry Autoanalyzer, Abbott, Chicago, IL, USA) was used for pretreatment measurements of fasting glucose, CRP, and albumin. The measurements were done following the manufacturer's instructions [23].

2.5. Chemoradiotherapy Protocol

The RT technique used for all patients was simultaneous integrated boost intensity-modulated RT (SIB-IMRT), as previously described [11]. Coregistered imaging modalities, including computed tomography (CT), 18-fluorodeoxyglucose–positron emission tomography/CT (18-FDG-PET-CT), and magnetic resonance imaging (MRI), were used to delineate target volumes. The RT dosages were as presented earlier [12]: high-, intermediate-, and low-risk planning target volumes (PTV) received 70 Gy, 59.4 Gy, and 54 Gy, respectively, delivered in 33 daily fractions without treatment on weekends. Along with RT (every 21 days), three cycles of concurrent chemotherapy using cisplatin and 5-fluorouracil were advised. After C-CRT, all patients were advised to undergo two additional cycles of the identical chemotherapy protocol as adjuvant therapy. Antiemetics, dietary recommendations, and other supportive care were provided when necessary.

2.6. Follow-Up Oral Examination

The method described in the "Baseline oral examination" section was followed, and subsequent oral and dental examinations were conducted according to the scheduled timeline or as determined by clinical indications. Each patient's clinical and radiological examination data were recorded at post-C-CRT 1, 3, 6, 9, and 12 months, and subsequently at every scheduled 6-month interval or whenever necessary. Based on the concepts highlighted in the "Baseline oral examination" section earlier, the treatment requirements for each patient were determined and reported.

2.7. Statistical Analysis

The primary endpoint was the connection between pretreatment GLUCAR index values and the requirement for tooth extractions during the post-C-CRT follow-up. The description of continuous variables included medians and ranges, while categorical variables were represented via percentage frequency distributions. Appropriate statistical analyses, such as the Chi-square test, Student's t-test, or Spearman correlation, were used to compare the groups of patients. We used receiver operating characteristic (ROC) curve analysis to identify the pre-C-CRT cutoff(s) that could divide the entire research cohort into two groups with different outcomes. A logistic regression analysis was performed to identify the variables with multivariate significance. All comparisons were two-tailed, and a $p \leq 0.05$ was considered significant.

3. Results

The current study examined 187 individuals diagnosed with LA-NPC who underwent C-CRT and fulfilled the necessary inclusion criteria. The baseline patient and disease characteristics of the entire study cohort are shown in Table 1. The age range for the total study was 18 to 78 years, with 56 years as the median age. The majority of study participants were male (67.4%), and the majority had T3–4 tumors (54.5%) and N2–3 nodal (63.6%) disease. In 67.9% and 57.8% of patients, respectively, there was a history of smoking or alcohol consumption. All patients underwent pre-C-CRT dental extractions, with a mean of 16 days (range: 10 to 22 days) between the tooth extractions and the initiation of C-CRT. Out of all the patients, 20.3% had diabetes. The median fasting glucose measure was 97 mg/dL (range: 71–194 mg/mL). The median CRP and albumin measures were 5.3 mg/dL (range: 0.4–39.4 mg/dL) and 37.2 g/dL (range: 23.4–51.7 g/dL), respectively.

Table 1. Baseline and treatment characteristics for the entire study cohort and per GLUCAR index groups.

Characteristics	All Patients (N = 187)	GLUCAR Index < 31.8 (N = 78)	GLUCAR Index ≥ 31.8 (N = 109)	p Value
Median age, years (range)	56 (18–78)	61 (18–77)	54 (18–78)	0.10
Age group				
≥56	99 (52.9)	30 (38.5)	69 (63.3)	0.001
<56	88 (47.1)	48 (61.5)	40 (36.7)	
Gender, N (%)				
Female	61 (32.6)	29 (37.2)	32 (29.4)	0.23
Male	126 (67.4)	49 (62.8)	77 (70.6)	
Smoking status, N (%)				
Yes	127 (67.9)	49 (62.8)	78 (71.6)	0.27
No	60 (32.1)	29 (37.2)	31 (28.4)	
Alcohol consumption, N (%)				
Yes	79 (42.2)	32 (53.8)	47 (43.1)	0.88
No	108 (57.8)	46 (46.2)	62 (56.9)	
Median number of pre-CCRT tooth extraction, N (%), (range)	4 (1–11)	4 (1–11)	4 (1–9)	0.3
Median tooth extraction time to C-CRT, days (range)	16 (10–22)	16 (10–22)	16 (12–22)	0.41
T-stage group, N (%)				
1–2	85 (45.5)	42 (53.8)	43 (39.4)	0.06
3–4	102 (54.5)	36 (46.2)	66 (60.6)	
N-stage group, N (%)				
0–1	68 (36.4)	31 (39.7)	37 (33.9)	0.44
2–3	119 (63.6)	47 (60.3)	72 (66.1)	
Median fasting glucose, mg/dL	97 (71–194)	93 (71–156)	104 (85–194)	0.03
Diabetes mellitus status, N (%)				
Yes	38 (20.3)	11 (14.1)	27 (24.8)	0.01
No	149 (79.7)	67 (85.9)	82 (75.2)	
Median CRP, mg/dL	5.3 (0.4–39.4)	3.4 (0.4–26.4)	6.1 (2.6–39.4)	0.002
Albumin, g/dL	37.2 (23.4–51.7)	41.7 (24.1–50.6)	32.2 (23.4–51.7)	0.008

Abbreviations: C-CRT, concurrent chemoradiotherapy; T, tumor; N, node; mg, milligram; dL, deciliter; g, gram.

The mean follow-up time was 48.3 months (range: 6–154.6 months). A total of 148 patients (79.1%) received two to three cycles of concurrent chemotherapy, while 136 patients (72.7%) received one to two cycles of adjuvant chemotherapy (Table 2). Tooth extraction was performed in 69.0% of patients during the follow-up period.

Table 2. The connection between postconcurrent chemoradiotherapy characteristics of the whole study group and two GLUCAR index groups.

Characteristics	All Patients (N = 187)	GLUCAR Index < 31.8 (N = 78)	GLUCAR Index ≥ 31.8 (N = 109)	p-Value
Concurrent chemoradiotherapy cycles, N (%)				
1	39 (20.9)	13 (16.7)	26 (23.9)	0.18
2–3	148 (79.1)	65 (83.3)	83 (76.1)	
Adjuvant chemoradiotherapy cycles, N (%)				
0	51 (27.3)	19 (24.4)	32 (29.3)	029
1–2	136 (72.7)	59 (75.6)	77 (707)	
Median MMPD; Gy (range)	46.8 (30.4–73.4)	46.3 (31.7–71.6)	47.4 (30.4–73.4)	0.51
Post-CCRT tooth extraction, N (%)				
Absent	58 (31.0)	41 (52.6)	17 (15.9)	<0.001
Present	129 (69.0)	37 (47.4)	92 (84.1)	
Median post-C-CRT extracted tooth, N (range)	1 (0–6)	0 (0–4)	1 (0–6)	<0.001
Median time from C-CRT to tooth extraction, mo. (range)	7 (2–19)	6 (5–18)	9 (2–19)	0.003
Time of post-CCRT tooth extraction, N (%) *				
≤6	68 (52.7)	19 (51.4)	49 (53.3)	0.50
>6	61 (47.3)	18 (48.7)	43 (46.7)	
MMD, Gy (range)	33.2 (10.1–50.4)	33.9 (10.7–50.4)	32.6 (10.1–50.1)	0.39
MMD group, N (%)				
<38.5 Gy	102 (54.5)	43 (55.1)	59 (54.1)	0.72
>38.5 Gy	85 (45.5)	35 (44.9)	50 (45.9)	
V55.2 Gy group, N (%)				
<40.5%	126 (67.4)	53 (67.9)	73 (67.0)	0.69
≥40.5%	61 (32.6)	25 (32.1)	36 (33.0)	

Abbreviations: MMPD, median maximum mandibular point dose; Gy, gray; C-CRT, concurrent chemoradiotherapy; MMD, mean mandibular dose; V, volume. Note: * For 129 patients who underwent post-C-CRT tooth extraction (for the GLUCAR index < 31.8 group (N = 37) and the GLUCAR index ≥31.8 group (N = 92)).

ROC curve analysis was used to determine fitting cutoff values for continuous variables, including the mean MMD, GLUCAR index, and Vx, for their potential interactions with post-C-CRT tooth extraction rates (Table 3). The GLUCAR index had an optimal cutoff point of 31.8 (AUC: 78.1%; sensitivity: 70.5%; specificity: 70.7%, Youden: 0.41), which divided the population into two groups with significantly different tooth extraction rates: the GLUCAR < 31.8 (N = 78) and GLUCAR ≥ 31.8 (N = 109) groups (Figure 1). Based on the data presented in Tables 1 and 2, it can be confidently stated that the distribution of pre-C-CRT characteristics and treatment features was almost identical between the two GLUCAR groups. However, a comparison between the two GLUCAR groups found that the rate of tooth extraction after C-CRT was significantly higher in patients with a GLUCAR ≥31.8 compared to those with a GLUCAR < 31.8 (84.4% vs. 47.4%; OR: 1.82; $p < 0.001$). Additional ROC analysis was executed to explore the existence of any potential correlations between the mean mandibular dose (MMD), Vx, and tooth extraction rates. The results indicated that the ideal cutoffs were 38.5 Gy (AUC: 74.6%; sensitivity: 73.7%; specificity: 70.4%; Youden: 0.44) for MMD and 40.5% for V55.2 Gy (AUC: 80.7%; sensitivity: 78.2%; specificity: 75.6%; Youden: 0.54). Highlighting the strong correlations between the dosimetric parameters and tooth losses after C-CRT, tooth extraction rates were significantly higher in the MMD 38.5 Gy and V55.2 Gy ≥ 40.5% groups as compared to their MMD < 38.5 Gy and V55.2 Gy < 40.5% counterparts, respectively.

Table 3. The univariate and multivariate results.

Factors	Post-C-CRT TE (%)	Univariate p-Value	Multivariate p-Value	OR
Age group (≥56 y vs. <56 y)	68.2 vs. 69.7	0.86	-	0.97 (0.91–1.15)
Gender (female vs. male)	67.7 vs. 73.0	0.94	-	0.83 (0.67–1.42)
Smoking status (yes vs. no)	70.1 vs. 66.7	0.74	-	1.06 (0.82–1.28)
Alcohol consumption (yes vs. no)	71.2 vs. 65.6	0.27	-	1.09 (0.92–1.23)
T-stage group (3–4 vs. 1–2)	70.4 vs. 67.8	0.33	-	1.11 (0.84–1.37)
N-stage group (2–3 vs. 0–1)	74.3 vs. 64.6	0.20	-	1.15 (0.94–1.38)
Concurrent chemotherapy cycles (2–3 vs.1)	70.3 vs. 59.4	0.026	0.084	1.28 (0.97–1.96)
Adjuvant chemotherapy cycles (1–2 vs. 0)	72.1 vs. 60.8	0.16	-	1.16 (0.93–1.37)
MMD group (≥38.5 Gy vs. <38.5 Gy)	76.5 vs. 54.9	0.008	0.014	1.45 (1.20–1.96)
Mandibular V55. 2 Gy group (≥40.5% vs. <40.5%)	80.3 vs. 63.5	0.004	<0.001	1.30 (1.10–1.6)
Diabetes mellitus group (present vs. absent)	71.8 vs.57.9	0.007	0.007	1.23 (1.12–1.4)
GLUCAR index group (≥31.8 vs. <31.8)	84.4 vs. 47.4	<0.001	<0.001	1.82 (1.47–2.33)

Abbreviations: C-CRT, concurrent chemoradiotherapy; TE, tooth extraction; y, year; T, tumor; N, node; MMD, mean mandibular dose; Gy, gray; V, volume; OR, odds ratio.

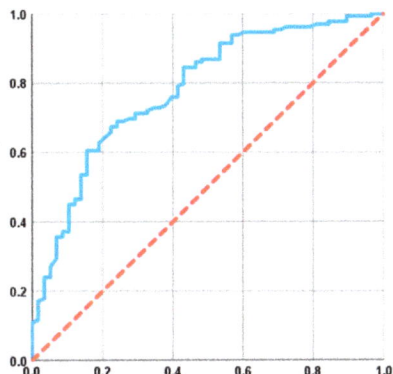

Figure 1. The results of a receiver operating characteristic (ROC) curve analysis investigating the relationship between pretreatment GLUCAR index values and tooth extraction rates after concurrent chemoradiotherapy (AUC: 78.1%; sensitivity: 70.5%; specificity: 70.7%, Youden: 0.41). Bule line represents Receiver Operating Curve; Red line represents no discrimination line.

In the univariate analysis, a statistically significant association was observed between the rates of tooth extraction after C-CRT and the MMD ≥ 38.5 Gy group (76.5% vs. 54.9% for <38.5 Gy, p = 0.008, OR: 1.45), the mandibular V55.2 Gy ≥ 40.5% group (80.3% vs. 63.5% for <40.5%, p = 0.004, OR: 1.30), and the presence of DM (71.8% vs. 57.9% for absent, p = 0.007, OR: 1.23). As shown in Table 3, the results of multivariate analyses indicated that each of the four characteristics examined remained significant and independent predictors of higher tooth extraction rates in patients with LA-NPC treated with definitive C-CRT (p < 0.05 for each) (Figure 2).

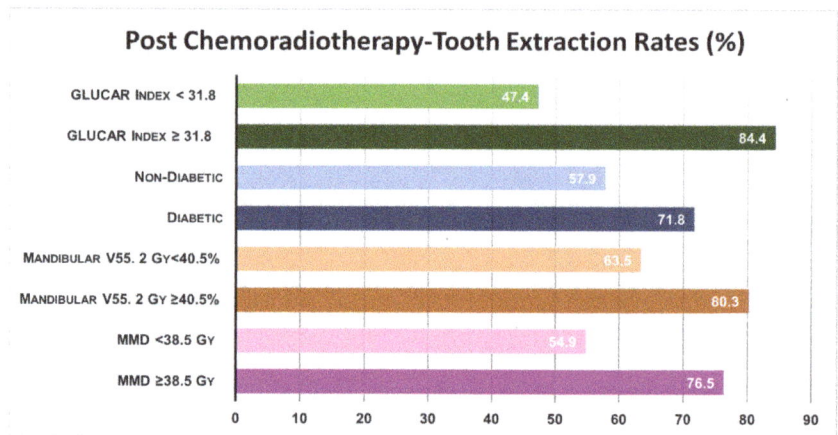

Figure 2. The bar chart showing post-C-CRT tooth extraction rates per factor demonstrated independent significance in multivariate analyses. Abbreviations: V, volume; Gy, gray; MMD, mean mandibular dose.

4. Discussion

The major objective of this study was to determine whether the incidence post-C-CRT-TE rates in patients with LA-NPC who had definitive C-CRT could be predicted using the GLUCAR index. In this research, we made a first attempt to investigate the association in this patient population. The findings of our study showed that the novel pretreatment GLUCAR index was successful in dividing LA-NPC patients into two groups based on their likelihood of requiring tooth extractions following C-CRT ($p < 0.001$).

The most significant finding of our investigation was the discovery of the pre-C-CRT GLUCAR index as a novel and efficacious biomarker for predicting tooth extractions after C-CRT in patients with LA-NPC. Accordingly, the incidence of C-CRT tooth extraction rates was significantly higher in GLUCAR ≥ 31.8 patients than in their GLUCAR < 31.8 counterparts (84.4 vs. 47.4%, OR: 1.82; $p < 0.001$). This finding suggests that the GLUCAR index can divide such patients into two risk groups for post-C-CRT tooth extractions, which may guide the prompt implementation of preventive measures in patients with a higher risk of tooth loss. Although it is a challenging task to discuss these first-of-its-kind results comparatively, studies on the effects of the components of this unique index may help form a rational scientific basis for them. Elevated glucose levels are correlated with persistent chronic infection, inflammation, periodontitis, and increased radiosensitivity in most tissues, including the mandible. Moreover, hyperglycemia leads to the overproduction of glycoproteins that coat the epithelial linings and have the potential to cause thickening and obstruction of blood vessels [24]. These factors contribute to compromised immune responses and delayed healing mechanisms in the affected tooth apex, root, and alveolar ligaments, ultimately resulting in tooth loss [25]. Hyperglycemic patients are at a higher risk of developing dental caries and experiencing tooth loss, even in the absence of RT, because of the reduced salivary flow rates and elevated glucose levels in the saliva, which are expected to be further exacerbated when RT is present [26,27]. In confirmation, a recent meta-analysis conducted by Weijdijk and colleagues confirmed that patients with DM have a 1.63 times ($p < 0.00001$) higher risk of tooth loss compared to individuals without diabetes [28]. Similarly, according to Kuo et al., patients with HNC and DM who received C-CRT were more susceptible to infection, hematological toxicity, weight loss, and treatment-related mortality than those without DM, indicating that DM causes hypersensitivity to RT [29]. Above findings are also supported by the observation of significantly higher tooth extractions in the DM group than their nondiabetic counterparts (71.8% vs. 57.9%; OR: 1.23; $p = 0.007$).

The second and third components of the GLUCAR index are CRP and albumin, which can be examined separately or as a combination of them, namely, the CRP-to-albumin ratio (CRP/albumin). The anabolic process of CRP is heightened under inflammatory conditions, in contrast to the catabolic breakdown of albumin. As a result, there is a well-established and robust inverse correlation between the levels of CRP and albumin. Indeed, it has been observed that the liver responds promptly to a single inflammatory stimulus by synthesizing CRP and causing a rapid increase in its levels [30]. However, the reactionary release of TNF-α and IL-6 in response to this stimulus leads to a decrease in serum albumin levels, which can be attributed to an increase in the breakdown of albumin and a reduction in its synthesis in the liver [31]. Previous investigations have revealed that CRP plays a vital role in the development of periodontitis, a significant cause of tooth loss, by causing the production of inflammatory mediators, such as IL-1, IL-6, and TNF-α [32–35]. Considering the albumin, previously, two studies by Yoshihara et al. established a significant connection between hypoalbuminemia and the number of missing teeth in 5 or 10 years [19], and the risk of root caries and related tooth loss [20]. Furthermore, Ando et al. [36] conducted a study using data from a large-scale community-based Japanese population, revealing a significant correlation between decreased albumin levels and an elevated likelihood of experiencing tooth loss. Low albumin levels that signify malnutrition and exacerbated inflammation may be the root cause of tooth extraction, as these two factors may adversely impact the teeth and supporting tissues, ultimately leading to the need for extraction [37,38]. The study conducted by Keinänen et al. investigated the influence of an elevated CRP/albumin ratio on patients. The findings revealed that those who had tooth loss exhibited a notably higher CRP/albumin ratio compared to those without tooth loss [39]. Therefore, although the exact mechanism may be more complex, available research findings and those presented here cumulatively suggest that the high GLUCAR levels may indicate a poorer inflammatory, immune, and nutritional status, which may lead to higher tooth loss rates after C-CRT in LA-NPC patients.

Another vital implication of our findings may be that a high pretreatment GLUCAR index may behave either as an early sign of occult tooth, periodontal tissue, or jaw bone pathologies, or a surrogate marker of radiation or chemoradiation hypersensitivity of these tissues in such patients. This remark is supported by an earlier study investigating the utility of pretreatment SII, another immune–inflammation marker, in predicting teeth caries and the need for tooth extraction after C-CRT in locally advanced HNC patients [12]. The researchers of this study discovered a positive correlation between a high pretreatment SII measure and a statistically significant rise in the post-treatment tooth extraction rates group (77.1% for SII > 558 vs. 51.4% for SII $\leq$ 558; r_s: 0.89; HR: 1.68; $p = 0.001$). In this particular context, it is possible that future research endeavors will validate these findings by performing correlative analyses between the radiomic and proteomic characteristics and immune–inflammation indices. This approach has the potential to improve the predictive capability of the results, particularly if it leads to the development of novel nomograms that exhibit high levels of predictive sensitivity and specificity.

The present investigation identified two additional parameters significantly associated with tooth extraction rates after C-CRT. These factors were MMD $\geq$ 38.5 Gy (76.5% vs. 54.9% for <38.5 Gy; OR: 1.45; $p = 0.008$) and mandibular V55.2 Gy $\geq$ 40.5% (80.3 vs. 63.5 for <40.5%; OR: 1.30; $p = 0.004$). Although the cutoff values differ, these results are well concordant with previous research suggesting higher tooth loss rates with increasing MMD and mandibular Vx values. The study carried out by Gomes-Silva et al. [40] examined the correlation between three distinct RT dosage levels (<30 Gy, 30–60 Gy, and >60 Gy) and the occurrence of tooth extraction after RT in patients with HNC. The likelihood of tooth extraction was found to be nearly three times higher with doses > 60 Gy compared to doses < 60 Gy ($p < 0.001$). Furthermore, an earlier investigation showed that the first degradation of the dental hard tissues became apparent even at doses between 30 and

60 Gy [41]. Research has indicated that the higher demand for tooth extraction following high RT doses can be attributed to several factors. RT leads to the development of porous areas in the enamel, resulting in a significant loss of the surface enamel and the protective coating it provides, which exposes the underlying dentin and impairs the natural remineralization process. Additionally, teeth may lose their resistance to acids and bacteria, as RT reduces the capacity of saliva to buffer acids, decreases the presence of antimicrobial antibodies and proteins, and diminishes salivary flow [40–42]. In addition, a study reported that most of the tooth loss occurring in the post-RT period occurred due to periodontal disease, apical periodontitis, and radiation caries, where high doses of RT may facilitate the development and progression of all these conditions [40]. While acknowledging the lack of a comparable study, the existing indirect evidence substantiates the findings of our investigation. In the research conducted by Yilmaz et al., it was observed that, out of 210 patients with LA-NPC, 174 individuals (84.8%) who underwent an MMD > 44.2 Gy had at least one tooth extraction during the post-C-CRT interval [43]. Similarly, a separate study demonstrated that 209 (79.5%) of 263 patients who underwent an MMD > 36.2 Gy and a V59.8 Gy > 36% reported tooth extraction in the post-C-CRT period [11]. Therefore, based on the findings of various studies, it is advisable to focus on minimizing the RT doses that affect the teeth and their surrounding structures, which can help reduce the likelihood of tooth loss after treatment, ultimately leading to an improved QoL for such patients.

The current investigation faces several limitations. First, the research relied on data obtained from retrospective analyses conducted inside a single institution with a relatively small study population. This characteristic introduces the possibility of inadvertent selection biases often associated with studies of this kind. Second, the lack of a validation cohort may have constrained our capacity to provide more robust interpretations of our findings. This limitation mainly stems from the restricted sample size of patients included in our study. Third, because our research only considered measurements taken at a single time point, the first day of C-CRT, it is crucial to assume that the existing cutoff values of GLUCAR may not accurately represent the optimal threshold for the best-fit risk stratification of LA-NPC patients. This is due to the potential for dramatic fluctuations of the blood albumin, CRP, and glucose levels during and after C-CRT. And fourth, we may have missed the opportunity to ascribe any plausible mechanistic associations between a cohort exhibiting an elevated GLUCAR score and the levels of cytokines/chemokines, nutritional status, and immune–inflammatory factors, such as IL-1, IL-6, and TNF-α. As a result, it is important to consider that the conclusions presented in this study should be seen as hypothetical rather than definitive recommendations until more well-designed large-scale research studies addressing these concerns provide supporting evidence. Nevertheless, the newly developed GLUCAR index components are easy to acquire and calculate, are affordable, and have reproducible factors, rendering it a suitable candidate biomarker for routine clinical use. Hence, despite the abovementioned constraints, the recently developed GLUCAR index can categorize LA-NPC patients into high- and low-risk groups based on their probability of experiencing tooth loss after C-CRT. Therefore, if confirmed with further research, its routine use may lead to close monitoring of high-risk patients and prompt implementation of proactive measures to avoid tooth loss at earlier stages.

5. Conclusions

The present research results demonstrate that the newly developed GLUCAR index is a dependable biomarker that successfully predicts the occurrence rates of post-C-CRT tooth extractions in patients with LA-NPC. This novel biological indicator may represent a significant milestone in identifying high-risk patients and may pave the way for the design of potent preventive measures and follow-up algorithms if further studies validate the results presented here.

Author Contributions: Conceptualization, E.S., E.T., B.Y., A.A.B., H.M. and U.S.; methodology, E.S., E.T., B.Y., A.A.B., H.M. and U.S.; software, E.S., E.T., B.Y., A.A.B., H.M. and U.S.; validation, E.S., E.T., B.Y., A.A.B., H.M. and U.S.; formal analysis, E.S., E.T., B.Y., A.A.B., H.M. and U.S.; investigation, E.S.,

E.T., B.Y., A.A.B., H.M. and U.S.; resources, E.S., E.T., B.Y., A.A.B., H.M. and U.S.; data curation, E.S., E.T., B.Y., A.A.B., H.M. and U.S.; writing—original draft preparation, E.S., E.T., B.Y., A.A.B., H.M. and U.S.; writing—review and editing, E.S., E.T., B.Y., A.A.B., H.M. and U.S.; visualization, E.S., E.T., B.Y., A.A.B., H.M. and U.S.; supervision, E.S., E.T., B.Y., A.A.B., H.M. and U.S.; project administration, E.S., E.T., B.Y., A.A.B., H.M. and U.S. All authors have read and agreed to the published version of the manuscript.

Funding: This research received no external funding.

Institutional Review Board Statement: The study was conducted in accordance with the Declaration of Helsinki, and approved by the Institutional Review Board (or Ethics Committee) of Baskent University Medical Faculty (protocol code DKA: 19/39 and 27 September 2019).

Informed Consent Statement: Informed consent was obtained from all subjects involved in the study.

Data Availability Statement: The datasets used and/or examined in the present work are available to qualified researchers who meet the requirements for accessing sensitive data. These datasets may be obtained from the Baskent University Department of Radiation Oncology Institutional Data Access by contacting adanabaskent@baskent.edu.tr.

Conflicts of Interest: The authors declare no conflict of interest.

References

1. Chang, E.T.; Ye, W.; Zeng, Y.X.; Adami, H.O. The Evolving Epidemiology of Nasopharyngeal Carcinoma. *Cancer Epidemiol. Biomark. Prev.* **2021**, *30*, 1035–1047. [CrossRef]
2. Cantù, G. Nasopharyngeal carcinoma. A "different" head and neck tumour. Part B: Treatment, prognostic factors, and outcomes. *Acta Otorhinolaryngol. Ital.* **2023**, *43*, 155–169. [CrossRef] [PubMed]
3. Lai, V.; Khong, P.L. Updates on MR imaging and ^{18}F-FDG PET/CT imaging in nasopharyngeal carcinoma. *Oral Oncol.* **2014**, *50*, 539–548. [CrossRef] [PubMed]
4. Lee, A.W.; Ma, B.B.; Ng, W.T.; Chan, A.T. Management of nasopharyngeal carcinoma: Current practice and future perspective. *J. Clin. Oncol.* **2015**, *33*, 3356–3364. [CrossRef] [PubMed]
5. Haksoyler, V.; Topkan, E. High Pretreatment Platelet-to-Albumin Ratio Predicts Poor Survival Results in Locally Advanced Nasopharyngeal Cancers Treated with Chemoradiotherapy. *Ther. Clin. Risk Manag.* **2021**, *17*, 691–700. [CrossRef] [PubMed]
6. Sroussi, H.Y.; Epstein, J.B.; Bensadoun, R.J.; Saunders, D.P.; Lalla, R.V.; Migliorati, C.A.; Heaivilin, N.; Zumsteg, Z.S. Common oral complications of head and neck cancer radiation therapy: Mucositis, infections, saliva change, fibrosis, sensory dysfunctions, dental caries, periodontal disease, and osteoradionecrosis. *Cancer Med.* **2017**, *6*, 2918–2931. [CrossRef] [PubMed]
7. Lajolo, C.; Rupe, C.; Gioco, G.; Troiano, G.; Patini, R.; Petruzzi, M.; Micciche, F.; Giuliani, M. Osteoradionecrosis of the Jaws Due to Teeth Extractions during and after Radiotherapy: A Systematic Review. *Cancers* **2021**, *13*, 5798. [CrossRef] [PubMed]
8. Koga, D.H.; Salvajoli, J.V.; Alves, F.A. Dental extractions and radiotherapy in head and neck oncology: Review of the literature. *Oral Dis.* **2008**, *14*, 40–44. [CrossRef]
9. Buurman, D.J.M.; Willemsen, A.C.H.; Speksnijder, C.M.; Baijens, L.W.J.; Hoeben, A.; Hoebers, F.J.P.; Kessler, P.; Schols, A.M.W.J. Tooth extractions prior to chemoradiation or bioradiation are associated with weight loss during treatment for locally advanced oropharyngeal cancer. *Support. Care Cancer* **2022**, *30*, 5329–5338. [CrossRef]
10. Ma, S.J.; Khan, M.; Chatterjee, U.; Santhosh, S.; Hashmi, M.; Gill, J.; Yu, B.; Iovoli, A.; Farrugia, M.; Wooten, K.; et al. Association of Body Mass Index with Outcomes Among Patients with Head and Neck Cancer Treated with Chemoradiotherapy. *JAMA Netw. Open.* **2023**, *6*, e2320513. [CrossRef]
11. Yilmaz, B.; Somay, E.; Topkan, E.; Pehlivan, B.; Selek, U. Pre-chemoradiotherapy low hemoglobin levels indicate increased osteoradionecrosis risk in locally advanced nasopharyngeal cancer patients. *Eur. Arch. Otorhinolaryngol.* **2023**, *280*, 2575–2584. [CrossRef] [PubMed]
12. Yilmaz, B.; Somay, E.; Selek, U.; Topkan, E. Pretreatment Systemic Immune-Inflammation Index Predict Needs for Teeth Extractions for Locally Advanced Head and Neck Cancer Patients Undergoing Concurrent Chemoradiotherapy. *Ther. Clin. Risk Manag.* **2021**, *17*, 1113–1121. [CrossRef] [PubMed]
13. Furukawa, T.; Wakai, K.; Yamanouchi, K.; Oshida, Y.; Miyao, M.; Watanabe, T.; Sato, Y. Associations of periodontal damage and tooth loss with atherogenic factors among patients with type 2 diabetes mellitus. *Intern. Med.* **2007**, *46*, 1359–1364. [CrossRef] [PubMed]
14. Suzuki, S.; Noda, T.; Nishioka, Y.; Imamura, T.; Kamijo, H.; Sugihara, N. Evaluation of tooth loss among patients with diabetes mellitus using the National Database of Health Insurance Claims and Specific Health Checkups of Japan. *Int. Dent. J.* **2020**, *70*, 308–315. [CrossRef] [PubMed]
15. Gomes-Filho, I.S.; Freitas Coelho, J.M.; da Cruz, S.S.; Passos, J.S.; Teixeira de Freitas, C.O.; Aragão Farias, N.S.; Amorim da Silva, R.; Silva Pereira, M.N.; Lima, T.L.; Barreto, M.L. Chronic periodontitis and C-reactive protein levels. *J. Periodontol.* **2011**, *82*, 969–978. [CrossRef] [PubMed]

16. Machado, V.; Botelho, J.; Escalda, C.; Hussain, S.B.; Luthra, S.; Mascarenhas, P.; Orlandi, M.; Mendes, J.J.; D'Aiuto, F. Serum C-Reactive Protein and Periodontitis: A Systematic Review and Meta-Analysis. *Front. Immunol.* **2021**, *12*, 706432. [CrossRef]
17. Escobar, G.F.; Abdalla, D.R.; Beghini, M.; Gotti, V.B.; Rodrigues Junior, V.; Napimoga, M.H.; Ribeiro, B.M.; Rodrigues, D.B.R.; Nogueira, R.D.; Pereira, S.A.L. Levels of Pro and Anti-inflammatory Cytokines and C-Reactive Protein in Patients with Chronic Periodontitis Submitted to Nonsurgical Periodontal Treatment. *Asian Pac. J. Cancer Prev.* **2018**, *19*, 1927–1933.
18. Moutsopoulos, N.M.; Madianos, P.N. Low-grade inflammation in chronic infectious diseases: Paradigm of periodontal infections. *Ann. N. Y. Acad. Sci.* **2006**, *1088*, 251–264. [CrossRef]
19. Yoshihara, A.; Iwasaki, M.; Ogawa, H.; Miyazaki, H. Serum albumin levels and 10-year tooth loss in a 70-year-old population. *J. Oral. Rehabil.* **2013**, *40*, 678–685. [CrossRef]
20. Yoshihara, A.; Takano, N.; Hirotomi, T.; Ogawa, H.; Hanada, N.; Miyazaki, H. Longitudinal relationship between root caries and serum albumin. *J. Dent. Res.* **2007**, *86*, 1115–1119. [CrossRef] [PubMed]
21. White, S.C.; Pharoah, M.J. *Oral Radiology-E-book: Principles and Interpretation*; Elsevier: St. Louis, MO, USA, 2018; pp. 808–832.
22. World Health Organization. *Oral Health Surveys: Basic Methods*, 4th ed.; World Health Organization: Geneva, Switzerland, 1997; Volume vii, p. 66.
23. Pauli, D.; Seyfarth, M.; Dibbelt, L. The Abbott Architect c8000: Analytical performance and productivity characteristics of a new analyzer applied to general chemistry testing. *Clin. Lab.* **2005**, *51*, 31–41.
24. Novotna, M.; Podzimek, S.; Broukal, Z.; Lencova, E.; Duskova, J. Periodontal Diseases and Dental Caries in Children with Type 1 Diabetes Mellitus. *Mediators Inflamm.* **2015**, *2015*, 379626. [CrossRef] [PubMed]
25. Ahmadinia, A.R.; Rahebi, D.; Mohammadi, M.; Ghelichi-Ghojogh, M.; Jafari, A.; Esmaielzadeh, F.; Rajabi, A. Association between type 2 diabetes (T2D) and tooth loss: A systematic review and meta-analysis. *BMC Endocr. Disord.* **2022**, *22*, 100. [CrossRef] [PubMed]
26. Jawed, M.; Shahid, S.M.; Qader, S.A.; Azhar, A. Dental caries in diabetes mellitus: Role of salivary flow rate and minerals. *J. Diabetes Complicat.* **2011**, *25*, 183–186. [CrossRef] [PubMed]
27. Mascarenhas, P.; Fatela, B.; Barahona, I. Effect of diabetes mellitus type 2 on salivary glucose—A systematic review and meta-analysis of observational studies. *PLoS ONE* **2014**, *9*, e101706. [CrossRef]
28. Weijdijk, L.P.M.; Ziukaite, L.; Van der Weijden, G.A.F.; Bakker, E.W.P.; Slot, D.E. The risk of tooth loss in patients with diabetes: A systematic review and meta-analysis. *Int. J. Dent. Hyg.* **2022**, *20*, 145–166. [CrossRef]
29. Kuo, H.C.; Chang, P.H.; Wang, C.H. Impact of Diabetes Mellitus on Head and Neck Cancer Patients Undergoing Concurrent Chemoradiotherapy. *Sci. Rep.* **2020**, *10*, 7702. [CrossRef]
30. Vigushin, D.M.; Pepys, M.B.; Hawkins, P.N. Metabolic and scintigraphic studies of radioiodinated human C-reactive protein in health and disease. *J. Clin. Investig.* **1993**, *91*, 1351–1357. [CrossRef]
31. Chojkier, M. Inhibition of albumin synthesis in chronic diseases: Molecular mechanisms. *J. Clin. Gastroenterol.* **2005**, *39*, S143–S146. [CrossRef]
32. Gupta, S.; Suri, P.; Patil, P.B.; Rajguru, J.P.; Gupta, P.; Patel, N. Comparative evaluation of role of hs C-reactive protein as a diagnostic marker in chronic periodontitis patients. *J. Family Med. Prim. Care* **2020**, *9*, 1340–1347. [CrossRef] [PubMed]
33. Zhang, Y.; Leveille, S.G.; Edward, J. Wisdom teeth, periodontal disease, and C-reactive protein in US adults. *Public Health* **2020**, *187*, 97–102. [CrossRef]
34. Bansal, T.; Pandey, A.; Deepa, D.; Asthana, A.K. C-Reactive Protein (CRP) and its Association with Periodontal Disease: A Brief Review. *J. Clin. Diagn. Res.* **2014**, *8*, ZE21-4.
35. Pirih, F.Q.; Monajemzadeh, S.; Singh, N.; Sinacola, R.S.; Shin, J.M.; Chen, T.; Fenno, J.C.; Kamarajan, P.; Rickard, A.H.; Travan, S.; et al. Association between metabolic syndrome and periodontitis: The role of lipids, inflammatory cytokines, altered host response, and the microbiome. *Periodontol. 2000* **2021**, *87*, 50–75. [CrossRef]
36. Ando, A.; Ohsawa, M.; Yaegashi, Y.; Sakata, K.; Tanno, K.; Onoda, T.; Itai, K.; Tanaka, F.; Makita, S.; Omama, S.; et al. Factors related to tooth loss among community-dwelling middle-aged and elderly Japanese men. *J. Epidemiol.* **2013**, *23*, 301–306. [CrossRef] [PubMed]
37. Iwasaki, M.; Yoshihara, A.; Hirotomi, T.; Ogawa, H.; Hanada, N.; Miyazaki, H. Longitudinal study on the relationship between serum albumin and periodontal disease. *J. Clin. Periodontol.* **2008**, *35*, 291–296. [CrossRef] [PubMed]
38. Musacchio, E.; Perissinotto, E.; Binotto, P.; Sartori, L.; Silva-Netto, F.; Zambon, S.; Manzato, E.; Corti, M.C.; Baggio, G.; Crepaldi, G. Tooth loss in the elderly and its association with nutritional status, socio-economic and lifestyle factors. *Acta Odontol. Scand.* **2007**, *65*, 78–86. [CrossRef]
39. Keinänen, A.; Uittamo, J.; Marinescu-Gava, M.; Kainulainen, S.; Snäll, J. Preoperative C-reactive protein to albumin ratio and oral health in oral squamous cell carcinoma patients. *BMC Oral Health* **2021**, *21*, 132. [CrossRef] [PubMed]
40. Gomes-Silva, W.; Morais-Faria, K.; Rivera, C.; Najas, G.F.; Marta, G.N.; da Conceição Vasconcelos, K.G.M.; de Andrade Carvalho, H.; de Castro, G., Jr.; Brandão, T.B.; Epstein, J.B.; et al. Impact of radiation on tooth loss in patients with head and neck cancer: A retrospective dosimetric-based study. *Oral Surg. Oral. Med. Oral Pathol. Oral Radiol.* **2021**, *132*, 409–417. [CrossRef] [PubMed]
41. Brennan, M.T.; Treister, N.S.; Sollecito, T.P.; Schmidt, B.L.; Patton, L.L.; Lin, A.; Elting, L.S.; Helgeson, E.S.; Lalla, R.V. Dental Caries Postradiotherapy in Head and Neck Cancer. *JDR Clin. Trans. Res.* **2023**, *8*, 234–243. [CrossRef] [PubMed]

42. Lieshout, H.F.J.; Bots, C.P. The effect of radiotherapy on dental hard tissue—A systematic review. *Clin. Oral Investig.* **2004**, *18*, 17–24. [CrossRef] [PubMed]
43. Yilmaz, B.; Somay, E.; Topkan, E.; Kucuk, A.; Pehlivan, B.; Selek, U. Utility of pre-chemoradiotherapy Pan-Immune-Inflammation-Value for predicting the osteoradionecrosis rates in locally advanced nasopharyngeal cancers. *Strahlenther. Onkol.* **2023**, *199*, 910–921. [CrossRef] [PubMed]

Disclaimer/Publisher's Note: The statements, opinions and data contained in all publications are solely those of the individual author(s) and contributor(s) and not of MDPI and/or the editor(s). MDPI and/or the editor(s) disclaim responsibility for any injury to people or property resulting from any ideas, methods, instructions or products referred to in the content.

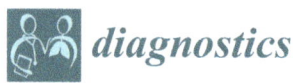

Article

Inflammatory Status Assessment by Machine Learning Techniques to Predict Outcomes in Patients with Symptomatic Aortic Stenosis Treated by Transcatheter Aortic Valve Replacement

Alexandru Stan [1,2,†], Paul-Adrian Călburean [1,2,*,†], Reka-Katalin Drinkal [1,2], Marius Harpa [1,2], Ayman Elkahlout [1], Viorel Constantin Nicolae [1], Flavius Tomșa [1], Laszlo Hadadi [1], Klara Brînzaniuc [2], Horațiu Suciu [1,2,‡] and Marius Mărușteri [2,‡]

[1] Emergency Institute for Cardiovascular Diseases and Transplantation Târgu Mureș, 540136 Târgu Mureș, Romania; alexandru.stan@umfst.ro (A.S.); reka_kata@yahoo.com (R.-K.D.)
[2] University of Medicine, Pharmacy, Science and Technology "George Emil Palade" of Târgu Mureș, 540139 Târgu Mureș, Romania
* Correspondence: calbureanpaul@gmail.com or paul.calburean@umfst.ro
[†] These authors contributed equally as first authors.
[‡] These authors contributed equally as senior authors.

Abstract: (1) Background: Although transcatheter aortic valve replacement (TAVR) significantly improves long-term outcomes of symptomatic severe aortic stenosis (AS) patients, long-term mortality rates are still high. The aim of our study was to identify potential inflammatory biomarkers with predictive capacity for post-TAVR adverse events from a wide panel of routine biomarkers by employing ML techniques. (2) Methods: All patients diagnosed with symptomatic severe AS and treated by TAVR since January 2016 in a tertiary center were included in the present study. Three separate analyses were performed: (a) using only inflammatory biomarkers, (b) using inflammatory biomarkers, age, creatinine, and left ventricular ejection fraction (LVEF), and (c) using all collected parameters. (3) Results: A total of 338 patients were included in the study, of which 56 (16.5%) patients died during follow-up. Inflammatory biomarkers assessed using ML techniques have predictive value for adverse events post-TAVR with an AUC-ROC of 0.743 and an AUC-PR of 0.329; most important variables were CRP, WBC count and Neu/Lym ratio. When adding age, creatinine and LVEF to inflammatory panel, the ML performance increased to an AUC-ROC of 0.860 and an AUC-PR of 0.574; even though LVEF was the most important predictor, inflammatory parameters retained their value. When using the entire dataset (inflammatory parameters and complete patient characteristics), the ML performance was the highest with an AUC-ROC of 0.916 and an AUC-PR of 0.676; in this setting, the CRP and Neu/Lym ratio were also among the most important predictors of events. (4) Conclusions: ML models identified the CRP, Neu/Lym ratio, WBC count and fibrinogen as important variables for adverse events post-TAVR.

Keywords: inflammatory markers; machine learning; transcatheter aortic valve replacement

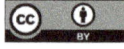

1. Introduction

Degenerative aortic valve stenosis (AS) is the most commonly acquired valvular heart disease and its prevalence increases with an ageing population [1]. Once AS becomes symptomatic, a poor prognosis is observed, with a survival rate of 30% at 5 years [2]. The only treatment option for decades was surgical aortic valve replacement (SAVR) with good long-term prognosis in ideal candidates. However, the operative risk is heterogenous, significantly increasing with old age and association of cardiac or non-cardiac comorbidities [3], leading to a deferral from SAVR in a third of the patients with symptomatic AS [4]. Transcatheter aortic valve replacement (TAVR) procedure, which was only relatively recently introduced in clinical practice, is nowadays generally accepted as the new standard of care for patients with symptomatic severe AS who are not candidates for open surgery [5]. Although TAVR significantly improves the long-term outcomes of symptomatic severe AS patients, reported 3-years mortality rates are roughly 40% [6,7]. Thus, identifying predictors of adverse events post-TAVR, especially modifiable parameters, is a major clinical desiderate.

Severe AS diagnosis is performed using transthoracic echocardiographic evaluation of the mean aortic transvalvular gradient, peak aortic transvalvular velocity, and aortic valve area [8]. In certain clinical conditions, echocardiography is not enough, and cardiac computed tomography contributes to the final diagnosis. Severe AS is diagnosed in the following three clinical presentations [8]: (1) High-gradient AS—mean aortic transvalvular gradient above 40 mmHg, peak aortic transvalvular velocity above 4.0 m/s, and aortic valve area less than 1 cm^2. All high-gradient AS cases are considered severe AS, irrespective of left ventricular ejection fraction (LVEF) or LV flow conditions. (2) Low-flow, low-gradient AS, reduced LVEF—mean aortic transvalvular gradient below 40 mmHg, aortic valve area less than 1 cm^2, a LVEF below 50% and an indexed stroke volume less than 35 mL/m^2. This clinical instance requires further investigation to determine whether the low aortic valve area is due to low-flow conditions and a dobutamine test should be performed. If under dobutamine, the aortic valve area remains under 1 cm^2 with a minimum of 20% increase in stroke volume, severe AS can be considered. (3) Low-flow, low-gradient AS, preserved LVEF—mean aortic transvalvular gradient below 40 mmHg, aortic valve area less than 1 cm^2, a LVEF above 50% and an indexed stroke volume less than 35 mL/m^2. The definite diagnosis of severe AS is relatively more difficult and prognosis of this clinical form of AS is similar to high-gradient AS [9], although this clinical instance is less frequent. High degrees of aortic valve calcifications at cardiac computed tomography provide important further diagnostic elements [8].

Machine learning (ML) techniques were described decades ago [10], but only recently gained exponential attention because of the increase in computational power and the availability of big data [11]. Machine learning techniques include, but are not limited to, algorithms such as random forest, gradient boosting machines or support vector machines [12]. Machine learning models differ from classical statistical methods such as logistical regression by their capacity to make predictions on unseen data [12]. Machine learning models can be used to perform either classification (binary or multiclass predictions) or regression (predicting a value). The use of ML techniques is appealing because it can effectively handle non-linearity and find complex interaction patterns among numerous variables, thus offering the potential to improve prediction accuracy [12,13]. However, due to its underlying mathematical complexity, ML models are difficult to interpret, being considered a black box [14]. In cardiovascular medicine, ML models can identify complex interactions among clinical variables and make an accurate event prediction [15]. The aim of our study was to identify potential inflammatory biomarkers with predictive capacity for post-TAVR event prediction from a wide panel of routine biomarkers by employing ML techniques.

2. Materials and Methods

All patients diagnosed with symptomatic severe AS and treated by TAVR since January 2016 at the Emergency Institute for Cardiovascular Diseases and Transplantation of Târgu Mureş were included in the present study. Patient data was retrospectively collected and included baseline demographic characteristics, cardiovascular risk factors, comorbidities, laboratory parameters on admission, echocardiographic parameters, coronary anatomy parameters, TAVR-related parameters, and clinical post-procedural evolution. A total of 93 clinical parameters were included in the ML analysis. Patients were not eligible for TAVR procedure if certain criteria were present, such as active infection, severe comorbidities, a high grade of frailty, severely reduced cognitive function, or limited life expectancy, consistent with our institutional TAVR protocol. The Romanian National Health Insurance System database supplied mortality rates for all the patients. For patients who had died during follow-up, the Regional Statistics Office of the Romanian National Institute of Statistics supplied the exact date and cause of death according to the tenth revision of the International Classification of Diseases (ICD-10). All included patients completed informed consent forms. The study was approved by the ethical committee of our institution. The protocol was carried out in accordance with the ethical principles for medical research involving human subjects established by the Declaration of Helsinki, protecting the confidentiality of personal information of the patients.

2.1. Machine Learning

A gradient boosting algorithm (XGBoost) was used to train (1) a model as a binary classifier for predicting 3-year all-cause cause mortality and (2) an accelerated failure time (AFT) model to predict survival. Open-source XGBoost native package was implemented in Python version 3.9. The model was trained using a 5-fold cross-validation technique. Predictions from the testing dataset for all 5 folds were pooled when performance was assessed. Hyperparameter optimization was obtained using grid search technique. No conversion of any data to a specific format was performed and one-hot encoding was used when dealing with categorical variables. Prediction interpretation and visualization was performed using open-source Shapley additive explanations (SHAP) framework that was also implemented in Python version 3.9. Three separate analyses were performed: (1) an analysis using only inflammatory biomarkers, (2) an analysis using inflammatory biomarkers, age, creatinine, and left ventricular ejection fraction (LVEF), and (3) an analysis using all collected parameters.

2.2. Statistical Analysis

A significance level α of 0.05 and a 95% confidence interval (CI) were considered. Continuous variables were evaluated for normal distribution using the Shapiro-Wilk test. Continuous variables with parametric distributions were reported as mean ± standard deviation and compared using a non-paired or paired Student t-test, while continuous variables with non-parametric distributions and discrete variables were reported as the median (interquartile range) and compared using a Mann–Whitney or Wilcoxon test. Categorical variables were reported as absolute and relative frequencies and compared using Fisher exact test for variables with frequencies of less than 5, and a Chi^2 test otherwise. The prediction performance of ML models were evaluated using multiple performance metrics: area under the receiver–operator characteristic (AUC-ROC), area under the precision–recall curve (AUC-PR). Statistical analysis was performed using R version 4.1.1 and R Studio version 1.4.17.

3. Results

A total number of 338 patients were included, of which 204 (60.3%) were males, with a median age of 76 (72–80) years and median body mass index of 29.01 ± 4.48 kg/m^2. The baseline characteristics of the studied population are reported in Table 1 and the survival curve is illustrated in Figure 1.

During follow-up, a total of 56 (16.5%) patients died, of which 3 (0.8%) patients suffered in-hospital death during their initial hospitalization for the TAVR procedure. There was no patient–prosthesis mismatch in the studied population.

Echocardiographic parameters are reported in Table 2. Among significant echocardiographic parameters besides LVEF, left ventricular end-diastolic diameter (LVEDD) was also higher among patients who died during follow-up, while baseline aortic gradients were not predictive of death.

Cardiac computed tomography parameters relevant for the TAVR population are reported in Table 3. Interestingly, none of the baseline LVOT or aortic root parameters were predictive of adverse events, while a higher calcium score of the left main coronary artery was predictive of impaired survival.

Table 1. Baseline characteristics of the studied population.

Parameter	Entire Population (n = 338)	Alive at 3 Years (n = 282)	Deceased at 3 Years (n = 56)	p
Age (years)	76 (71–80)	76 (71–80)	78 ± 6	0.01
BMI (kg/m^2)	29.01 ± 4.48	29.28 ± 4.52	26.02 ± 2.65	0.08
Male sex	204 (60.3%)	171 (60.6%)	33 (58.9%)	0.88
LVEF (%)	50 (40–60)	50 (40–60)	40 (35–55)	0.001
DCM	33 (9.76%)	22 (7.8%)	11 (19.64%)	0.01
CAD	202 (59.76%)	165 (58.51%)	37 (66.07%)	0.37
Previous MI	21 (6.21%)	16 (5.67%)	5 (8.93%)	0.36
Previous PCI	183 (54.1%)	151 (53.5%)	32 (57.1%)	0.66
Previous CABG	12 (3.55%)	10 (3.55%)	2 (3.57%)	0.99
Hypertension	270 (79.88%)	229 (81.21%)	41 (73.21%)	0.20
Diabetes mellitus	104 (30.77%)	79 (28.01%)	25 (44.64%)	0.01
Atrial fibrillation	99 (29.29%)	79 (28.01%)	20 (35.71%)	0.26
Stroke	19 (5.62%)	15 (5.32%)	4 (7.14%)	0.26
COPD	22 (6.51%)	19 (6.74%)	3 (5.36%)	0.99

BMI—body mass index; CABG—coronary artery bypass graft; CAD—coronary artery disease; COPD—chronic obstructive pulmonary disease; DCM—dilated cardiomyopathy; LVEF—left ventricular ejection fraction; MI—myocardial infarction; PCI—percutaneous coronary intervention.

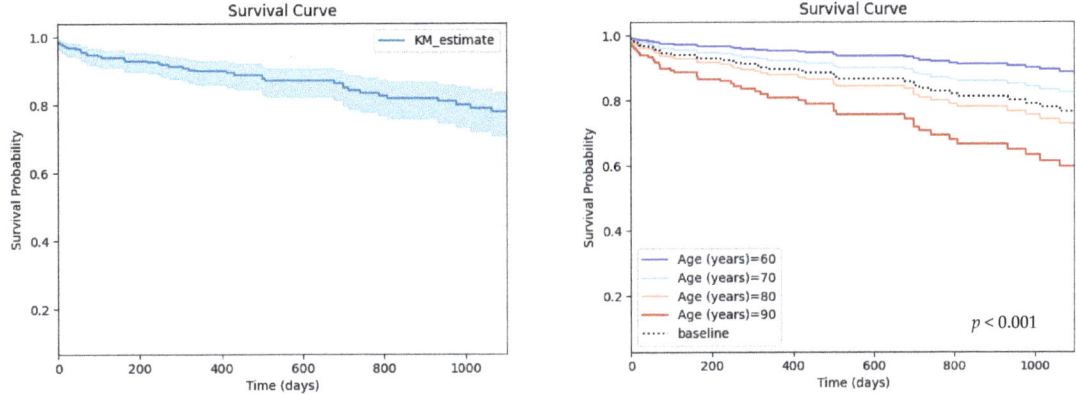

Figure 1. Survival curve for the studied population (**left**) and partial effects of age on survival (**right**).

Table 2. Comparison between pre-procedural echocardiographic parameters among studied groups.

Parameter	Entire Population (n = 338)	Alive at 3 Years (n = 282)	Deceased at 3 Years (n = 56)	p
LVEDD (mm)	50 (45–55.75)	50 (45–55)	54.05 ± 7.41	0.03
RVEDD (mm)	28 (24.75–32)	28 (24–31.25)	28.98 ± 6.22	0.45
PWT (mm)	13 (11–14)	13 (11–13.25)	12 (11.75–14)	0.23
IVST (mm)	14 (12–16)	14 (12–16)	14 (12–15)	0.65
Aortic annulus (mm)	21 (19–22)	21 (19–22)	21 (20–22)	0.49
Ascending aorta (mm)	33 (27–36)	33 (21–36)	33 (30.75–36.25)	0.98
LVOT diameter (mm)	20 (18–21)	20 (18–21)	20.65 ± 1.93	0.07

Table 2. Cont.

Parameter	Entire Population (n = 338)	Alive at 3 Years (n = 282)	Deceased at 3 Years (n = 56)	p
LA diameter (mm)	43 (37.75–47)	43 (36.75–47)	45 (39–49.25)	0.06
RA diameter (mm)	20 (15–30.75)	20 (15–29)	27.6 ± 16.31	0.23
Maximum gradient (mmHg)	71 (52.5–81)	72 (54.5–81.5)	66 (43.25–75.25)	0.42
PHT (ms)	300 (50–461)	270 (51.5–459)	335 (48.25–472.5)	0.44

LA—left atrium; LVEDD—left ventricular end-diastolic diameter; LVOT—left ventricular outflow tract; IVST—interventricular septum thickness; PHT—aortic pressure half-time; PWT—posterior wall thickness; RA—right atrium; RVEDD—right ventricular end-diastolic diameter.

Table 3. Comparison between cardiac computed tomography parameters among studied groups.

Parameter	Entire Population (n = 338)	Alive at 3 Years (n = 282)	Deceased at 3 Years (n = 56)	p
Annulus area (mm^2)	510 (448.5–577.5)	509 (439–573)	573.67 ± 88.64	0.63
Annulus perimeter (mm)	82.36 ± 9.14	82 ± 9.27	86.37 ± 6.83	0.15
LVOT perimeter (mm)	81.2 (73.8–88.9)	80.6 (73.8–88.5)	85.23 ± 5.61	0.95
LVOT area (mm)	493 (414.5–591.25)	486.5 (405.75–585.75)	551.5 ± 69.39	0.29
Sinotubular diameter (mm)	28.79 ± 3.5	28.1 (26.9–30.7)	29.92 ± 4.57	0.78
LCA height (mm)	13.6 (12.4–16)	13.6 (12.7–16)	13.45 ± 2.89	0.81
RCA height (mm)	15.5 (13.25–18.4)	15.5 (13.4–18.2)	16.95 ± 4.55	0.44
LM calcium score	0 (0–111)	55 (0–72)	161 ± 61	0.02
LAD calcium score	246 (93–655)	239 (106–654)	403 ± 324	0.80
CX calcium score	13 (0–254)	10 (0–271)	136 ± 116	0.19
RCA calcium score	157 (24–444)	155 (21–441)	123 ± 44	0.17
Total coronary calcium score	689 (212–1336)	644 (213–1281)	983 ± 748	0.13

CX—circumflex artery; LCA—left coronary artery; LM—left main artery; LVOT—left ventricular outflow tract; RCA—right coronary artery.

A wide range of routinely performed laboratory parameters were determined. Of those, inflammatory related parameters (Table 4) had a predictive value for clinical evolution after TAVR.

Table 4. Comparison between inflammatory markers among studied groups.

Parameter	Entire Population (n = 338)	Alive at 3 Years (n = 282)	Deceased at 3 Years (n = 56)	p
WBC count ($\times 10^3/\mu$L)	6.86 (5.94–8.36)	6.91 (6.06–8.35)	6.33 (5.44–8.46)	0.22
Neu ($\times 10^3/\mu$L)	4.91 (4.08–5.96)	4.91 (4.11–5.95)	4.87 (3.9–6.53)	0.89
Lym ($\times 10^3/\mu$L)	1.43 (1.14–1.87)	1.45 (1.15–1.89)	1.24 (0.81–1.59)	0.006
Neu (%)	66.3 (61.17–71.03)	66.28 (61–70.8)	68.03 (63.56–72.84)	0.98
Lym (%)	20 (16.3–24.01)	20.14 (16.42–24.17)	17.84 (12.75–22.03)	0.03
Neu/Lym ratio	3.43 (2.61–4.51)	3.41 (2.57–4.46)	3.99 (2.99–5.88)	0.04
Plt/Lym ratio	115.1 (91.4–150.1)	113.9 (90.8–147.6)	140.3 ± 66.4	0.12
CRP (mg/dL)	0.59 (0.16–1.39)	0.55 (0.15–1.33)	1.18 (0.52–2.39)	0.006
Fibrinogen (mg/dL)	371.9 (322.5–432.7)	371.9 (322.5–427.9)	392.6 ± 104.5	0.20

Table 4. Cont.

Parameter	Entire Population (n = 338)	Alive at 3 Years (n = 282)	Deceased at 3 Years (n = 56)	p
ESR (s)	27.7 (15–45)	28.3 (15–45)	28.0 ± 23.1	0.97

CRP—C-reactive protein; ESR—erythrocyte sedimentation rate; WBC—white blood cells.

Biochemical parameters with potentially important survival effects are reported in Table 5. Serum creatinine and serum albumin were significantly higher and lower, respectively, in patients who suffered all-cause death during follow-up.

Table 5. Comparison between biochemical parameters among studied groups.

Parameter	Entire Population (n = 338)	Alive at 3 Years (n = 282)	Deceased at 3 Years (n = 56)	p
Creatinine (mg/dL)	1.05 (0.88–1.31)	1.04 (0.88–1.29)	1.27 (0.98–1.53)	0.001
Total serum proteins (mg/dL)	6.6 (6.16–6.95)	6.57 ± 0.6	6.22 (5.98–6.91)	0.06
Serum albumin (mg/dL)	3.89 ± 0.44	3.93 ± 0.4	3.55 ± 0.54	0.001
Total serum CK (U/L)	80.67 (55.38–124.06)	81.5 (57.5–122.5)	78.4 (49.33–140)	0.73
Serum CK-MB (U/L)	19.42 (15.31–24.38)	19.42 (16–24)	19.25 (12.38–30.38)	0.81
Total bilirubin (mg/dL)	0.68 (0.51–0.88)	0.67 (0.51–0.87)	0.81 (0.56–1.23)	0.06
Cholesterol (mg/dL)	147 (125–180.75)	149.8 (127–181.12)	145.77 ± 41.66	0.10
LDL-cholesterol (mg/dL)	88.75 (72–115.25)	89.75 (72–115.62)	89.21 ± 30.57	0.35
HDL-cholesterol (mg/dL)	36.5 (30.83–44)	36.65 (31–44)	37.19 ± 12.14	0.43
Triglyceride (mg/dL)	98 (74.5–130.5)	99 (74.5–131)	92 (77.35–121.25)	0.26

CK-MB—Creatine kinase; CK-MB—Creatine kinase–MB isoform; HDL—high-density lipoprotein; LDL—low-density lipoprotein.

Machine Learning Assessment

Inflammatory biomarkers assessed using ML techniques had a predictive value for adverse events post-TAVR, with an AUC-ROC of 0.743 and an AUC-PR of 0.329 (Figure 2). When adding age, creatinine and LVEF to the inflammatory panel, the ML performance increased to an AUC-ROC of 0.860 and an AUC-PR of 0.574 (Figure 2). If using the entire dataset (inflammatory parameters and complete patient characteristics), the ML performance was the highest with an AUC-ROC of 0.916 and an AUC-PR of 0.676 (Figure 2).

Of note, the tuned hyperparameters of the final models included (1) a total of 300 decision trees aggregated, (2) a tree depth of four levels and (3) a learning rate of 0.01. The ML decision process can be understood using Shapley values [16]. Initially, the ML model ranks the most important variables for the prediction of mortality (Figure 3). On the dataset with only inflammatory markers, C-reactive protein (CRP), white blood cells (WBC) count and Neu/Lym ratio were the three most important features (Figure 3A). On the dataset with inflammatory markers, age, creatinine and left ventricular ejection fraction (LVEF), LVEF, CRP and WBC were the three most important features (Figure 3B). On the dataset with complete patient characteristics, left ventricular end-diastolic diameter (LVEDD), LVEF, CRP and Neu/Lym ratio were the most important features (Figure 3C). Afterwards, each variable was assigned a SHAP value for a particular variable value. A lower SHAP value is protective, while a higher score reflects impaired prognosis. In Figure 3, the x-axis reflects SHAP values, while each parameter has a blue and red side reflecting lower and higher parameter values, respectively. For instance, the blue side of the LVEDD parameter reflects lower LVEDD values and is on negative side of SHAP values; thus, there is a better prognosis when the LVEDD is lower. In contrast, the blue side of the LVEF parameter reflects higher LVEF values and is on the positive side of SHAP values;

thus, there is a worse prognosis when the LVEF is lower. The dependence plots between predictor value and SHAP value for the most important variables are illustrated in Figure 4.

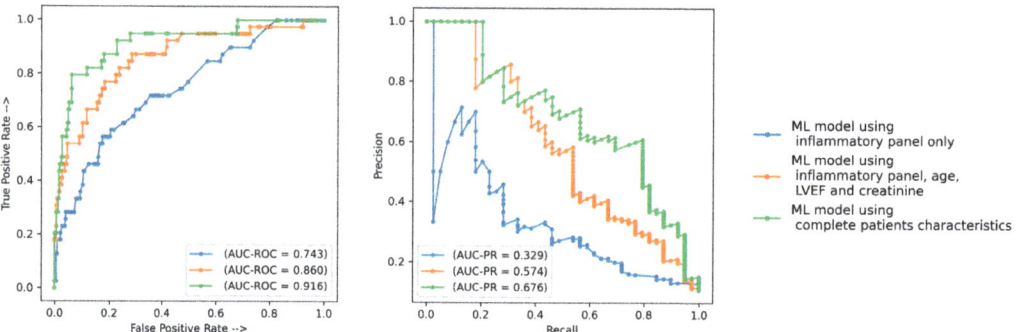

Figure 2. Prediction performance of the ML models. AUC-PR—area under precision recall curve; AUC-ROC—area under receiver operator curve; ML—machine learning.

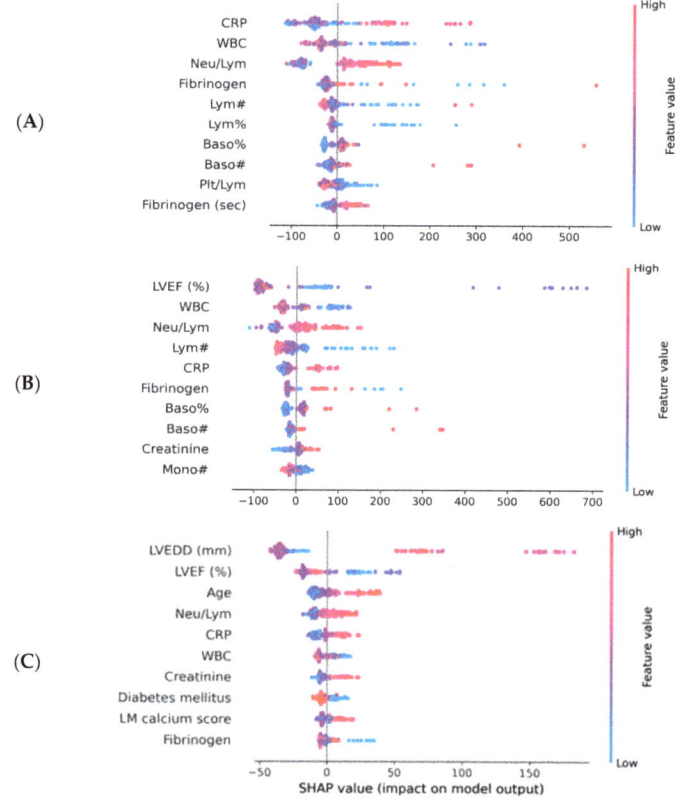

Figure 3. Importance plots for the ML models. CRP—C reactive protein; LM—left main artery; LVEF—left ventricular ejection fraction; LVEDD—left ventricular end diastolic diameter; ML—machine learning; WBC—white blood cells. (**A**) Importance plot for ML model applied to dataset with inflammatory markers. (**B**) Importance plot for ML model applied to dataset with inflammatory markers, LFEV, age and creatinine. (**C**) Importance plot for ML model applied to entire dataset.

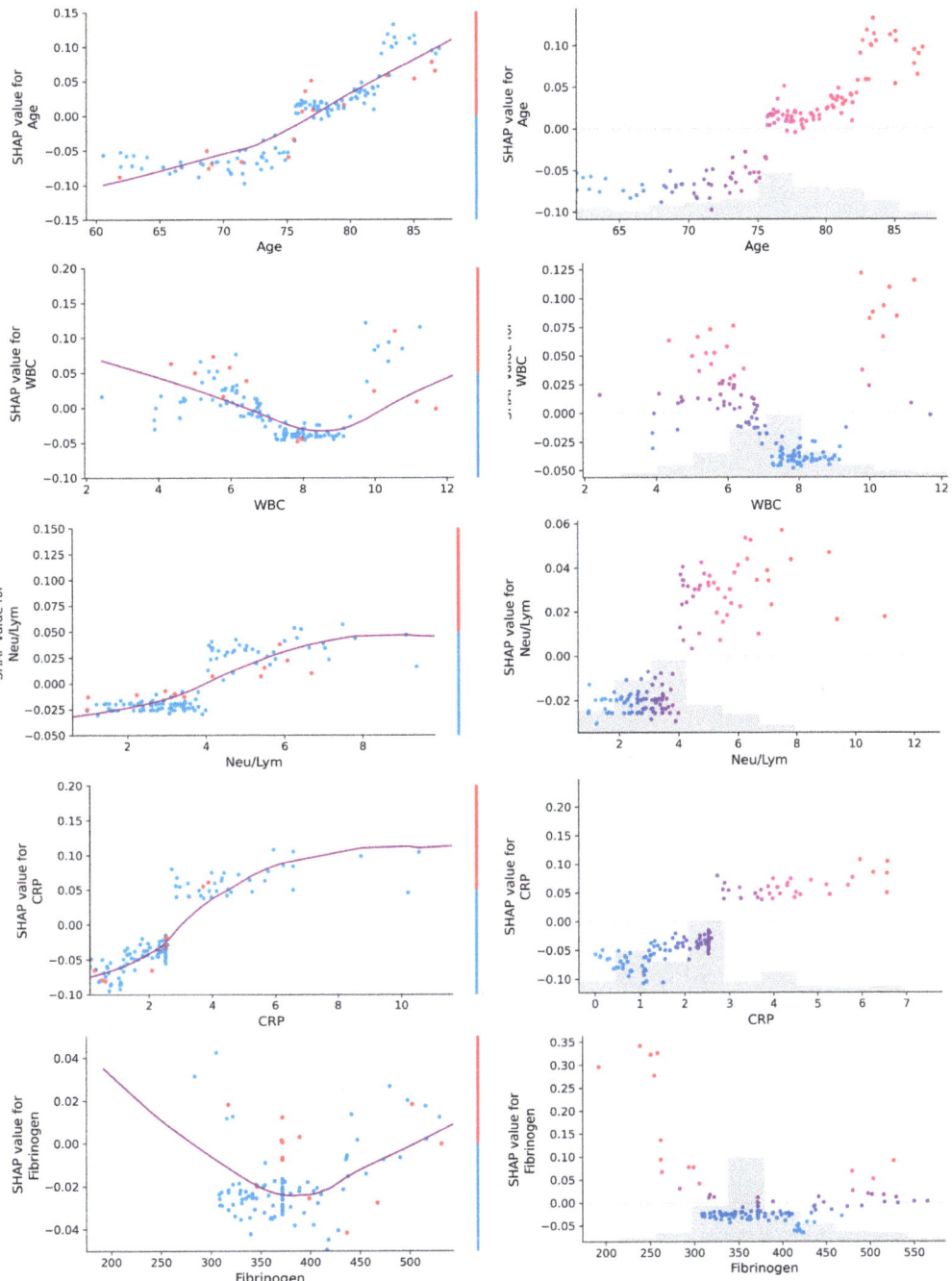

Figure 4. Dependance plot (**left**) and scatter plot (**right**) for age and inflammatory parameters. A linear relationship can be observed between values of age, CRP and Neu/Lym ratio and their SHAP values, while a bimodal relationship can be observed between values of WBC and fibrinogen and their SHAP values.

4. Discussion

The main findings of our study can be summarized as follows: (1) inflammatory biomarkers assessed using ML techniques have predictive value for adverse events post-TAVR, with an AUC-ROC of 0.743 and an AUC-PR of 0.329; the most important variables were CRP, WBC count and the Neu/Lym ratio. (2) When adding age, creatinine and LVEF to an inflammatory panel, the ML performance increased to an AUC-ROC of 0.860 and an AUC-PR of 0.574; even though the LVEF was the most important predictor, inflammatory parameters retained their value. (3) When using the entire dataset (inflammatory parameters and complete patient characteristics), the ML performance was the highest, with an AUC-ROC of 0.916 and an AUC-PR of 0.676; in this setting, the CRP and Neu/Lym ratio were also among the most important predictors of events. (4) When using SHAP values to explain the outcomes, with the increase in age, CRP and Neu/Lym ratio, an increase in event risk was also observed, while for WBC count and fibrinogen levels, a bimodal relationship was observed—the event risk was higher for both low and high levels of both WBC and fibrinogen. Even though numerous echocardiographic and cardiac computed tomography parameters were also included in the final analysis, only the LVEF and LVEDD were among the most important predictors. Besides inflammatory markers, it is not surprising that age, echocardiographic parameters, and creatinine are other important clinical parameters, as it is commonly known that they are the main survival determinants of heart disease populations. Our study supports the concept of precision phenotyping—AI and ML techniques can find complex patterns and interactions among clinical parameters that are invisible or unimportant to the clinician. The performance analysis of the ML models showed that an accurate prognosis estimate was given from routine biomarkers. The performance in survival prediction was reflected not only by the AUC-ROC, but also by the AUC-PR, a better metric for imbalanced datasets (e.g., deceased patients were fewer than alive patients) [17–19].

Undisputedly, TAVR offers both short-term and long-term advantages over SAVR, especially in high-risk patients, but post-TAVR evolution does not lack adverse events. Growing evidence suggests that inflammation status both before and after TAVR is an important predictor of adverse outcomes. High levels of biomarkers such as CRP, GDF-15 or IL-8 were associated with a 1-year mortality after TAVR [20]. Similarly, impaired platelet activity after TAVR was also a predictor of mortality [21]. In our study, the CRP and Neu/Lym ratio were higher in patients who died during follow-up. Moreover, by employing ML models, a bimodal relationship was observed for WBC count—lower and higher values were associated with impaired survival (Table 3). This relationship was not observed when alive versus deceased patients were compared (Table 2). All included patients in the present study underwent transfemoral TAVR approach. A recent study reported that the inflammatory response was significantly lower in transfemoral TAVR compared to both SAVR and apical TAVR [22]. This reduced response in the context of transfemoral TAVR may also be responsible for the improved evolution of patients treated with this strategy. Noteworthy, patients were not subjected to TAVR procedure if there was an active infection or inflammation as per our institutional protocol and clinical guidelines. Our findings suggest that even subclinical inflammation assessed by routine biomarkers has important prognostic value.

Inflammation is an important element in atherosclerotic disease that leads to aortic valve degeneration, thus being a potential and attractive pharmacologic target. In current clinical practice, pharmacological treatment in the context of symptomatic AS is directed to treating comorbidities since no pharmacological agent improves the clinical course of AS per se. The same principle is applied post-TAVR, with the exception of empirical double antiplatelet therapy for 3–6 months followed by indefinite single platelet inhibitor treatment [23]. Our observations, along with other evidence from literature, could sustain the hypothesis of a beneficial effect exerted by anti-inflammatory medication. Indeed, certain anti-inflammatory agents reduced the risk of cardiovascular events, such as colchicine, in the context of coronary artery disease [24].

The 3-year all-cause mortality or stroke rate was roughly 9% lower in TAVR versus SAVR high-risk patients [25]. However, TAVR mortality during follow-up was still high, at 32.9% in the same study [25]. In our study, mortality during follow-up was lower; however, the included population was also smaller. Nevertheless, the ML model, using all the clinical characteristics, predicted mortality with an AUC-ROC of 0.916. Low LVEF and high LVEDD were the two most important predictors, followed by a CRP and Neu/Lym ratio. A large meta-analysis also showed the impaired prognosis associated with low LVEF [26]. This is not surprising, since LVEF is the most important parameter of cardiac systolic function.

Our study is limited by the relatively small size of the study population, using all-cause instead of cardiovascular-cause mortality, and a lack of frailty scores. Including more patients would increase the statistical power of the study. However, some clear trends were observed for the studied parameters (Table 3).

5. Conclusions

Identifying predictors, especially modifiable ones, for impaired survival after TAVR for symptomatic severe AS is an important objective in contemporary cardiovascular medicine, since post-TAVR mortality is still relatively high. Inflammatory status assessment could provide such predictors. In our study, the ML models identified the CRP, Neu/Lym ratio, WBC count and fibrinogen as important variables for adverse events.

Author Contributions: Conceptualization, M.M.; methodology, P.-A.C.; software, P.-A.C.; formal analysis, P.-A.C., M.M. and A.S.; investigation, A.S. and H.S.; resources, A.S. and H.S.; data curation, R.-K.D.; writing—original draft preparation, P.-A.C. and A.S.; writing—review and editing, all authors; visualization, P.-A.C.; supervision, M.M. and H.S.; project administration, H.S. All authors have read and agreed to the published version of the manuscript.

Funding: This research received no external funding.

Institutional Review Board Statement: This study was conducted in accordance with the Declaration of Helsinki and approved by the Institutional Ethics Committee of the Emergency Institute for Cardiovascular Diseases and Transplantation Târgu Mureș, Târgu Mureș, Romania (1397/20 February 2023).

Informed Consent Statement: Informed consent was obtained from all subjects involved in the study.

Data Availability Statement: Data available on request. The data and scripts underlying this article will be shared upon reasonable request by the corresponding author.

Conflicts of Interest: The authors declare no conflict of interest.

References

1. Nkomo, V.T.; Gardin, J.M.; Skelton, T.N.; Gottdiener, J.S.; Scott, C.G.; Enriquez-Sarano, M. Burden of valvular heart diseases: A population-based study. *Lancet Lond Engl.* **2006**, *368*, 1005–1011. [CrossRef]
2. Ross, J.; Braunwald, E. Aortic stenosis. *Circulation* **1968**, *38*, 61–67. [CrossRef] [PubMed]
3. Otto, C.M. Valvular aortic stenosis: Disease severity and timing of intervention. *J. Am. Coll. Cardiol.* **2006**, *47*, 2141–2151. [CrossRef] [PubMed]
4. Iung, B.; Baron, G.; Butchart, E.G.; Delahaye, F.; Gohlke-Bärwolf, C.; Levang, O.W.; Tornos, P.; Vanoverschelde, J.-L.; Vermeer, F.; Boersma, E.; et al. A prospective survey of patients with valvular heart disease in Europe: The Euro Heart Survey on Valvular Heart Disease. *Eur. Heart J.* **2003**, *24*, 1231–1243. [CrossRef]
5. Webb, J.G.; Wood, D.A. Current Status of Transcatheter Aortic Valve Replacement. *J. Am. Coll. Cardiol.* **2012**, *60*, 483–492. [CrossRef] [PubMed]
6. Gurvitch, R.; Wood, D.A.; Tay, E.L.; Leipsic, J.; Ye, J.; Lichtenstein, S.V.; Thompson, C.R.; Carere, R.G.; Wijesinghe, N.; Nietlispach, F.; et al. Transcatheter Aortic Valve Implantation. *Circulation* **2010**, *122*, 1319–1327. [CrossRef] [PubMed]
7. Ussia, G.P.; Barbanti, M.; Petronio, A.S.; Tarantini, G.; Ettori, F.; Colombo, A.; Violini, R.; Ramondo, A.; Santoro, G.; Klugmann, S.; et al. Transcatheter aortic valve implantation: 3-year outcomes of self-expanding CoreValve prosthesis. *Eur. Heart J.* **2012**, *33*, 969–976. [CrossRef]
8. Vahanian, A.; Beyersdorf, F.; Praz, F.; Milojevic, M.; Baldus, S.; Bauersachs, J.; Capodanno, D.; Conradi, L.; De Bonis, M.; De Paulis, R.; et al. 2021 ESC/EACTS Guidelines for the management of valvular heart disease: Developed by the Task Force for the management of valvular heart disease of the European Society of Cardiology (ESC) and the European Association for Cardio-Thoracic Surgery (EACTS). *Eur. Heart J.* **2022**, *43*, 561–632. [CrossRef]

9. Tribouilloy, C.; Rusinaru, D.; Maréchaux, S.; Castel, A.-L.; Debry, N.; Maizel, J.; Mentaverri, R.; Kamel, S.; Slama, M.; Lévy, F. Low-Gradient, Low-Flow Severe Aortic Stenosis With Preserved Left Ventricular Ejection Fraction. *J. Am. Coll. Cardiol.* **2015**, *65*, 55–66. [CrossRef]
10. Breiman, L. *Classification and Regression Trees*; Routledge: New York, NY, USA, 1984; ISBN 978-1-315-13947-0. [CrossRef]
11. Hussain, I.; Park, S.J. Big-ECG: Cardiographic Predictive Cyber-Physical System for Stroke Management. *IEEE Access* **2021**, *9*, 123146–123164. [CrossRef]
12. Jordan, M.I.; Mitchell, T.M. Machine learning: Trends, perspectives, and prospects. *Science* **2015**, *349*, 255–260. [CrossRef] [PubMed]
13. Ghahramani, Z. Probabilistic machine learning and artificial intelligence. *Nature* **2015**, *521*, 452–459. [CrossRef] [PubMed]
14. Savage, N. Breaking into the black box of artificial intelligence. *Nature* **2022**. [CrossRef] [PubMed]
15. Călburean, P.-A.; Grebenișan, P.; Nistor, I.-A.; Pal, K.; Vacariu, V.; Drincal, R.-K.; Țepes, O.; Bârlea, I.; Șuș, I.; Somkereki, C.; et al. Prediction of 3-year all-cause and cardiovascular cause mortality in a prospective percutaneous coronary intervention registry: Machine learning model outperforms conventional clinical risk scores. *Atherosclerosis* **2022**, *350*, 33–40. [CrossRef] [PubMed]
16. Lundberg, S.; Lee, S.-I. A Unified Approach to Interpreting Model Predictions. *arXiv* **2017**, arXiv:1705.07874.
17. Saito, T.; Rehmsmeier, M. The Precision-Recall Plot Is More Informative than the ROC Plot When Evaluating Binary Classifiers on Imbalanced Datasets. *PLoS ONE* **2015**, *10*, e0118432. [CrossRef]
18. Călburean, P.-A.; Osorio, T.G.; Sorgente, A.; Almorad, A.; Pannone, L.; Monaco, C.; Miraglia, V.; Al Housari, M.; Mojica, J.; Bala, G. High vagal tone predicts pulmonary vein reconnection after cryoballoon ablation for paroxysmal atrial fibrillation. *Pacing Clin. Electrophysiol.* **2021**, *44*, 2075–2083. [CrossRef]
19. Călburean, P.-A.; Pannone, L.; Sorgente, A.; Gauthey, A.; Monaco, C.; Strazdas, A.; Almorad, A.; Bisignani, A.; Bala, G.; Ramak, R.; et al. Heart rate variability and microvolt T wave alternans changes during ajmaline test may predict prognosis in Brugada syndrome. *Clin. Auton. Res.* **2023**, *33*, 51–62. [CrossRef]
20. Sinning, J.-M.; Wollert, K.C.; Sedaghat, A.; Widera, C.; Radermacher, M.-C.; Descoups, C.; Hammerstingl, C.; Weber, M.; Stundl, A.; Ghanem, A.; et al. Risk scores and biomarkers for the prediction of 1-year outcome after transcatheter aortic valve replacement. *Am. Heart J.* **2015**, *170*, 821–829. [CrossRef]
21. Sexton, T.R.; Wallace, E.L.; Chen, A.; Charnigo, R.J.; Reda, H.K.; Ziada, K.M.; Gurley, J.C.; Smyth, S.S. Thromboinflammatory response and predictors of outcomes in patients undergoing transcatheter aortic valve replacement. *J. Thromb. Thrombolysis* **2016**, *41*, 384–393. [CrossRef]
22. Uhle, F.; Castrup, C.; Necaev, A.-M.; Grieshaber, P.; Lichtenstern, C.; Weigand, M.A.; Böning, A. Inflammation and Its Consequences After Surgical Versus Transcatheter Aortic Valve Replacement. *Artif. Organs* **2018**, *42*, E1–E12. [CrossRef] [PubMed]
23. Guedeney, P.; Mehran, R.; Collet, J.-P.; Claessen, B.E.; ten Berg, J.; Dangas, G.D. Antithrombotic Therapy After Transcatheter Aortic Valve Replacement. *Circ. Cardiovasc. Interv.* **2019**, *12*, e007411. [CrossRef] [PubMed]
24. Nidorf, S.M.; Fiolet, A.T.L.; Mosterd, A.; Eikelboom, J.W.; Schut, A.; Opstal, T.S.J.; The, S.H.K.; Xu, X.-F.; Ireland, M.A.; Lenderink, T.; et al. Colchicine in Patients with Chronic Coronary Disease. *N. Engl. J. Med.* **2020**, *383*, 1838–1847. [CrossRef] [PubMed]
25. Deeb, G.M.; Reardon, M.J.; Chetcuti, S.; Patel, H.J.; Grossman, P.M.; Yakubov, S.J.; Kleiman, N.S.; Coselli, J.S.; Gleason, T.G.; Lee, J.S.; et al. 3-Year Outcomes in High-Risk Patients Who Underwent Surgical or Transcatheter Aortic Valve Replacement. *J. Am. Coll. Cardiol.* **2016**, *67*, 2565–2574. [CrossRef]
26. Sannino, A.; Gargiulo, G.; Schiattarella, G.G.; Brevetti, L.; Perrino, C.; Stabile, E.; Losi, M.A.; Toscano, E.; Giugliano, G.; Scudiero, F.; et al. Increased mortality after transcatheter aortic valve implantation (TAVI) in patients with severe aortic stenosis and low ejection fraction: A meta-analysis of 6898 patients. *Int. J. Cardiol.* **2014**, *176*, 32–39. [CrossRef]

Disclaimer/Publisher's Note: The statements, opinions and data contained in all publications are solely those of the individual author(s) and contributor(s) and not of MDPI and/or the editor(s). MDPI and/or the editor(s) disclaim responsibility for any injury to people or property resulting from any ideas, methods, instructions or products referred to in the content.

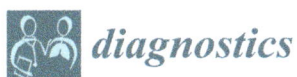

Article

Serum Adropin Levels and Body Mass Composition in Kidney Transplant Recipients—Are There Sex Differences?

Josipa Radić [1,2], Sanja Lovrić Kojundžić [3,4,5,*], Andrea Gelemanović [6], Marijana Vučković [1], Danijela Budimir Mršić [3,4,5], Daniela Šupe Domić [5,7], Maja Dodig Novaković [8] and Mislav Radić [2,9]

1. Department of Nephrology and Dialysis, University Hospital of Split, 21000 Split, Croatia; josiparadic1973@gmail.com (J.R.); mavuckovic@kbsplit.hr (M.V.)
2. Department of Internal Medicine, School of Medicine, University of Split, 21000 Split, Croatia; mislavradic@gmail.com
3. Department of Diagnostic and Interventional Radiology, University Hospital of Split, 21000 Split, Croatia; danijelabudimir@gmail.com
4. School of Medicine, University of Split, 21000 Split, Croatia
5. Department of Health Studies, University of Split, 21000 Split, Croatia; daniela.supe.domic@ozs.unist.hr
6. Biology of Robustness Group, Mediterranean Institute for Life Sciences (MedILS), 21000 Split, Croatia; andrea.gelemanovic@gmail.com
7. Department of Medical Laboratory Diagnostics, University Hospital of Split, 21000 Split, Croatia
8. Department of Radiology, General Hospital Šibenik, 22000 Šibenik, Croatia; dodig.maja@gmail.com
9. Department of Rheumatology and Clinical Immunollogy, University Hospital of Split, 21000 Split, Croatia
* Correspondence: lovric.sanja@gmail.com

Abstract: Adropin is a secretory peptide that regulates glucose, lipid, and protein metabolism, which is closely related to obesity, insulin resistance, dyslipidemia, and atherogenesis. The serum adropin level is related to sex and depends upon nutritional preferences. This study aims to determine the association between serum adropin levels and body composition parameters in kidney transplant recipients (KTRs), especially emphasizing sex differences. Our case–control study involved 59 KTRs (28 postmenopausal women and 31 men) who were divided into two groups according to sex, and each group of those KTRs was further divided into higher or lower adropin values than the mean value in each sex group. Univariate regression showed a negative association of adropin levels with most anthropometric and body composition parameters in men's KTRs. Contrary to this, the serum adropin level was negatively associated only with phase angle in postmenopausal female KTRs. Multivariate regression showed that skeletal muscle mass and phase angle were the only negative predictors in women's KTRs, whereas in men, negative predictors were BMI and body water. These findings imply that adropin could have a different impact on metabolic homeostasis in KTRs regarding sex and could be considered a negative predictor of body composition in KTRs.

Keywords: adropin; kidney transplant recipients; nutritional status; body composition

1. Introduction

Adropin is a recently identified regulatory protein, encoded by energy balance-related genes (Enho) and involved in the maintenance of energy homeostasis [1,2]. This peptide hormone is mainly expressed in the liver and brain but is also present in other tissues such as the heart, cerebellum, lung, kidney, muscles, and pancreas [3–5].

Recent studies have shown that adropin is involved in the regulation of glucose, lipid, and protein metabolism, which is closely related to obesity, insulin resistance, dyslipidemia, and atherogenesis [2,3,6]. Animal studies confirmed that adropin levels in serum are low in mice with high-fat diet-induced obesity and that adropin knock-out mice (AdrKO) displayed increased adiposity despite normal food intake [7].

However, studies investigating plasma adropin concentrations in humans have indicated some differences between sexes. For example, women have lower serum adropin

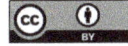

levels compared to men [2]. Although most investigations have shown a negative correlation between body mass index (BMI) and adropin levels, this rule has sometimes not been shown to be statistically significant or applicable to both sexes. In the study of St-Onge, high plasma adropin concentrations were found only in male patients and associated with the lean phenotype at a younger age [8]. On the contrary, this association is completely reversed to an increased risk of obesity later in life [8].

Moreover, the relationship between plasma adropin concentrations and the levels of low-density lipoprotein cholesterol (LDL-C) is also sex-dependent and is only found in men [9]. This effect on cholesterol homeostasis is more evident in overweight to obese men patients and limited to atherogenic LDL-C without influence on very-low-density lipoprotein cholesterol (VLDL-C) or high-density lipoprotein cholesterol (HDL-C) levels [9]. Furthermore, the association of adropin levels with nutritional preferences was only confirmed in female patients. Plasma adropin levels showed a positive correlation with fat intake [8] and a negative correlation with the consumption of carbohydrates [10].

Several studies have investigated adropin, focusing on the female population in the generative period. A study based on polycystic ovary syndrome (PCOS), which is associated with obesity, dyslipidemia, and insulin resistance, showed lower serum and follicular fluid (FF) adropin levels in PCOS women compared to control patients of similar age and BMI [11]. Contrary to this, a study based on a younger androgenic PCOS group did not find any correlation between adropin or any other anthropometric parameters, but they observed a positive correlation between adropin and androstenedione levels [12].

A recent study investigating the role of adropin in autoimmune disease—primary Sjogren syndrome (pSS), which is more common in women—showed that these patients have significantly higher serum adropin levels compared to healthy controls [13]. Also, adropin was positively correlated with HDL-C and anti-SSA/Ro52 antibodies in patients with pSS.

Accordingly, there is no study investigating the role of adropin and parameters of body composition in immunocompromised populations as in KTRs. Therefore, our study aimed to assess serum adropin levels and body mass composition parameters in KTRs and to assess sex differences between men and postmenopausal women who are not influenced by hormonal disturbances.

2. Materials and Methods

2.1. Study Design and Population

This cross-sectional study was conducted at the Outpatient Clinic for Clinical Nutrition, Nephrology and Dialysis Division, Internal Medicine Clinic, University Hospital of Split, Croatia, between July 2020 and October 2020.

The study comprised 59 KTRs, aged over 18, with functional graft, no mobility issues, and follow-up for more than a year following kidney transplantation (28 women and 31 men). The exclusion criteria were active inflammatory or malignant disease, history of stroke and myocardial infarction, implanted pacemaker or cardioverter defibrillator, stents, or limb amputation.

2.2. Medical History and Clinical and Laboratory Parameters

Baseline clinical data included the patient's age and sex, smoking status, presence of chronic kidney disease, cardiovascular risk factors (hyperlipidemia, arterial hypertension, and diabetes mellitus), presence of cardiovascular and cerebrovascular disease, duration, and type of dialysis treatment before kidney transplantation.

In terms of laboratory parameters, all study participants received standard peripheral blood sampling on the same day as the body composition and blood pressure measurements. Peripheral venous blood samples were collected following overnight fasting and handled according to standard laboratory practice by an experienced medical biochemist blinded to group assignments. The conventional hematological and biochemical parameters were analyzed on the same day. The samples for adropin analysis were centrifuged and maintained at −80 °C until analysis.

We measured the following parameters: urea (mmol/L), creatinine (mmol/L), uric acid (mmol/L), serum albumin (g/L), phosphates (mmol/L), C-reactive protein (CRP; mg/L), calcium (mmol/L), glucose (mmol/L), triglycerides (TG; mmol/L), total cholesterol (TC; mmol/L), LDL-C, (mmol/L), erythrocytes (10^{12}), hemoglobin (g/L), mean cellular volume (MCV; fL), sodium (mmol/L), potassium (mmol/L), and estimated glomerular filtration rate (eGFR; mL/min/1.73 m^2) using Chronic Kidney Disease Epidemiology Collaboration (CKD-EPI). A complete blood count was obtained using a hematology analyzer (Advia 120, Siemens, Erlangen, Germany).

Serum adropin levels were determined using a commercially available dual enzyme-linked immunosorbent assay (ELISA) kit (Phoenix Pharmaceuticals, Burlingame, CA, USA) according to the manufacturer's instructions. The test range was 0.3–20 ng/mL and sensitivity of 0.08 ng/m, and inter-assay and intra-assay coefficients of variation (CV) within the probe were less than 10%.

2.3. Body Composition and Anthropometric Measurements

Each participant's body composition was analyzed using bioelectrical impedance measurement (BIA) with a Tanita MC-780 Multi Frequency Segmental Body Analyzer (Tokyo, Japan). BIA included analysis of these data: body mass (kg), muscle mass (kg and %), skeletal muscle mass (kg and %), fat mass (kg and %), fat-free mass (kg and %), visceral fat, trunk fat mass (kg and %), skeletal muscle mass (kg and %), sarcopenic muscle index (SMI), phase angle (PhA (◦)), total body water (TBW, kg), extracellular water (EW, kg) and intracellular water (IW, kg).

All patients were requested to refrain from eating or drinking anything for at least three hours before the measurement, to urinate right before the analysis, and to abstain from alcohol, excessive eating or drinking, and excessive training for at least one day before the body composition assessment [14]. Anthropometric measurements included information on each study participant's height, weight, BMI, waist circumference, mid-upper arm circumference, and waist to height ratio (WHtR).

2.4. Central Blood Pressure and Arterial Stiffness Measurement

Using an Agedio B900 (IEM, Stolberg, Germany) oscillometry-based equipment, peripheral and central blood pressure and arterial stiffness were measured. The correct-sized cuff was chosen and precisely placed based on the upper arm circumference. All participants were analyzed while calmly seated, with their backs and arms supported, feet flat on the floor, their legs uncrossed, and their bladders empty. We collected information on peripheral systolic blood pressure (pSBP, mmHg), peripheral diastolic blood pressure (pDBP, mmHg), peripheral mean arterial pressure (pMAP, mmHg), peripheral pulse pressure (pPP), central systolic blood pressure (cSBP, mmHg), central diastolic blood pressure (cDBP, mmHg), central mean arterial pressure (cMAP, mmHg), central pulse pressure (cPP), mmHg), and pulse wave velocity (PWV; m/s).

2.5. Statistical Analysis

The normality of the data was first evaluated using the Shapiro–Wilks test. In cases where the data were normally distributed, it was presented with mean and standard deviation (SD), whereas if the data were not normally distributed, it was presented with median and interquartile range (IQR). Categorical data were presented as numbers with percentages. To test the differences between the groups, the chi-square test, T-test, or Mann–Whitney test were applied as appropriate. To evaluate the predictors of serum adropin levels, first, a univariate linear regression was performed, after which all parameters with p-values less than 0.1 were entered into the LASSO regression model, which was used to select the most relevant variables. Finally, a multivariate linear regression model was applied with selected variables after LASSO regression to identify the strongest predictors for serum adropin levels and to obtain beta coefficients, standard errors, and p-values.

3. Results

3.1. Baseline Clinical, Anthropometric, Laboratory, Body Composition, and Blood Pressure Parameters of the Study Population

The study included 59 KTRs of which 31 (53%) were men and 28 (47%) were women. All studied KTR women were in the postmenopausal period.

Table 1 presents data about baseline clinical characteristics; anthropometric, laboratory, body composition, and blood pressure parameters; and sex differences in all those parameters. Generally, most of the sex differences were observed between body composition parameters. Men had significantly more muscle mass and body water, and women had significantly more fat content. Also, several sex differences were shown regarding laboratory parameters (hemoglobin, cholesterol, and phosphates). Men's and women's KTRs did not differ in other observed parameters, including serum adropin levels, as shown in Table 1.

To determine whether there are sex differences depending on higher and lower adropin values, we divided both sex groups into two subgroups depending on the mean adropin value (≤mean value and >mean value). Therefore, we obtained two subgroups in female KTRs regarding the adropin value: those with lower adropin values (n = 11 (39%)) and women with higher adropin values (n = 17 (61%)). We used the same methodology to categorize men into two subgroups: those with lower adropin values (N = 14 (45%)) and male patients with higher adropin values than the mean value (n = 17 (55%)).

Table 1. Baseline and observed parameter characteristics of the study population including sex differences.

Predictor	Women	Men	p
	n = 28 (47%)	n = 31 (53%)	
Transplantation (years), median (IQR)	5 (7.5)	5 (7)	0.993
PD, n (%)	13 (48.15)	9 (31.03)	0.394
HD, n (%)	12 (44.44)	18 (62.07)	0.394
PD + HD, n (%)	2 (7.41)	2 (6.9)	0.394
Dialysis (years), median (IQR)	1.75 (4)	3 (3.58)	0.379
Age (years), median (IQR)	60 (13.5)	65 (11.5)	0.168
Arterial hypertension—no n (%)	4 (14.29)	5 (16.67)	1.000
Arterial hypertension—yes n (%)	24 (85.71)	25 (83.33)	1.000
Diabetes Mellitus—no, n (%)	23 (85.19)	24 (77.42)	0.676
Diabetes Mellitus—yes, n (%)	4 (14.81)	7 (22.58)	0.676
Cardiovascular Disease—no, n (%)	22 (84.62)	24 (80)	0.920
Cardiovascular Disease—yes, n (%)	4 (15.38)	6 (20)	0.920
Cerebrovascular Disease—no, n (%)	25 (96.15)	27 (90)	0.710
Cerebrovascular Disease—yes, n (%)	1 (3.85)	3 (10)	0.710
Nonsmoker, n (%)	10 (40)	12 (50)	0.652
Former smoker, n (%)	7 (28)	7 (29.17)	0.652
Smoker, n (%)	8 (32)	5 (20.83)	0.652
Anthropometric parameters			
Height (cm), mean (SD)	165.04 (5.97)	178.38 (8.67)	<0.001
Weight (kg), mean (SD)	73.9 (14.15)	80.34 (15.17)	0.123
BMI (kg/m^2), mean (SD)	27.07 (4.73)	25.19 (4.02)	0.132
Waist circumference, mean (SD)	97.78 (14.75)	100.22 (11.49)	0.567
WHtR, mean (SD)	0.59 (0.09)	0.56 (0.06)	0.191

Table 1. Cont.

Predictor	Women	Men	p
	n = 28 (47%)	n = 31 (53%)	
Laboratory parameters			
Albumin (g/L), mean (SD)	41.5 (3.05)	40.75 (3.43)	0.421
Calcium (mmol/L), median (IQR)	2.47 (0.22)	2.43 (0.16)	0.416
CRP (mg/L), median (IQR)	2.5 (4.22)	2.25 (3.65)	0.769
Erythrocyte count ($\times 10^{12}$), mean (SD)	4.48 (0.47)	4.64 (0.61)	0.077
Fasting blood glucose (mmol/L), median (IQR)	5.1 (0.75)	5.2 (0.85)	0.566
Hemoglobin (g/L), median (IQR)	130.44 (10.8)	139.1 (12.93)	0.009
Potassium (mmol/L), mean (SD)	4.02 (0.46)	4.21 (0.56)	0.169
Cholesterol (mmol/L), mean (SD)	6.13 (1.06)	5.35 (1.27)	0.028
Creatinine (mmol/L), median (IQR)	112 (57)	123 (40)	0.231
LDL-C (mmol/L), mean (SD)	3.66 (0.89)	3.18 (1.05)	0.107
MCV (fL), mean (SD)	88.79 (5.38)	88.71 (5.54)	0.954
Sodium (mmol/L), median (IQR)	141.85 (1.69)	141.5 (1.56)	0.470
Phosphate (mmol/L), mean (SD)	1.1 (0.22)	0.97 (0.23)	0.042
Triglycerides (mmol/L), median (IQR)	1.6 (1.1)	1.9 (1.67)	0.652
Uric acid (mmol/L), mean (SD)	387.44 (67.36)	389.86 (70.72)	0.896
Urea (mmol/L), median (IQR)	9.15 (3.65)	9.6 (2.6)	0.679
eGFR (mL/min/1.73 m^2), mean (SD)	48.73 (21.28)	53.92 (19.38)	0.344
Adropin, mean (SD)	2.37 (0.36)	2.37 (0.47)	0.974
Body composition parameters			
Fat mass (kg), median (IQR)	21.8 (13.7)	12.6 (11.55)	0.003
Fat mass (%), mean (SD)	29.31 (7.95)	17.1 (7.52)	<0.001
Fat free mass (kg), mean (SD)	51.51 (7.82)	66.52 (9.22)	<0.001
Visceral fat, mean (SD)	7.4 (2.9)	9.62 (3.63)	0.021
Metabolic age (years), median (IQR)	50 (13)	50.5 (12)	0.817
Muscle mass (kg), mean (SD)	48.9 (7.44)	63.12 (8.94)	<0.001
Skeletal muscle mass (kg), median (IQR)	26 (4.4)	37.8 (7.63)	<0.001
Skeletal muscle mass (%), mean (SD)	37.43 (5.55)	46.52 (7.5)	<0.001
Body mass (kg), mean (SD)	2.61 (0.38)	3.31 (0.43)	<0.001
Body water (kg), mean (SD)	36.52 (5.62)	46.85 (6.84)	<0.001
Body water (%), mean (SD)	50.1 (5.7)	58.41 (6.14)	<0.001
Phase angle (°), mean (SD)	5.26 (0.6)	5.35 (0.91)	0.682
ECW, mean (SD)	16.21 (2.37)	19.45 (2.24)	<0.001
ICW, median (IQR)	19.4 (3.3)	28.2 (5.72)	<0.001
Trunk visceral fat, mean (SD)	9.76 (4.65)	8.22 (5.72)	0.307
Blood pressure parameters			
pSBP (mmHg), mean (SD)	132.67 (18.38)	137.74 (14.05)	0.254
pDBP (mmHg), mean (SD)	86.61 (11.77)	87.48 (12.78)	0.793
pMAP (mmHg), mean (SD)	108.32 (12.92)	110.57 (11.76)	0.537
pPP (mmHg), mean (SD)	48.32 (14.67)	50.8 (11.97)	0.533
cSBP (mmHg), mean (SD)	126.38 (16.25)	130.36 (13.42)	0.376
cDBP (mmHg), mean (SD)	87.14 (12.27)	89.02 (12.01)	0.603
cMAP (mmHg), mean (SD)	100.22 (12.29)	102.8 (11.26)	0.465
cPP (mmHg), mean (SD)	35.8 (11.26)	39.24 (11.01)	0.303
AIx, mean (SD)	21.72 (13.77)	19.98 (12.22)	0.654
PWV (m/s), mean (SD)	8.83 (1.61)	9.15 (1.77)	0.502

Abbreviations: n—number, PD—peritoneal dialysis, HD—hemodialysis, BMI—body mass index, WHtR—waist to height ratio, CRP—C-reactive protein, LDL—C —low density lipoprotein cholesterol, MCV—mean cellular volume, eGFR—estimated glomerular filtration rate using CKD-EPI, ECW—extracellular water, ICW—intracellular water, p—peripheral, c—central, SBP—systolic blood pressure, DBP—diastolic blood pressure, MAP—mean arterial pressure, PP—pulse pressure, AIx—augmentation index, PWV—pulse wave velocity.

There was no statistically significant difference within the adropin subgroups in the time since transplantation, the type of dialysis, comorbidities, and smoking status. We observed significant differences in both sexes between the adropin subgroups for body weight (in women $p = 0.015$; men $p = 0.012$), BMI (women $p = 0.035$; men $p = 0.005$), and waist circumference (in women $p = 0.020$; men $p = 0.036$). Therefore, we observed significant differences between the sexes in the relation of adropin levels to body composition. We found only in male KTRs that serum adropin level was significantly related to fat tissue mass ($p = 0.003$), the percentage of fat tissue ($p = 0.009$), and visceral fat ($p = 0.021$). Contrary to this, the serum adropin levels in female KTRs were associated with overall muscle mass and skeletal muscle mass ($p = 0.044$ and $p = 0.033$, respectively), as shown in Table 2. Considering the sex differences in the relation of adropin to the proportion of water, we found a significant difference in the mass of water in men ($p = 0.019$), while in women, this difference was noticed only in the percentage of body water ($p = 0.039$). As shown in Table 2, regarding the relation of adropin levels to laboratory parameters, we found significant differences for creatinine ($p = 0.035$), triglycerides ($p = 0.037$), and urate ($p = 0.028$) in the male group. Among female KTRs, a significant difference was detected only for potassium ($p = 0.026$).

Table 2. Difference regarding adropin categories in each sex group.

	Total Number of KTRs with Measured Adropin (n = 59)					
	Women (n = 28)			Men (n = 31)		
	Adropin ≤ Mean Value (n = 11)	Adropin > Mean Value (n = 17)	p	Adropin ≤ Mean Value (n = 14)	Adropin > Mean Value (n = 17)	p
Time since transplantation (years) median (IQR)	3.5 (3.75)	6 (8)	0.236	5 (8)	5 (6.5)	0.567
Dialysis type, n (%)						
PD	5 (50)	8 (47.06)	0.893	6 (46.15)	3 (18.75)	0.257
HD	4 (40)	8 (47.06)	0.893	6 (46.15)	12 (75)	0.257
PD+HD	1 (10)	1 (5.88)	0.893	1 (7.69)	1 (6.25)	0.257
Dialysis duration (years) median (IQR)	1.25 (1.5)	2 (4)	0.517	2 (3.5)	4 (3)	0.256
Age (years) median (IQR)	54.45 (9.98)	60.71 (9.53)	0.108	62.5 (16.75)	65 (13)	0.361
Presence of chronic kidney disease, n (%)						
No	4 (40)	3 (17.65)	0.409	3 (23.08)	6 (37.5)	0.666
Yes	6 (60)	14 (82.35)	0.409	10 (76.92)	10 (62.5)	0.666
Presence of arterial hypertension, n (%)						
No	2 (18.18)	2 (11.76)	1.000	2 (15.38)	3 (17.65)	1.000
Yes	9 (81.82)	15 (88.24)	1.000	11 (84.62)	14 (82.35)	1.000
Presence of diabetes mellitus, n (%)						
No	9 (90)	14 (82.35)	1.000	10 (71.43)	14 (82.35)	0.770
Yes	1 (10)	3 (17.65)	1.000	4 (28.57)	3 (17.65)	0.770
Presence of cardiovascular disease, n (%)						
No	8 (88.89)	14 (82.35)	1.000	11 (78.57)	13 (81.25)	1.000
Yes	1 (11.11)	3 (17.65)	1.000	3 (21.43)	3 (18.75)	1.000
Presence of cerebrovascular disease, N (%)						
No	8 (88.89)	17 (100)	0.742	12 (85.71)	15 (93.75)	0.903
Yes	1 (11.11)	NA	0.742	2 (14.29)	1 (6.25)	0.903
Smoking status, N (%)						
Nonsmoker	2 (22.22)	8 (50)	0.290	5 (41.67)	7 (58.33)	0.713
Former smoker	4 (44.44)	3 (18.75)	0.290	4 (33.33)	3 (25)	0.713
Smoker	3 (33.33)	5 (31.25)	0.290	3 (25)	2 (16.67)	0.713
Anthropometric parameters						
Height (cm), mean (SD)	167.11 (6.75)	163.88 (5.35)	0.199	178.75 (6.52)	178.07 (10.41)	0.847
Weight (kg), mean (SD)	82.82 (12.2)	68.89 (12.9)	0.015	88.15 (17)	73.65 (9.67)	0.012
BMI (kg/m^2), mean (SD)	29.69 (4.04)	25.59 (4.54)	0.035	27.47 (4.27)	23.24 (2.58)	0.005
Upper arm circumference (cm), median (IQR)	30.67 (3.57)	28.57 (3.5)	0.179	28 (10)	27 (2.75)	0.510
Waist circumference (cm), mean (SD)	106.44 (8.78)	92.21 (15.35)	0.020	105.78 (12.01)	94.67 (8.17)	0.036
WHtR, mean (SD)	0.64 (0.05)	0.56 (0.09)	0.043	0.59 (0.05)	0.54 (0.06)	0.074

Table 2. Cont.

	Total Number of KTRs with Measured Adropin (n = 59)					
	Women (n = 28)			Men (n = 31)		
	Adropin ≤ Mean Value (n = 11)	Adropin > Mean Value (n = 17)	p	Adropin ≤ Mean Value (n = 14)	Adropin > Mean Value (n = 17)	p
	Laboratory parameters					
Albumin (g/L), mean (SD)	41.78 (2.77)	41.33 (3.29)	0.738	40.18 (3.03)	41.17 (3.74)	0.478
Calcium (mmol/L), median (IQR)	2.53 (0.16)	2.41 (0.15)	0.055	2.44 (0.17)	2.42 (0.16)	0.645
CRP (mg/L), median (IQR)	3.85 (5.75)	2.1 (3.72)	0.218	3.9 (5.3)	1.9 (2.55)	0.612
Erythrocyte count ($\times 10^{12}$), mean (SD)	4.6 (0.45)	4.39 (0.4)	0.229	4.53 (0.42)	4.9 (0.65)	0.091
Fasting blood glucose (mmol/L), median (IQR)	5.1 (0.78)	5.11 (0.66)	0.967	5 (1)	5.3 (0.95)	0.258
Hemoglobin (g/L), median (IQR)	132.9 (11.05)	129 (10.71)	0.375	134.38 (12.71)	142.94 (12.16)	0.076
Potassium (mmol/L), mean (SD)	4.27 (0.4)	3.87 (0.44)	0.026	4.6 (0.9)	3.95 (0.45)	0.061
Cholesterol (mmol/L), mean (SD)	5.92 (1.97)	6.2 (0.67)	0.619	5.6 (1.53)	5.14 (1)	0.365
Creatinine (mmol/L), median (IQR)	105.5 (84)	113 (40)	0.581	149 (59)	116 (34.5)	0.035
LDL-C (mmol/L), mean (SD)	3.3 (0.8)	3.7 (1)	0.363	3.34 (1.29)	3.05 (0.83)	0.500
MCV (fL), mean (SD)	87.29 (4.82)	89.73 (5.65)	0.269	89.3 (3.37)	88.19 (6.99)	0.607
Sodium (mmol/L), median (IQR)	141.12 (1.55)	142.33 (1.67)	0.121	141.64 (1.86)	141.4 (1.35)	0.710
Phosphate (mmol/L), mean (SD)	1.06 (0.27)	1.12 (0.18)	0.478	1.06 (0.27)	0.82 (0.2)	0.016
Triglycerides (mmol/L), median (IQR)	1.8 (1.1)	1.6 (0.9)	0.591	2.65 (1.55)	1.16 (1.33)	0.037
Uric acid (mmol/L), mean (SD)	385.2 (78.47)	388.76 (62.48)	0.897	421.23 (63.17)	364.38 (67.8)	0.028
Urea (mmol/L), median (IQR)	9 (4.7)	9.3 (3.2)	1.000	11.42 (4.08)	9.32 (2.2)	0.087
eGFR (mL/min/1.73 m^2), mean (SD)	54.54 (25.77)	45.32 (18.14)	0.286	46.68 (20.87)	59.8 (16.44)	0.069
Adropin, mean (SD)	2.01 (0.26)	2.6 (0.16)	0.000	1.94 (0.24)	2.73 (0.27)	0.000
	Body composition parameters					
Fat mass (kg), median (IQR)	26.69 (8.76)	19.99 (8.72)	0.079	20.1 (8.82)	9.45 (6.72)	0.003
Fat mass (%), mean (SD)	31.8 (7.42)	27.91 (8.12)	0.249	21.65 (6.15)	13.85 (6.82)	0.009
Fat free mass (kg), mean (SD)	56.3 (4.2)	47.95 (5.67)	0.044	70.75 (6.95)	63.49 (9.67)	0.055
Visceral fat, mean (SD)	8.44 (3)	6.81 (2.76)	0.182	11.6 (2.27)	8.21 (3.83)	0.021
Metabolic age (years), median (IQR)	50.56 (14.29)	48.25 (12.76)	0.682	51.5 (7.5)	49.5 (14.25)	0.907
Muscle mass (kg), mean (SD)	53.5 (4)	45.5 (5.4)	0.044	67.25 (6.61)	60.18 (9.42)	0.054
Skeletal muscle mass (kg), mean (SD)	29.1 (3.1)	25.2 (2.75)	0.033	38.97 (4.85)	35.09 (6.95)	0.144
Skeletal muscle mass (%), median (IQR)	36.19 (5.39)	38.13 (5.68)	0.412	43.03 (3.31)	49.01 (8.71)	0.052
Body mass (kg), mean (SD)	2.8 (0.2)	2.45 (0.28)	0.056	3.5 (0.34)	3.17 (0.44)	0.060
Body water (kg), mean (SD)	40.2 (2.8)	33.9 (3.82)	0.039	49.76 (5.47)	44.77 (7.14)	0.077
Body water (%), mean (SD)	48.42 (5.31)	51.05 (5.86)	0.278	55.03 (4.08)	60.82 (6.33)	0.019
Phase angle (°), median (IQR)	5.49 (0.72)	5.14 (0.5)	0.164	5.72 (0.79)	5.09 (0.92)	0.095
ECW, mean (SD)	17.67 (2.33)	15.39 (2.03)	0.018	20.68 (1.93)	18.58 (2.08)	0.020
ICW, mean (SD)	21.7 (2.3)	18.8 (2.07)	0.033	29.08 (3.62)	26.19 (5.18)	0.144
ECW/ICW, mean (SD)	0.8 (0.07)	0.8 (0.07)	0.911	0.72 (0.04)	0.72 (0.09)	0.796
Trunk visceral fat, median (IQR)	12.08 (4.16)	8.46 (4.51)	0.060	12.45 (6.03)	4.75 (4.77)	0.003
	Blood pressure parameters					
pSBP (mmHg), mean (SD)	132.68 (18.47)	132.66 (18.92)	0.997	139.19 (11.87)	136.29 (16.26)	0.594
pDBP (mmHg), mean (SD)	88.41 (11.09)	85.38 (12.42)	0.521	91.14 (14.48)	83.82 (10.02)	0.132
pMAP (mmHg), mean (SD)	108.28 (13.09)	108.34 (13.25)	0.991	111.82 (10.24)	109.32 (13.49)	0.630
pPP (mmHg), mean (SD)	43 (15.39)	51.31 (13.84)	0.179	45.64 (12.54)	55.95 (9.23)	0.040
cSBP (mmHg), mean (SD)	122.22 (17.47)	128.72 (15.61)	0.348	130.25 (9.65)	130.45 (16.62)	0.973
cDBP (mmHg), mean (SD)	89.72 (12.44)	85.69 (12.33)	0.442	93.4 (12.76)	85.05 (10.25)	0.113
cMAP (mmHg), mean (SD)	100.57 (12.85)	100.03 (12.39)	0.918	105.68 (10.56)	100.18 (11.72)	0.275
cPP (mmHg), mean (SD)	30.83 (13.19)	38.59 (9.32)	0.099	36 (12.09)	42.18 (9.53)	0.207
PWV (m/s), median (IQR)	8.1 (1.71)	9.24 (1.45)	0.091	9.4 (2.15)	9.6 (1.4)	0.460

Abbreviations: KTRs—kidney transplant recipients, n—number, PD—peritoneal dialysis, HD—hemodialysis, BMI—body mass index, WHtR—waist to height ratio, CRP—C-reactive protein, LDL—C —low density lipoprotein cholesterol, MCV—mean cellular volume, eGFR—estimated glomerular filtration rate using CKD-EPI, ECW—extracellular water, ICW—intracellular water, p—peripheral, c—central, SBP—systolic blood pressure, DBP—diastolic blood pressure, MAP—mean arterial pressure, PP—pulse pressure, PWV—pulse wave velocity.

3.2. The Association of Serum Adropin Levels and Clinical, Anthropometric, Laboratory, Body Composition, and Blood Pressure Parameters

As presented in Table 3, univariate linear regression analysis showed that age ($p = 0.022$) and PhA ($p = 0.025$) were significant predictors of serum adropin levels in female KTRs.

Table 3. Comparison between men and women related to significant predictors that determine the serum adropin level.

Predictor	Univariate Linear Regression					
	Women (n = 28)			Men (n = 31)		
	Beta	SE	p	Beta	SE	p
Age (years)	0.015	0.006	0.022	0.011	0.006	0.105
Anthropometric parameters						
Weight (kg)	−0.006	0.005	0.169	−0.023	0.005	0.000
BMI (kg/m^2)	−0.023	0.013	0.098	−0.082	0.018	0.000
Upper arm circumference (cm)	−0.010	0.019	0.608	−0.066	0.023	0.010
Waist circumference (cm)	−0.005	0.005	0.306	−0.026	0.009	0.010
Laboratory parameters						
Phosphate (mmol/L)	0.236	0.329	0.480	−0.814	0.375	0.039
Triglycerides (mmol/L)	−0.019	0.084	0.822	−0.177	0.074	0.026
Body composition parameters						
Fat mass (kg)	−0.007	0.007	0.348	−0.039	0.009	0.000
Fat mass (%)	−0.003	0.008	0.742	−0.037	0.012	0.005
Fat free mass (kg)	−0.012	0.008	0.165	−0.034	0.009	0.001
Visceral fat	−0.003	0.023	0.897	−0.065	0.026	0.021
Muscle mass (kg)	−0.012	0.009	0.164	−0.036	0.009	0.001
Skeletal muscle mass (kg)	−0.021	0.014	0.147	−0.043	0.014	0.006
Body mass (kg)	−0.234	0.168	0.176	−0.739	0.198	0.001
Body water (kg)	−0.017	0.011	0.150	−0.044	0.013	0.002
Body water (%)	0.003	0.012	0.808	0.040	0.015	0.015
Phase angle	−0.238	0.100	0.025	−0.300	0.100	0.006
ECW	−0.036	0.027	0.199	−0.151	0.035	0.000
ICW	−0.028	0.018	0.146	−0.058	0.019	0.006
Trunk visceral fat	−0.010	0.014	0.499	−0.061	0.014	0.000
Blood pressure parameters						
pDBP (mmHg)	−0.004	0.006	0.494	−0.017	0.007	0.019
cDBP (mmHg)	−0.005	0.005	0.334	−0.018	0.008	0.041

Abbreviations: n—number, BMI—body mass index, ECW—extracellular water, ICW—intracellular water, p—peripheral, c—central, DBP—diastolic blood pressure.

In contrast, in male KTRs, serum adropin levels were negatively associated with weight ($p < 0.001$), BMI ($p < 0.001$), upper arm circumference ($p = 0.010$), and waist circumference ($p = 0.010$). Considering the body composition parameters, we found a significant negative association for most of the parameters for male KTRs. Male KTRs showed a significant negative association of adropin with the percentage of fat mass ($p = 0.005$), fat-free mass ($p = 0.001$), visceral fat ($p = 0.021$), muscle mass ($p = 0.001$), skeletal muscle mass, ($p = 0.002$), body water ($p = 0.019$), the percentage of body water ($p = 0.015$), PhA ($p = 0.002$), and trunk visceral fat ($p = 0.002$). When observing blood pressure parameters, the only significant and negative association was found for pDBP ($p = 0.019$) and cDBP ($p = 0.041$) in male KTRs, as shown in Table 3.

3.3. Multivariate Linear Regression Analysis Showed Association of Adropin with Age and BMI

The whole sample showed only a significant positive correlation of adropin values with age ($p = 0.020$) and a negative value with BMI ($p < 0.001$) as shown in Figure 1.

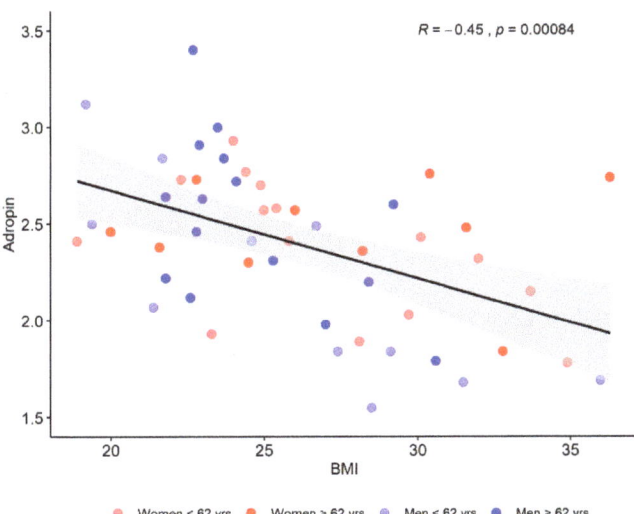

Figure 1. Associations between serum adropin levels and BMI regarding age and sex. Abbreviations: BMI—body mass index.

After selecting the strongest predictors for serum adropin levels following the multivariate LASSO regression model, for female KTRs, the only significant negative predictors were skeletal muscle mass (kg; beta = −0.024, SE = 0.011, p = 0.043) and PhA (beta = −0.207, SE = 0.099, p = 0.046), whereas for male KTRs, the only significant negative predictors were BMI (beta = −0.403, SE = 0.072, p < 0.001) and body water (kg; beta = −0.022, SE = 0.008, p = 0.003).

4. Discussion

The main result of our study in KTRs showed that most of the anthropometric and body composition parameters, as well as some of the laboratory and blood pressure parameters, differed between the high and low serum adropin groups, which was more pronounced in men compared to postmenopausal women. In men, most of these anthropometric and body composition parameters also remained negative predictors of serum adropin levels. In male KTRs, adropin was not a predictor of almost all measured parameters, except for PhA. Multivariate analysis showed that independent predictors were also different between men and women. These results confirmed substantial sex differences in adropin levels in the KTRs cohort.

The study confirmed that lower adropin levels were related to higher body weight and fat content, which was estimated with the following anthropometric parameters: weight, waist circumference, WHtR, and BMI. Although the mentioned parameters differed between high and low adropin groups in both sexes, they were significant predictors of adropin levels only in men. The negative association between adropin, weight gain, and BMI was well confirmed in the previous studies conducted in different cohorts and settings [15,16]. The adropin levels were shown to be lower in overweight and obese vs. normal weight populations, suggesting a possible role of this hormone in the development of obesity. BIA has become established over the past four decades as a widespread technique for the assessment of body composition. In our study, adropin was associated with several body composition parameters estimated by BIA, such as fat mass, visceral fat, body, and extracellular water in men, while in women, only skeletal muscle and muscle mass were significantly higher in the group with lower adropin levels. Similar results were obtained in a study by Yosaee et al. [15], which compared patients with metabolic syndrome, obese, and normal weight patients, including more than 86% of men of younger age in the population sample. It seems that higher body fat amounts are related to a negative impact on serum adropin levels. However, the exact role of adropin in the pathogenesis of obesity is not fully understood. It remains unclear whether overexpression of adropin merely delays body weight gain or prevents it. Also, the exact mechanism of the lowering of serum adropin concentrations while raising excess body fat amounts remains unexplained. Laboratory parameters examined in our study were generally not associated with serum adropin levels, especially in women. Previous studies have shown that high adropin levels can improve lipid metabolism, and a negative association between adropin and cholesterol levels, LDL - C and TG, and a positive association with HDL- C have been described [17,18]. Low adropin was associated with dyslipidemia in hemodialysis patients only in unadjusted analysis [19], but after excluding confounders, the lipid levels were shown not to be related to adropin levels. Similarly, regression analysis in a study by Hu et al. in patients with diabetes mellitus type 2 showed no association between lipids and adropin levels [20]. In our cohort, no association was found either, except for the case of the independent negative prediction of TG levels of adropin in men. This suggests that an association may exist, although it may be weak. Future studies will better explain the involvement of adropin in lipid homeostasis.

Blood pressure parameters generally showed the least association with serum adropin levels, except for cDBP and pDBP in male KTRs, which differed between high and low adropin level groups and remained negative predictors of adropin levels. Previous studies have shown that adropin concentrations are lower in hypertension [21]. Adropin was propped to be an inductor of nitric oxide (NO) production, which acts as a vasodilator [22]. It was also shown that adropin is involved in controlling the functions of endothelial cells [5]. Adropin may influence blood pressure by protecting endothelial function, and low adropin levels are related to endothelial dysfunction [23], which could partially explain the connection.

In female KTRs, skeletal muscle mass and PhA were found to be negative predictors of adropin. The PhA is a body composition measure of cellular stability. It was shown to be lower in obesity and metabolic syndrome. In a previous study, PhA was positively associated with body fat percent, free fat mass, upper arm circumference, and muscle mass [24], thus explaining the connection. Previous research showed in general a weaker association between female sex and adropin levels compared to male sex, which could be partially explained by the influence of estrogens [25]. However, in our cohort of KTRs postmenopausal women, in whom hormones could not influence adropin levels, the weaker association of adropin with all parameters remained in women.

Finally, kidney transplantation is the treatment of choice for end-stage renal disease (ESRD). However, KTRs are at risk of developing metabolic disorders. The increasing use of immunosuppressive therapy, which is potentially diabetogenic and atherogenic, can worsen pre-existing medical conditions or induce the development of other problems including bone disease, infections, and malignancies [26]. The pathogenesis of cardiovascular disease as a major cause of death in this population is multifactorial and can be reduced through numerous lifestyle modifications. The modification and adjustment of drug therapy by reducing the use of glucocorticoids, calcineurin inhibitors, or other drugs in patients with major risk factors for cardiovascular disease, as well as the consistent and timely treatment of diabetes, hypertension, and/or hyperlipidemia and anemia can also reduce cardiovascular morbidity in the KTRs population [27].

So far, there are several studies conducted on ESRD patients, which showed lower levels of adropin in patients receiving dialysis treatment compared to controls [18,19]. The study based on a rat model of chronic kidney failure showed that adropin had a protective effect on inflammation and chronic kidney damage progression [28]. In another study, reduced levels of adropin were associated with renal dysfunction in patients with type 2 diabetes mellitus, and adropin was proposed to be used as a biomarker for the early diagnosis of diabetic nephropathy [29]. The latest study confirmed that type 2 diabetics with chronic heart failure with lower adropin values were more likely to develop chronic kidney disease [30]. Moreover, recent studies have proposed a possible immunomodulatory effect of adropin. Also, autoimmune disorders such as pSS, or rheumatoid arthritis were shown to be associated with lower adropin levels [13,31]. This shows how low adropin level accompanies these conditions and has a potential role in the pathogenesis of the disease. To the best of our knowledge, there are no studies on immunocompromised populations that were investigated like in our study. Immunosuppressants administered to KTRs could potentially interfere with and disrupt the protective immunomodulatory effects of adropin, but the exact mechanism remains to be elucidated.

The main strength of the study, to the best of our knowledge, is that this was the first research that investigated associations of serum adropin levels and body composition in an immunocompromised KTRs cohort. Furthermore, it is important to note that this KTRs cohort is specific for its low incidence of diabetes, obesity, and cardiovascular disease. It is important to underline that women in our cohort were all postmenopausal, which is another confirmation of the sex dependence of adropin in the KTRs population. The results of this research will provide new insights into the possible role of serum adropin in the pathophysiology of cardiovascular risk in these susceptible immunocompromised KTRs. The limitations of this study are a relatively small number of KTRs and a lack of healthy control. The cross-sectional study design did not allow for the definition of any causal relations.

5. Conclusions

The present study shows that higher adropin levels are associated with different metabolic abnormalities in male KTRs compared to postmenopausal women. This confirms sex-dependent adropin differences in the immunocompromised KTRs population.

Author Contributions: J.R., S.L.K. and M.V. contributed equally to this paper. Conceptualization, S.L.K. and J.R.; methodology, J.R. software, A.G.; validation, M.V., M.D.N., M.R. and D.B.M.; formal analysis, A.G.; investigation, M.V., D.Š.D. and M.D.N.; resources, J.R. and S.L.K.; data curation, D.Š.D.; writing—original draft preparation, S.L.K.; writing—review and editing, D.B.M., J.R., M.V. and AG.; visualization, M.R.; supervision, S.L.K.; project administration, J.R. All authors have read and agreed to the published version of the manuscript.

Funding: This research is part of the project "Digitalization and improvement of nutritional care for patients with chronic diseases" co-financed by the European Regional Development Fund through the Operational Program "Competitiveness and Cohesion 2014–2020" KK.01.1.1.04.0115.

Institutional Review Board Statement: The study was conducted according to the guidelines of the Declaration of Helsinki and approved by the Ethics Committee of the University Hospital of Split on 30 August 2019 (Ur. No. 2181-147-01/06/M.S.-19-2, Class: 500-03/19-01/72).

Informed Consent Statement: Informed consent was obtained from all subjects involved in the study.

Data Availability Statement: Data are available upon request to the corresponding author via e-mail.

Conflicts of Interest: The authors declare no conflict of interest.

References

1. Kumar, K.G.; Trevaskis, J.L.; Lam, D.D.; Sutton, G.M.; Koza, R.A.; Chouljenko, V.N.; Kousoulas, K.G.; Rogers, P.M.; Kesterson, R.A.; Thearle, M.; et al. Identification of adropin as a secreted factor linking dietary macronutrient intake with energy homeostasis and lipid metabolism. *Cell Metab.* **2008**, *8*, 468–481. [CrossRef]
2. Butler, A.A.; Zhang, J.; Price, C.A.; Stevens, J.R.; Graham, J.L.; Stanhope, K.L.; King, S.; Krauss, R.M.; Bremer, A.A.; Havel, P.J. Low plasma adropin concentrations increase risks of weight gain and metabolic dysregulation in response to a high-sugar diet in men nonhuman primates. *J. Biol. Chem.* **2019**, *294*, 9706–9719. [CrossRef] [PubMed]
3. Gao, S.; McMillan, R.P.; Jacas, J.; Zhu, Q.; Li, X.; Kumar, G.K.; Casals, N.; Hegardt, F.G.; Robbins, P.D.; Lopaschuk, G.D.; et al. Regulation of substrate oxidation preferences in muscle by the peptide hormone Adropin. *Diabetes* **2014**, *63*, 3242–3252. [CrossRef]
4. Aydin, S.; Kuloglu, T.; Aydin, S.; Eren, M.N.; Yilmaz, M.; Kalayci, M.; Sahin, I.; Kocaman, N.; Citil, C.; Kendir, Y. Expression of adropin in rat brain, cerebellum, kidneys, heart, liver, and pancreas in streptozotocin-induced diabetes. *Mol. Cell. Biochem.* **2013**, *380*, 73–81. [CrossRef]

5. Lovren, F.; Pan, Y.; Quan, A.; Singh, K.K.; Shukla, P.C.; Gupta, M.; Al-Omran, M.; Teoh, H.; Verma, S. Adropin is a novel regulator of endothelial function. *Circulation* **2010**, *122*, S185–S192. [CrossRef]
6. Butler, A.A.; Tam, C.S.; Stanhope, K.L.; Wolfe, B.M.; Ali, M.R.; O'Keeffe, M.; St-Onge, M.-P.; Ravussin, E.; Havel, P.J. Low circulating adropin concentrations with obesity and aging correlate with risk factors for metabolic disease and increase after gastric bypass surgery in humans. *J. Clin. Endocrinol. Metab.* **2012**, *97*, 3783–3791. [CrossRef]
7. Ganesh-Kumar, K.; Zhang, J.; Gao, S.; Rossi, J.; McGuinness, O.P.; Halem, H.H.; Culler, M.D.; Mynatt, R.L.; Butler, A.A. Adropin deficiency is associated with increased adiposity and insulin resistance. *Obes. Silver Spring* **2012**, *20*, 1394–1402. [CrossRef]
8. St-Onge, M.-P.; Shechter, A.; Shlisky, J.; Tam, C.S.; Gao, S.; Ravussin, E.; Butler, A.A. Fasting plasma adropin concentrations correlate with fat consumption in human females. *Obesity* **2014**, *22*, 1056–1063. [CrossRef] [PubMed]
9. Ghoshal, S.; Stevens, J.R.; Billon, C.; Girardet, C.; Sitaula, S.; Leon, A.S.; Rao, D.C.; Skinner, J.S.; Rankinen, T.; Bouchard, C.; et al. Adropin: An endocrine link between the biological clock and cholesterol homeostasis. *Mol. Metab.* **2018**, *8*, 51–64. [CrossRef] [PubMed]
10. Stevens, J.R.; Kearney, M.L.; St-Onge, M.-P.; Stanhope, K.L.; Havel, P.J.; Kanaley, J.A.; Thyfault, J.P.; Weiss, E.P.; Butler, A.A. Inverse association between carbohydrate consumption and plasma adropin concentrations in humans. *Obesity* **2016**, *24*, 1731–1740. [CrossRef]
11. Bousmpoula, A.; Kouskouni, E.; Benidis, E.; Demeridou, S.; Kapeta-Kourkouli, R.; Chasiakou, A.; Baka, S. Adropin levels in women with polycystic ovaries undergoing ovarian stimulation: Correlation with lipoprotein lipid profiles. *Gynecol. Endocrinol.* **2018**, *34*, 153–156. [CrossRef]
12. Kuliczkowska-Płaksej, J.; Mierzwicka, A.; Jończyk, M.; Stachowska, B.; Urbanovych, A.; Bolanowski, M. Adropin in women with polycystic ovary syndrome. *Endokrynol. Polska* **2019**, *70*, 151–156. [CrossRef]
13. Danolić, M.J.; Perković, D.; Petrić, M.; Barišić, I.; Gugo, K.; Božić, J. Adropin Serum Levels in Patients with Primary Sjögren's Syndrome. *Biomolecules* **2021**, *11*, 1296. [CrossRef]
14. Available online: https://tanita.eu/media/wysiwyg/manuals/medical-approved-body-composition-monitors/mc-780-portable-instruction-manual.pdf (accessed on 29 June 2023).
15. Yosaee, S.; Khodadost, M.; Esteghamati, A.; Speakman, J.R.; Shidfar, F.; Nazari, M.N.; Bitarafan, V.; Djafarian, K. Metabolic Syndrome Patients Have Lower Levels of Adropin When Compared with Healthy Overweight/Obese and Lean Subjects. *Am. J. Men's Health* **2017**, *11*, 426–434. [CrossRef] [PubMed]
16. Soltani, S.; Kolahdouz-Mohammadi, R.; Aydin, S.; Yosaee, S.; Clark, C.C.T.; Abdollahi, S. Circulating levels of adropin and overweight/obesity: A systematic review and meta-analysis of observational studies. *Hormones* **2022**, *21*, 15–22. [CrossRef] [PubMed]
17. Akcılar, R.; Emel Koçak, F.; Şimşek, H.; Akcılar, A.; Bayat, Z.; Ece, E.; Kökdaşgil, H. The effect of adropin on lipid and glucose metabolism in rats with hyperlipidemia. *Iran. J. Basic Med. Sci.* **2016**, *19*, 245–251. [PubMed]
18. Boric-Skaro, D.; Mizdrak, M.; Luketin, M.; Martinovic, D.; Tokic, D.; Vilovic, M.; Supe-Domic, D.; Kurir, T.T.; Bozic, J. Serum Adropin Levels in Patients on Hemodialysis. *Life* **2021**, *11*, 337. [CrossRef]
19. Grzegorzewska, A.E.; Niepolski, L.; Mostowska, A.; Warchoł, W.; Jagodziński, P.P. Involvement of adropin and adropin-associated genes in metabolic abnormalities of hemodialysis patients. *Life Sci.* **2016**, *160*, 41–46. [CrossRef]
20. Hu, W.; Chen, L. Association of Serum Adropin Concentrations with Diabetic Nephropathy. *Mediat. Inflamm.* **2016**, *2016*, 6038261. [CrossRef]
21. Gu, X.; Li, H.; Zhu, X.; Gu, H.; Chen, J.; Wang, L.; Harding, P.; Xu, W. Inverse Correlation Between Plasma Adropin and ET-1 Levels in Essential Hypertension: A Cross-Sectional Study. *Medicine* **2015**, *94*, e1712. [CrossRef]
22. Fujie, S.; Hasegawa, N.; Sato, K.; Fujita, S.; Sanada, K.; Hamaoka, T.; Iemitsu, M. Aerobic exercise training-induced changes in serum adropin level are associated with reduced arterial stiffness in middle-aged and older adults. *Am. J. Physiol.* **2015**, *309*, H1642–H1647. [CrossRef] [PubMed]
23. Bozic, J.; Kumric, M.; Kurir, T.T.; Mens, I.; Borovac, J.A.; Martinovic, D.; Vilovic, M. Role of Adropin in Cardiometabolic Disorders: From Pathophysiological Mechanisms to Therapeutic Target. *Biomedicines* **2021**, *9*, 1407. [CrossRef]
24. Bučan Nenadić, D.; Radić, J.; Kolak, E.; Vučković, M.; Novak, I.; Selak, M.; Radić, M. Phase Angle Association with Dietary Habits and Metabolic Syndrome in Diabetic Hypertensive Patients: A Cross-Sectional Study. *Nutrients* **2022**, *14*, 5058. [CrossRef] [PubMed]
25. Meda, C.; Dolce, A.; Vegeto, E.; Maggi, A.; Della Torre, S. ERα-Dependent Regulation of Adropin Predicts Sex Differences in Liver Homeostasis during High-Fat Diet. *Nutrients* **2022**, *14*, 3262. [CrossRef]
26. Gupta, G.; Unruh, M.L.; Nolin, T.D.; Hasley, P.B. Primary care of the renal transplant patient. *J. Gen. Intern. Med.* **2010**, *25*, 731–740. [CrossRef]
27. Reggiani, F.; Moroni, G.; Ponticelli, C. Cardiovascular Risk after Kidney Transplantation: Causes and Current Approaches to a Relevant Burden. *J. Pers. Med.* **2022**, *12*, 1200. [CrossRef]
28. Yazgan, B.; Avcı, F.; Memi, G.; Tastekin, E. Inflammatory response and matrix metalloproteinases in chronic kidney failure: Modulation by adropin and spexin. *Exp. Biol. Med.* **2021**, *246*, 1917–1927. [CrossRef] [PubMed]
29. Es-Haghi, A.; Al-Abyadh, T.; Mehrad-Majd, H. The Clinical Value of Serum Adropin Level in Early Detection of Diabetic Nephropathy. *Kidney Blood Press. Res.* **2021**, *46*, 734–740. [CrossRef]

30. Berezina, T.A.; Obradovic, Z.; Boxhammer, E.; Berezin, A.A.; Lichtenauer, M.; Berezin, A.E. Adropin Predicts Chronic Kidney Disease in Type 2 Diabetes Mellitus Patients with Chronic Heart Failure. *J. Clin. Med.* **2023**, *12*, 2231. [CrossRef]
31. Simac, P.; Perkovic, D.; Bozic, I.; Bilopavlovic, N.; Martinovic, D.; Bozic, J. Serum Adropin Levels in Patients with Rheumatoid Arthritis. *Life* **2022**, *12*, 169. [CrossRef]

Disclaimer/Publisher's Note: The statements, opinions and data contained in all publications are solely those of the individual author(s) and contributor(s) and not of MDPI and/or the editor(s). MDPI and/or the editor(s) disclaim responsibility for any injury to people or property resulting from any ideas, methods, instructions or products referred to in the content.

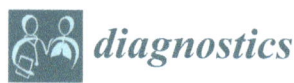

Article

Prognosis Predictive Markers in Patients with Chronic Obstructive Pulmonary Disease and COVID-19

Nicoleta Ștefania Motoc [1], Iulia Făgărășan [1], Andrada Elena Urda-Cîmpean [2,*] and Doina Adina Todea [1]

[1] Department of Medical Sciences-Pulmonology, Faculty of Medicine, "Iuliu Hațieganu" University of Medicine and Pharmacy, 8 Victor Babeș Street, 400012 Cluj-Napoca, Romania
[2] Department of Medical Informatics and Biostatistics, Faculty of Medicine, "Iuliu Hațieganu" University of Medicine and Pharmacy, Louis Pasteur Str. No. 6, 400349 Cluj-Napoca, Romania
* Correspondence: aurda@umfcluj.ro

Abstract: Some studies have reported that chronic respiratory illnesses in patients with COVID-19 result in an increase in hospitalization and death rates, while other studies reported to the contrary. The present research aims to determine if a predictive model (developed by combing different clinical, imaging, or blood markers) could be established for patients with both chronic obstructive pulmonary disease (COPD) and COVID-19, in order to be able to foresee the outcomes of these patients. A prospective observational cohort of 165 patients with both diseases was analyzed in terms of clinical characteristics, blood tests, and chest computed tomography results. The beta-coefficients from the logistic regression were used to create a score based on the significant identified markers for poor outcomes (transfers to an intensive care unit (ICU) for mechanical ventilation, or death). The severity of COVID-19, renal failure, diabetes, smoking status (current or previous), the requirement for oxygen therapy upon admission, high lactate dehydrogenase (LDH) and C-reactive protein level (CRP readings), and low eosinophil and lymphocyte counts were all identified as being indicators of a poor prognosis. Higher mortality was linked to the occurrence of renal failure, the number of affected lobes, the need for oxygen therapy upon hospital admission, high LDH, and low lymphocyte levels. Patients had an 86.4% chance of dying if their mortality scores were −2.80 or lower, based on the predictive model. The factors that were linked to a poor prognosis in patients who had both COPD and COVID-19 were the same as those that were linked to a poor prognosis in patients who had only COVID-19.

Keywords: COPD; COVID-19; SARS-CoV-2 infection; biomarkers; predictive model; mortality; intensive care unit; mechanical ventilation

Citation: Motoc, N.Ș.; Făgărășan, I.; Urda-Cîmpean, A.E.; Todea, D.A. Prognosis Predictive Markers in Patients with Chronic Obstructive Pulmonary Disease and COVID-19. Diagnostics 2023, 13, 2597. https://doi.org/10.3390/diagnostics13152597

Academic Editor: Koichi Nishimura

Received: 31 May 2023
Revised: 28 July 2023
Accepted: 30 July 2023
Published: 4 August 2023

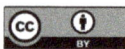

Copyright: © 2023 by the authors. Licensee MDPI, Basel, Switzerland. This article is an open access article distributed under the terms and conditions of the Creative Commons Attribution (CC BY) license (https://creativecommons.org/licenses/by/4.0/).

1. Introduction

The coronavirus disease of 2019 (COVID-19) was declared a public health emergency in January 2020 and was officially categorized as a pandemic in March 2020 [1]. The presentation of COVID-19 was extremely heterogeneous, ranging from the absence of symptoms to severe, and sometimes fulminant, disease that was associated with high mortality [2,3]. Factors associated with poor outcomes, according to Center for Disease Control and Prevention, were age, cancer, cerebrovascular disease, preexisting conditions (such as chronic kidney disease, chronic respiratory disease, chronic liver disease, diabetes mellitus, heart conditions, HIV, mental health disorders, and neurologic conditions), obesity (body mass index (BMI) ≥ 30 kg/m^2) and being overweight (BMI ranging from 25 to 29 kg/m^2), physical inactivity, pregnancy or recent pregnancy, primary immunodeficiencies, smoking (current and former), and the use of corticosteroids or other immunosuppressive medications [4–7].

The prevalence of respiratory chronic diseases among COVID-19 patients varied greatly in various studies and according to the periods of time when such studies were published. In the initial reports, chronic respiratory conditions such as chronic obstructive pulmonary disease (COPD) and asthma had a lower prevalence in COVID-19 patients than in the general population [8], while in more recent studies, the prevalence was higher than it was in the general population [9,10]. The impact of respiratory chronic diseases on COVID-19 remains an intensely debated subject. While there were studies that showed poorer outcomes among patients with coexisting chronic respiratory disease, in terms of mortality and hospitalization, there were other studies that reported no significant difference in SARS-CoV-2 infection, hospital admission, or death between patients with chronic respiratory disease and patients without chronic respiratory disease [11,12]. In addition, some chronic respiratory conditions, such as asthma, were associated with a lower risk of death than other chronic respiratory conditions [13].

Some authors even suggested a certain protection from COVID-19 among asthma patients [14]. On the other hand, COPD has consistently been a risk factor for adverse outcomes of COVID-19. The high expression levels of ACE2 in the small airway epithelium of smokers and COPD patients have indicated that both COPD and smoking were indicators of a greater risk of adverse outcomes of COVID-19. In COVID-19 patients, the presence of COPD was associated with a greater probability of intensive-care-unit admission, mechanical ventilation, and death [15]. COPD prevalence in patients with severe acute respiratory syndrome coronavirus 2 (SARS-CoV-2) infection varied among the studies from 1.1% to 38%, based on the selection of patients and the time when the studies were performed. Such patients seemed to have a more severe form of COVID-19, a higher risk of death, a higher hospitalization rate, an increased chance of being admitted to an intensive care unit, and a higher likelihood of being mechanically ventilated [16]. As in the case of respiratory diseases and COVID-19, there were data supporting the contrary: i.e., that COPD does not have an impact on the development of a SARS-CoV-2 infection [17–19]. Considering the higher susceptibility of COPD patients to developing COVID-19, due to greater expression of ACE, and the reduced lung reserve usually found in such patients, the majority of the studies seemed to favor the first hypothesis: i.e., that COPD has a negative affect on the outcomes of COVID-19 patients.

The primary objective of the current study was to determine markers (clinical, imaging, or blood tests) that could anticipate the outcomes in patients with COPD and COVID-19 As a secondary objective, we wanted to investigate whether a prediction model for poor outcomes could be created using such indicators. Such a model could help clinicians in their daily practice to quicky evaluate, based on certain markers at the time of hospital admission, a patient's chances of a poor outcome, and then take the necessary measures to ensure the best possible recovery.

2. Materials and Methods

This prospective observational study took place in the "Leon Daniello" Clinical Hospital of Pulmonology in Cluj-Napoca (Romania), a first-line hospital in the battle against COVID-19.

Study population: In our study, 180 patients with a confirmed SARS-CoV-2 infection were included; they had previously been diagnosed with COPD and been consecutively admitted to the hospital from 27 March 2020 to September 2021. We used a patient sample of convenience, as we had access to only this hospital and we included all patients who had both diseases. COVID-19 diagnostics were confirmed using a real-time reverse-transcriptase polymerase-chain-reaction (RT-PCR) assay to test nasal and pharyngeal swab specimens, according to World Health Organization guidance. COPD had already been diagnosed by a clinician according to Global Initiative for Chronic Obstructive Lung Disease (GOLD) guidelines. In Romania, hospitalization was compulsory for all patients diagnosed with COVID-19, regardless of the disease's clinical severity. Therefore, the patients had a mild, moderate, or severe form of COVID-19. Inclusion criteria consisted of all hospitalized patients with confirmed COVID-19 and COPD who gave their consent to participate in the study. Exclusion criteria included patients with confirmed COVID-19 and cancer, hematological diseases, severe cardiac disease (NYHA III and IV cardiac failure, recent myocardial infarction in the last three months, unstable arrhythmia), liver disease, systemic diseases, or pulmonary fibrosis. In addition, patients who did not wish to not participate and patients with missing data were excluded.

Study design: We collected patients' demographic, clinical, laboratory, and treatment data (if available) at hospital admission. If such data were not available, we extracted the data from the hospital's electronic medical records. At the time of hospital entry (i.e., before any intervention), we collected samples from all patients for laboratory tests and recorded the test results.

Blood examinations involved measuring complete blood cell counts and differential values. Serum bio-chemical tests were carried out, and erythrocyte sedimentation rates, C-reactive protein levels, procalcitonin levels, D-dimer levels, and serum ferritin levels were determined for the COVID-19 patients. All laboratory tests were carried out in the hospital laboratory with standard procedures. The laboratory reference values for white blood cells, neutrophils, lymphocytes, and eosinophils were 4.2–10, 1.8–7.3, 1.5–4, and 0.05–0.35 $\times 10^3/\mu L$, respectively. For ferritin, the values were 30–220 μg/la, and D-dimers were considered positive if they were above 500 ng/mL FEU (25–5000 ng/mL FEU). For procalcitonin, a value above 0.5 ng/mL was considered suggestive of bacterial infection.

The NLR ratio was calculated as the absolute count of neutrophils divided by the total count of lymphocytes. The PLR ratio was defined as: the absolute count of platelets divided by the absolute count of lymphocytes.

We also collected the following: clinical markers (age, number of days from the onset of symptoms until hospitalization, number of hospitalization days, smoking status, BMI, previous medication, previous oxygen therapy, and type of oxygen therapy administered at admission), imaging markers (severity of lung involvement, the presence of consolidation), and paraclinical parameters (blood tests). We assessed COVID-19 disease severity in all cases, using the following criteria [20]:

- mild disease: mild symptoms without dyspnea or pneumonia;
- moderate disease: evidence of lower respiratory disease by clinical assessment or imaging and a saturation of oxygen (SaO_2) $\geq$ 94 percent in room air at sea level;
- severe disease: tachypnea (respiratory rate > 30 breaths/minute), hypoxia (oxygen saturation $\leq$93% in room air or PaO_2/FiO_2 < 300 mmHg), or >50% lung involvement on imaging;
- critical care: involving respiratory failure, shock, or multiorgan dysfunction.

The types of oxygen therapy administered at admission were No O_2 (no mask), nasal canula (NC), simple O_2 mask (SM), ventury mask (VM), non-rebreathable mask (NRM), and high flow oxigen therapy(HFOT).

Regardless of disease severity, we performed chest computer tomographies (CTs) in the hospital radiology department for all the patients. Subsequently, the images were reviewed by a radiologist and a pulmonologist (the same radiologist and the same pulmonologist were involved throughout the entire study). Typical imaging findings in COVID-19 patients included ground-glass opacities (GGO) with peripheral and subpleural distribution, usually involving lower lobes. The CT severity score used in our study was the total severity score (TSS) proposed by Li et al. It has five grades of severity of involvement for five lung lobes: 0%, 1–25%, 26–50%, 51–75%, and 75–100%. The higher the score, the more severe the lung involvement [21]. Consolidation on thoracic CT in COVID-19 patients might be a sign of bacterial infection; therefore, those situations were noted separately.

Poor outcomes were defined as a patient's transfer to the intensive care unit (ICU) for mechanical ventilation (invasive or noninvasive) and death of a patient.

A good outcome was defined as discharge of a patient who was either completely healed or whose health had improved.

Statistical analysis was performed using the IBM (Richmond, VA, USA) SPSS STATISTICS 25 application. Qualitative data were presented using frequencies and percentages. The Kolmogorov–Smirnov test was used to test data distribution. Median values (25th percentile to 75th percentile) were calculated for quantitative variables with a non-normal distribution; means and standard deviations were calculated for quantitative variables with a normal distribution. The comparison of independent samples was tested with the Kruskal–Wallis test for non-normally distributed data. Frequencies were compared with the Chi-square test or the Fisher exact test. The significance level was set at $p < 0.05$. The event considered was the recovery of the patient (a good outcome), which was the opposite of the poor outcomes (transfer to the intensive care unit for mechanical ventilation or death). We used this variable as dependent in a multivariate logistic regression. All significant variables from the univariate analysis were introduced into the entered model as independent variables. A p-value < 0.05 was regarded as statistically significant. A logistic regression was performed to develop a model that might help in predicting outcomes in these patients. To evaluate the correctness of the fit of the logistic regression model, the Nagelkerke's R-squared value was computed (the model's power of explanation). For each possible model, a formula with specific biomarkers was presented in detail. The area under the curve (AUC) with a 95% confidence interval and the score cutoff points were calculated, based on the patients' score result and on the poor/good outcomes.

3. Results

Among the patients hospitalized with COVID-19 in the hospital, COPD prevalence was 7% (180 out of 2570 patients). All relevant data was available for only 165 patients. The patients' demographics characteristics are shown in Table 1. Most patients were male and over 65 years old, with a cardiovascular disease.

Table 1. Distribution of demographic characteristics and comorbidities for patients with COVID-19 and COPD.

Factors $n = 165$	n (%)	Factors $n = 165$	n (%)
Location		Smoking status	
• Rural	82 (49.7)	• Active smoker	40 (24.3)
• Urban	83 (50.3)	• Former smoker	42 (25.4)
		• Never-smoker data	83 (50.3)
Gender		Comorbidities present n(%)	
• Masculine	127 (77)	1. Cardiovascular disease	136 (82.4)
• Feminine	38 (23)	2. Arterial hypertension	136 (82.4)
		3. Diabetes	61 (36.9)
Age		4. Renal failure	22 (13.3)
• <65 years	42 (25.45)	5. Respiratory failure	55 (33.3)
• ≥65 years	123 (74.5)	6. Treatment	118 (71.52)
Spirometry parameters	m ± SD	50% (25–75%)	
FVC%	73.98 ± 22.68	72.4 (61.9–89.1)	
FEV1%	66.89 ± 26.49	63.9 (50.15–83.58)	
FEV1 (L)	1.78 ± 0.53	1.77 (1.42–2.07)	
MEF 50	43.71 ± 30.99	36.2 (19.73–60.23)	

3.1. Markers (Clinical, Imaging, or Blood Tests) That Could Predict the Outcomes in Patients with Both COPD and COVID-19

3.1.1. Risk Factors for Non-Invasive Ventilation Prognosis

To identify the significant risk factors, univariate logistic regression was used and one factor at a time was introduced into the modeling (Tables 2 and 3). The dependent variable was the binary variable for non-invasive ventilation (Yes/No).

Table 2. Qualitative markers for non-invasive ventilation.

Qualitative Markers		Non-Invasive Ventilation		p-Value
		Present (n = 42) n (%)	Absent (n = 123) n (%)	
COVID-19 severity	Severe	39 (92.9%)	79 (64.2%)	0.025 [a]
	moderate	2 (4.8%)	25 (20.3%)	
	light	1 (2.4%)	19 (15.4%)	
Consolidation		28 (66.7%)	51 (41.5%)	0.005 [a]
Number of affected lobes = 0		17 (40.5%)	76 (61.8%)	<0.001 [a]
Cardiovascular disease present		34 (81%)	102 (82.9%)	0.468 [b]
Arterial hypertension present		37 (88.1%)	99 (80.5%)	0.263 [a]
Diabetes present		22 (52.4%)	39 (31.7%)	0.017 [a]
Renal failure present		10 (23.8%)	12 (9.8%)	0.021 [a]
Respiratory failure present		16 (38.1%)	39 (31.7%)	0.448 [a]
Pre-existing treatment present		31 (73.8%)	87 (70.7%)	0.703 [a]
O₂-therapy type at admission	No O₂	3 (7.2%)	21 (17.1%)	<0.01 [a]
	NC	0 (0%)	32 (26.1%)	
	SM	3 (7.2%)	19 (15.5%)	
	VM	8 (19.1%)	25 (20.4%)	
	NRM	25 (59.6%)	24 (19.6%)	
	HFOT	3 (7.2%)	2 (1.7%)	
Smoker status	Non-smoker	27 (64.3%)	56 (45.5%)	0.044 [a]
	Former smoker	5 (11.9%)	37 (30.1%)	
	Active smoker	10 (23.8%)	30 (24.4%)	
	Non-smoker and former smoker	32 (76.2%)	93 (75.6%)	0.940 [a]
	Active smoker	10 (23.8%)	30 (24.4%)	
	Non-smoker	27 (64.3%)	56 (45.5%)	0.036 [a]
	Active smoker and former smoker	15 (35.7%)	67 (54.5%)	
ICU and invasive mechanical ventilation present		13 (31%)	5 (4.1%)	<0.001 [b]
Death		13 (31%)	12 (9.8%)	0.001 [a]

[a] Chi-square test; [b] Fisher exact test. Bold values were statistically significant.

Table 3. Quantitative markers for non-invasive ventilation.

Quantitative Markers	Present (n = 42) Median (Q1–Q3)	Absent (n = 123) Median (Q1–Q3)	Mann–Whitney U: p-Value
Age	72 (65.75–75)	70 (64–78)	0.752
LDH	425 (326.5–695)	336 (240–482)	0.003
PCR	60.1 (9.88–111.33)	15.88 (6.5–57)	0.004
Eosinophile	0 (0–0.01)	0.01 (0–0.08)	0.002
Lymphocytes	0.75 (0.54–1.13)	0.98 (0.72–1.35)	0.017
Leucocytes	8.73 (5.68–11.72)	7.66 (5.92–10.12)	0.429
Thrombocytes	202.5 (157.75–286)	225 (174–300)	0.483
Neutrophiles	7.08 (4.43–9.71)	6.12 (4.32–8.27)	0.346
PLR	257.13 (171.03–452.69)	221.54 (162.1–321.84)	0.109
NLR	10.37 (4.44–14.85)	6.12 (4.07–9.88)	0.020

The logistic regression included COVID-19 severity, consolidation, number of affected lung lobes, eosinophiles, PCR, LDH, neutrophiles, lymphocytes, leucocytes, thrombocytes, diabetes, renal failure, respiratory failure, pre-existing treatment present, O_2-therapy type at admission, smoker status, and non-invasive ventilations.

In this predictive model, 61.7% (Nagelkerke's R-squared value) of the variance of non-invasive ventilation were explained by the number of affected pulmonary lobes (1 lobe), high PCR values, and the presence of diabetes.

Based on these significant markers, a score was computed for each patient, using the beta-coefficients from the logistic regression model:

Non-invasive ventilation score =
  if 1 lobe was affected, then −3.39, otherwise 0
  + PCR value * 0.02
  + if diabetes present, then 1.15, otherwise 0
  − 6.2 (constant).

The area under the curve (AUC) for the non-invasive ventilation score and non-invasive ventilation was 66.7% (95% CI [57.8–75.6%], $p < 0.001$) (Figure 1).

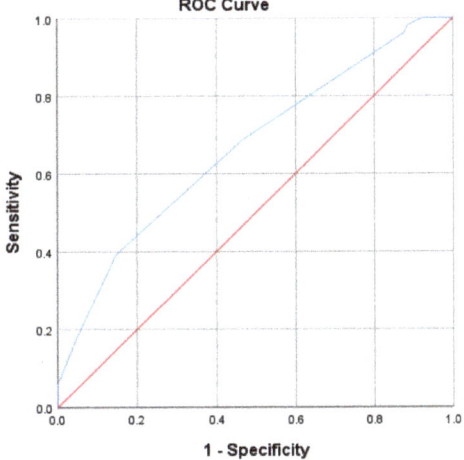

Figure 1. ROC curve (blue line) for predicting non-invasive ventilation using the non-invasive ventilation score.

A patient with a non-invasive ventilation score of −4.5 or lower had an 85% chance of being placed on non-invasive ventilation.

3.1.2. Risk Factors for ICU and Invasive Mechanical Ventilation Prognosis

To identify the significant risk factors, univariate logistic regression was used and one factor at a time was introduced into the modeling (Tables 4 and 5). The dependent variable was the binary variable for ICU and invasive mechanical ventilation (Yes/No).

The logistic regression included COVID-19 severity, consolidation, number of affected lung lobes, eosinophiles, PCR, LDH, neutrophiles, lymphocytes, leucocytes, thrombocytes, renal failure, diabetes, O_2 therapy type at admission, smoker status, non-invasive ventilation, and pre-existing treatment.

In this predictive model, 78% (Nagelkerke's R-squared value) of the variance of invasive mechanical ventilation in the ICU was explained by the number of affected pulmonary lobes (two lobes), active smoker status, pre-existing pulmonary treatment, and existing non-invasive ventilation.

Table 4. Qualitative markers for invasive mechanical ventilation in the ICU.

		Invasive Ventilation		
Qualitative Markers		Present (*n* = 18) *n* (%)	Absent (*n* = 147) *n* (%)	*p*-Value
COVID-19 severity	severe	14 (77.8%)	104 (70.7%)	>0.05 [b]
	moderate	2 (11.1%)	25 (17%)	
	light	2 (11.1%)	18 (12.2%)	
Consolidation		12 (66.7%)	67 (45.6%)	0.091 [a]
Number of affected lobes = 0		8 (44.8%)	85 (57.8%)	
Number of affected lobes ≥ 3		8 (44.8%)	18 (12.3%)	**0.002** [b]
Cardio-vascular disease present		16 (88.9%)	120 (81.6%)	0.742 [b]
Arterial hypertension present		14 (77.8%)	122 (83%)	0.526 [b]
Diabetes present		7 (38.9%)	54 (36.7%)	0.858 [a]
Renal failure present		4 (22.2%)	18 (12.2%)	0.267 [b]
Respiratory failure present		6 (33.3%)	49 (33.3%)	>0.05 [b]
Pre-existing treatment present		6 (33.3%)	112 (76.2%)	**<0.001** [a]
O$_2$-therapy type at admission	No O$_2$	4 (22.2%)	20 (13.6%)	>0.05 [b]
	NC	0 (0%)	32 (21.8%)	
	SM	4 (22.2%)	18 (12.2%)	
	VM	1 (5.6%)	32 (21.8%)	
	NRM	7 (38.9%)	42 (28.6%)	
	HFOT	2 (11.1%)	3 (2%)	
Smoker status	Non-smoker	13 (72.2%)	70 (47.6%)	>0.05 [b]
	Former smoker	1 (5.6%)	41 (27.9%)	
	Active smoker	4 (22.2%)	36 (24.5%)	
	Non-smoker and former smoker	14 (77.8%)	111 (75.5%)	>0.05 [b]
	Active smoker	4 (22.2%)	36 (24.5%)	
	Non-smoker	13 (72.2%)	70 (47.6%)	**0.049** [a]
	Active-smoker and former smoker	5 (27.8%)	77 (52.4%)	
Non-invasive ventilation present		13 (72.2%)	29 (19.7%)	**<0.001** [b]

[a] Chi-square test; [b] Fisher exact test. Bold values were statistically significant.

Table 5. Quantitative markers for invasive mechanical ventilation in the ICU.

Quantitative Markers	Present (*n* = 18) Median (Q1–Q3)	Absent (*n* = 147) Median (Q1–Q3)	Mann–Whitney U: *p*-Value
Age	69 (62.25–74.5)	71 (64–78)	0.430
LDH	425 (326.5–717.25)	349 (244–506)	0.053
PCR	16.44 (7.78–93.03)	20.6 (7.19–70)	0.576
Eosinophile	0 (0–0.01)	0.01 (0–0.07)	0.031
Lymphocytes	0.69 (0.57–0.91)	0.98 (0.71–1.34)	0.012
Leucocytes	8.88 (6.28–14.67)	7.77 (5.84–10.12)	0.234
Thrombocytes	222 (152.25–324)	222 (172–298)	0.724
Neutrophiles	7.86 (5.67–13.06)	6.29 (4.31–8.35)	0.083
PLR	291.89 (212.83–476.66)	232.97 (162.6–354.08)	0.123
NLR	11.73 (6.73–17.2)	6.13 (4.07–10.33)	0.006

Based on these significant markers, a score was computed for each patient, using the beta-coefficients from the logistic regression model:
Invasive ventilation score =
　　if two lobes were affected, then −14, otherwise 0
　　+ if active smoker, then −13.4, otherwise 0
　　+ if with non-invasive ventilation, then +8, otherwise 0
　　+ if with existing pulmonary medication, then −8.3, otherwise 0.
The area under the curve (AUC) for the invasive ventilation score and invasive mechanical ventilation in the ICU and was 83.8% (95% CI [76.8–90.8%], $p < 0.001$) (Figure 2).

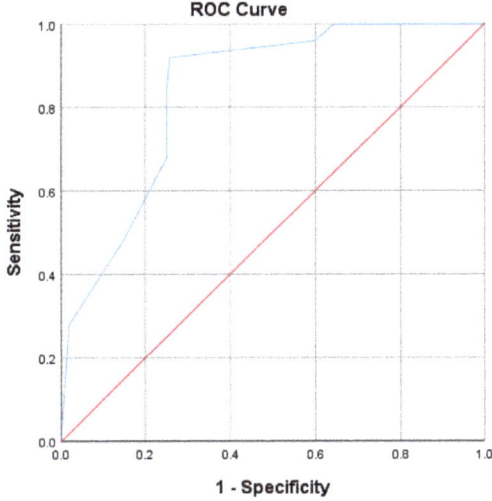

Figure 2. ROC curve for predicting ICU and invasive mechanical ventilation using the invasive ventilation score.

A patient with an invasive ventilation score of −7.15 or lower had a 74.2% chance of being transferred to the ICU and being placed on invasive mechanical ventilation.

3.1.3. Risk Factors for Death Prognosis

To identify the significant risk factors for a prognosis of death, univariate logistic regression was used one factor at a time and introduced into the modeling (Tables 6 and 7). The dependent variable was the binary variable of death (Yes/No).

The logistic regression included renal failure, non-invasive ventilation, invasive mechanical ventilation in the ICU, lymphocytes, and pre-existing treatment.

In this predictive model, only 38.7% (Nagelkerke's R-squared value) of the variance of death were explained by the presence of renal failure and existing mechanical ventilation in the ICU.

Based on these significant markers, a score was computed for each patient, using the beta-coefficients from the logistic regression model:
Mortality Score =
　　if renal failure present, then 1.36, otherwise 0
　　+ if with mechanical ventilation in the ICU, then +3.75, otherwise 0
　　− 3.48 (constant).

The area under the curve (AUC) for mortality score and death was 83.8% (95% CI [74.3–93.2%], $p < 0.001$) (Figure 3).

Table 6. Qualitative markers for death (univariate logistic regression).

Qualitative Markers		Death Present (n = 25) n (%)	Death Absent (n = 140) n (%)	p-Value
COVID-19 severity	Severe	21 (84%)	97 (69.3%)	>0.05 [b]
	moderate			
	light	2 (8%)	25 (17.9%)	
Consolidation		15 (60%)	64 (45.7%)	0.188 [a]
Number of affected lobes ≥ 3		9 (36%)	17 (12.1%)	**<0.01 [b]**
Cardio-vascular disease present		23 (92%)	113 (80.7%)	0.255 [b]
Arterial hypertension present		20 (80%)	116 (82.9%)	0.776 [b]
Diabetes present		10 (40%)	51 (36.4%)	0.733 [a]
Renal failure present		7 (28%)	15 (10.7%)	**0.048 [b]**
Respiratory failure present		11 (44%)	44 (31.4%)	0.219 [a]
Pre-existing treatment present		15 (60%)	103 (73.6%)	0.166 [a]
O_2-therapy type at admission	No O_2	4 (16%)	20 (14.3%)	≥0.05 [b]
	NC	0 (0%)	32 (22.9%)	
	SM	3 (12%)	19 (13.6%)	
	VM	3 (12%)	30 (21.4%)	
	NRM	12 (48%)	37 (26.4%)	
	HFOT	3 (12%)	2 (1.4%)	
Smoker status	Non-smoker	16 (64%)	67 (47.9%)	0.308 [a]
	Former smoker	4 (16%)	38 (27.1%)	
	Active smoker	5 (20%)	35 (25%)	
	Non-smoker and former smoker	20 (80%)	105 (75%)	0.591 [a]
	Active smoker	5 (20%)	35 (25%)	
	Non-smoker	16 (64%)	67 (47.9%)	0.137 [a]
	Active smoker and former smoker	9 (36%)	73 (52.1%)	
ICU and Invasive mechanical ventilation present		13 (52%)	5 (3.6%)	**<0.001 [b]**
Non-invasive ventilation present		13 (52%)	29 (20.7%)	**0.001 [a]**

[a] Chi-square test; [b] Fisher exact test. Bold values were statistically significant.

Table 7. Quantitative markers for death.

Quantitative Markers	Present (n = 25) Median (Q1–Q3)	Absent (n = 140) Median (Q1–Q3)	Mann–Whitney U: p-Value
Age	71 (66.5–76.5)	71 (64–77.75)	0.457
LDH	427 (351–737.5)	343.5 (244–503.75)	0.031
PCR	24 (9.18–95.3)	20.25 (6.53–65.88)	0.233
Eosinophile	0 (0–0.03)	0.01 (0–0.06)	0.221
Lymphocytes	0.77 (0.6–0.99)	0.99 (0.68–1.34)	0.036
Leucocytes	8.61 (5.15–11.82)	7.68 (5.88–10.33)	0.757
Thrombocytes	198 (133.5–277)	225 (174–299.5)	0.139
Neutrophiles	6.47 (3.65–8.75)	6.36 (4.5–9.01)	0.849
PLR	232.97 (157.79–418.86)	239.78 (167.85–359.88)	0.794
NLR	8.61 (4.45–12.54)	6.44 (4.03–10.88)	0.304

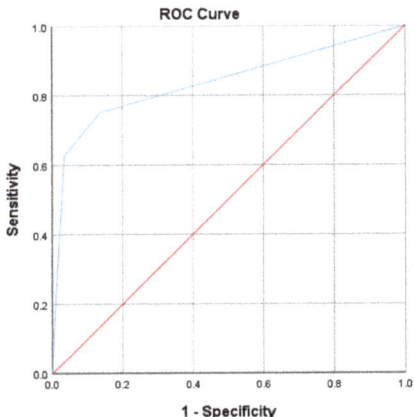

Figure 3. ROC curve for predicting death, using the mortality score.

A patient with a mortality score of −2.80 or lower had an 86.4% chance of dying.

For example, a male patient with declining health was initially prescribed non-invasive ventilation, then invasive mechanical ventilation, but then he died. He had three affected lobes, a PCR = 8.8, no renal failure, an existing pulmonary medication, was a non-smoker, and had diabetes, with the following scores:

- Non-invasive ventilation score = −4.87 (power of predictive model 61.7%, chance of non-invasive ventilation), which was lower than −4.5; thus, he had an 85% chance of being placed on non- invasive ventilation.
- Invasive ventilation score = −0.3 (power of predictive model 78%, chance of invasive mechanical ventilation), which was greater than −7.15, and he had a 74.2% chance of being transferred to the ICU and being placed on invasive ventilation.
- Mortality score = 0.27, which was higher than −2.80. Since there were only 25 deaths in the sample, this model had low precision and only 38.7% of the variance of death was explained by the above markers.

3.2. Good versus Poor Prognosis

Non-invasive ventilation was prescribed to 25.45% (42/165) of the hospitalized patients, but for 30.1% (13/42) of those non-invasive ventilated patients needed to be transferred to the ICU for mechanical ventilation (invasive) and, in the end, 9 of those 13 patients died (Table 8).

Table 8. Distribution of patients according to their oxygen-ventilation type and death outcome.

Ventilation	ICU and Invasive Mechanical Ventilation						Total
	Mechanical Ventilation		Mechanical Ventilation Total	No Mechanical Ventilation		No Mechanical Ventilation Total	
	Death	Survival		Death	Survival		
Non-invasive ventilation	9	4	13	4	25	29	42
No ventilation	4	1	5	8	110	118	123
Total	13	5	18	12	133	147	165

Poor outcome = death (YES) OR ICU + IMV(YES) OR NIV (YES) = 18 + 12 + 25 = 55. Good outcome = 110 (survival with no ventilation OR survival with no invasive mechanical ventilation).

4. Discussion

The present study analyzed prognosis predictive markers in patients hospitalized with concomitant COPD and SARS-CoV-2 infection. Out of 165 patients with complete data, 55 had a poor prognosis (non-invasive/invasive mechanically ventilation or death), and 110 patients survived with no ventilation at all. We used a sample of all patients from the beginning of the pandemic in March 2020 until September 2021, during which period COVID-19 patients were hospitalized in Romania, regardless of the COVID-19 severity. Therefore, the sample was varied and random.

The negative prognostic factors identified in the present research were COVID-19 severity, the presence of renal failure, the presence of diabetes, smoking status (active or former), the requirement of oxygen therapy at admission, high values of LDH and CRP, and low values of eosinophils and lymphocytes. The presence of renal failure, the number of affected lobes, the requirements of oxygen therapy at admission, high LDH, and low lymphocytes values were associated with higher mortality. Based on the significant discovered markers for each defined prognosis (non-invasive ventilation, invasive ventilation, or death), a score was computed using the beta-coefficients from the logistic regression.

Although the predictive models were all statistically significant ($p < 0.05$), the power of each prediction model to explain the model differed. Of the three prediction models using biomarkers, the invasive ventilation score description was the most accurate (78%). Furthermore, its AUC of 83.8% (95% CI [76.8–90.8%]) demonstrated a moderate-to-good prediction of patients being provided with invasive mechanical ventilation in the ICU.

A non-invasive ventilation score of −4.5 or lower indicated an 85% likelihood of a patient being placed on non-invasive ventilation. A patient's risk of being admitted to the ICU and receiving invasive mechanical ventilation was 74.2% if their invasive ventilation score was −7.15 or below. A patient had an 86.4% probability of dying if the patient's mortality score was −2.80 or lower. Models for predicting non-invasive and invasive ventilation scores took into account the number of affected lobes, which reflected the severity of a SARS-CoV-2 infection. The most important parameter for the mortality score, as expected, was invasive mechanical ventilation. Based on the results, we assumed that the prognosis of patients with both COPD and COVID-19 depended mostly on the severity of COVID-19 rather than on COPD status. Since our study did not address the evaluation of COPD severity—a study limitation—we were unable to provide any definitive conclusions.

The identified poor-prognosis risk factors in our study were the same as the risk factors for poor prognosis in COVID-19 cases: i.e., certain comorbidities (renal failure and diabetes), active or former smoker status, and the extension of pulmonary lesions [4–6]. Our findings were consistent with those that suggested that COPD had no impact on the outcomes for COVID-19 patients [17–19]. As patients with pre-existing chronic diseases may be more vulnerable to organ failure, as a result of their altered previous status, this factor may encourage the development of more severe types of COVID-19. The prevalence of COPD in our study was 7%. According to a study carried out by the Romanian Society of Pulmonology in 2019, the prevalence of COPD in the general population was 8.3% in patients over 40 years old [22].

Thus, COPD was more prevalent in the general population than it was among COVID-19 patients. In a retrospective cohort, the prevalence of respiratory disease among COVID-19 patients at the beginning of pandemic was very low—1.6% for chronic obstructive pulmonary disease (COPD) and 0.6% for asthma—lower even than the prevalence of such respiratory diseases in the general population (8.6% and 4.2%, respectively) [8]. The low prevalence was confirmed by other studies [23–25]. This was in contrast with the UK study of the International Severe Acute Respiratory and Emerging Infection Consortium (ISARIC), World Health Organization Clinical Characterization Protocol (UK study), which reported a higher proportion of patients with asthma (10.4%) and non-asthmatic chronic pulmonary diseases (18%) among patients with COVID-19, as compared with the general population [9].

There are, however, a few factors that must be taken into consideration when considering the differences among these observational studies. First, there could have been some under-reporting of data, as the first studies focused on hospitalized and intensive-care-unit (ICU) patients, rather than on mild outpatient cases. Second, the means used by clinicians to collect data in the beginning of the pandemic, when everything was new and unknown, plus the lack of a nationwide standardized electronic data registry system in all countries, contributed to these differences. Finally, there was an underdiagnosis of COPD in many countries (including Romania) during the pandemic, as spirometry was not performed, to avoid contamination.

The patients included in the present study had stage 2 COPD (a moderate form) and most of them (71.52%) were receiving inhaled treatment. Compliance with the treatment was, unfortunately, not determined. This could explain why previous medication administration, as a parameter, was associated with poor prognosis in patients who were invasively ventilated. Another explanation could be that those patients had more severe or symptomatic forms of COPD. We did not find any relationship between GOLD-stage COPD and outcomes; it would have been useful to determine the outcome by including a consideration of COPD severity. Most of our patients were typical of the general population with respect to COPD and COVID-19: i.e., male, over 65 years old, and former-or-active smokers. Age and sex are known prognostic factors for many chronic diseases. For COVID-19, age was a prognostic factor related to hospitalization and mortality, presenting a linear dose–response association with mortality. Although large between-study heterogeneity was observed, in most studies, the risk of severe disease rose steadily with age, with more than 93% of deaths occurring among adults $\geq$ 50 years and 74% of deaths occurring in adults $\geq$65 years [6]. Sex was identified as a prognostic factor for ICU admission, acute kidney injury, invasive mechanical ventilation, and a composite outcome (defined as ICU admission and death). In these situations, small or moderate between-study heterogeneity was observed, but 95% of the prediction intervals included a null value for acute kidney injury and a composite outcome. We did not find any relationship with COPD severity, as assessed by lung function. In a recent study published by Yeung et al., which looked into the association of smokers' lung function and COPD in COVID-19, the authors did not find any relationship between lung function and COPD, while they found that smoking increased the risk of COVID-19, compared with population controls, for overall COVID-19, including the life-time smoking index odds ratio (OR) of 1.19 with a 95% confidence interval (CI) [1.11–1.27], hospitalization with COVID-19 (OR = 1.67, 95% CI [1.42–1.97]), and severe COVID-19 (OR = 1.48, 95% CI [1.10–1.98]), with directionally consistent effects based on sensitivity analyses [26].

In another study, smoking was an important risk factor for poor outcomes in COVID-19 patients. SARS-CoV-2 bears an envelope spike protein that is primed by the cellular serine protease TMPRSS2 to facilitate fusion of the virus with the cell's angiotensin-converting enzyme 2 (ACE-2) receptor and subsequent cell entry [27,28]. ACE-2 expression was significantly elevated in COPD patients, compared to control subjects. Current smoking was also associated with higher ACE-2 expression, compared with that of former smokers or patients who had never smoked, an observation that has subsequently been validated by other groups in separate reports on lung tissue and airway epithelial samples and supported by additional evidence linking ACE-2 expression to nicotine exposure [27,29].

Nonetheless, there was increasing evidence that COPD may be a risk factor for more severe COVID-19 disease. An analysis of comorbidities in 1590 COVID-19 patients found that COPD carried an odds ratio of 2.681 (95% CI [1.424–5.048]; p = 0.002) for ICU admission, mechanical ventilation, or death, even after adjustment for age and smoking; 62.5% of the severe cases had a history of COPD (compared with only 15.3% of the non-severe cases), and 25% of those patients who died were COPD patients (compared with only 2.8% of those who survived). In a multicenter study, COPD patients made up 15.7% of the critically ill patients, but only 2.3% of the moderately ill patients (p < 0.001) [15]. Other studies found similar, but statistically weaker, differences in COPD rates between ICU-admission patients and non-ICU-admission patients (8.3% versus 1.0%; p = 0.054) [9], between severe and non-severe cases (4.8% versus 1.4%; p = 0.026) [16]; and between non-survivors and survivors (7% versus 1%; p = 0.047). The same conclusion was drawn from the research performed by Lee et al., in which they concluded that even though COPD was not a risk factor for respiratory failure, it was a significant independent risk factor for all-cause mortality (OR = 1.80, 95% CI [1.11–2.93]) [30]. Among COVID-19 patients, relatively greater proportions of patients with COPD received mechanical ventilation and intensive critical care [16,30,31].

Acute severe respiratory failure associated with COVID-19 was characterized by severe hypoxemia, with good lung compliance [16]. Similar risk factors have been described by Bellou et al. in a recent systematic review that evaluated, in over 400 articles (observational studies, meta-analyses), prognostic factors for adverse outcomes in patients with COVID-19. The following parameters were associated with a poor outcome: age, sex, smoking status, the presence of dyspnea, oxygen saturation at admission, obstructive sleep apnea, venous thromboembolism, cardiovascular disease, chronic kidney disease, chronic lung disease, diabetes mellitus, obesity, cancer, chronic liver disease, COPD, dementia, peripheral arterial disease, and rheumatological disease [32].

We decided to mark the consolidation cases separately, as those cases could be a sign of bacterial infection. Consolidation is defined as a homogenous high density (area of increased attenuation) that obscures the bronchial and vascular markings (airway walls and blood vessels). It is caused by the filling of the alveolar spaces with fluid, exudates, transudate, blood, or neoplastic cells. In this condition, alveolar air is replaced by other materials (e.g., pathological fluids, cells, or tissues), with a subsequent increase in pulmonary parenchymal density. It has bilateral, multifocal, and subsegmental distribution. The presence of consolidation is considered a sign of progressive COVID-19 disease, as it develops in the second week after the onset of symptoms. It is seen more in patients who are over 50 years old; therefore, consolidation could serve as a clue for an illness that necessitates greater vigilance in management [33].

According to another review, consolidation in COVID-19 pneumonia tended to be patchy or segmental, irregular, or nodular, and mainly subpleural and peripheral, with a reported incidence of 2–64%, depending on the duration of the illness. It usually appears 10 to 12 days after the onset of symptoms—after the appearance of GGO. One study reported high mortality in patients with consolidation. Another study of 83 patients reported consolidation in patients with severe or advanced disease. In a different study, the incidence of consolidation was significantly higher in older patients (>50 years) and significantly higher in patients who had symptoms for more than 4 days [34].

Air bronchogram, which is defined as air-filled bronchi in areas with high density, has variable incidence in different reports, ranging from 28% to 80% of patients. It is usually a sign of advanced disease and is usually seen after the second week from the onset of symptoms. It can be seen in both GGO and consolidation cases [21,34].

As COVID-19 and bacterial pneumonia are different clinical entities from COPD acute exacerbation (although they might/frequently coexist), we decided to describe the consolidation as if they are very frequent, as they might suggest that COPD increases the risk of bacterial complication in patients with SARS-CoV-2 infection. Bacterial infection was not very common in COVID-19 patients, especially not at the beginning of the disease. Since it could appear later, as a complication of the disease or because of medical care (especially invasive medical care), it is worth reflecting on the innate altered immune response that is involved in severe forms of COVID-19 [34].

If bacterial pneumonia could coexist with COPD, why would COVID-19 not coexist—especially if we consider SARS-CoV-2 a virus that could be a trigger for exacerbation?

An acute exacerbation of COPD represents the aggravation of respiratory symptoms beyond day-to-day variation that requires a change in medication. Eighty percent of the acute exacerbations were linked either to bacterial or viral pathogens. More than half of them had a bacterial etiology [35,36]. The most frequent germs that have been isolated during COPD exacerbation were streptococcus pneumoniae, hemophilus influenza and moraxella catharalis, but we must consider that microorganisms are commonly detected in the airways in stable COPD cases and are considered to be "colonizers" in the absence of acute infective symptoms [37].

The term "colonization" is debatable, as the microorganisms identified in stable COPD cases are not necessarily benign. As a subset of COPD patients has frequent exacerbations, the concept of the inherent susceptibility to acute infection in COPD cases subsequently triggering AECOPD events has been developed. The impaired innate immune response favored by smoking results in bacterial colonization, which promotes airway and systemic inflammation, leading to COPD progression and exacerbation. To this, we add the antibiotic-mediated lung dysbiosis during therapy [37]. Defects in innate immunity could also play a role in increased susceptibility to viruses. Recognition of viral infection by the innate immune system is essential for coordinating an effective antiviral response in the airways; however, in patients with COPD, the cascade from recognition to response falters, due to exposure to cigarette smoke that diminishes the antiviral response [38]. Furthermore, mucociliary clearance, which is key for the removal of virus from the airways, appears to be perturbed in COPD, as cigarette smoking exposure reduces both the number and the length of cilia, while goblet cell hyperplasia in COPD leads to more viscous mucus in the airways, further impeding proper ciliary motion [38–40].

Since the SARS-CoV-2 virus shares common pathobiological and clinical features with other viral agents, it could trigger COPD exacerbation, with the potential for a more long-term adverse impact. Nevertheless, COVID-19 and AECOPD are different clinical entities, although they could coexist, making it very difficult to differentiate the two. When an exacerbation of COPD occurred during COVID-19, the usual guidelines called for initiation of systemic glucocorticoids, as recommend by the GOLD guidelines. For patients hospitalized with COVID-19, the use of nebulized medications should be avoided or limited to negative pressure rooms because of the risk of aerosolizing SARS-CoV-2 and enhancing the spread of disease. Clinical outcomes, including mortality, are worse in males, older individuals, and patients with comorbidities. COPD patients are included in shielding strategies because of their susceptibility to virus-induced exacerbations, compromised pulmonary function, and a high prevalence of associated comorbidities [39]. Most of our patients had corticosteroids (ICS) in their treatment, in a fixed combination with a bronchodilator. In case of diagnostic uncertainty, we advise physicians to be careful about initiating ICS or ICS/long-acting β-agonist in patients in the absence of clear objective evidence of asthma. Similarly, there was no evidence to suggest a change in the advice that the dose of ICS for asthma patients be increased at the onset of exacerbation [16].

However, we believe that our findings are pertinent, as they demonstrate the significance of COVID-19 severity in patients' outcomes for chronic respiratory disorders. A medical team should act more quickly and take more drastic measures as a result of the presence of observed poor prognosis variables in patients with COPD and COVID-19. We believe that it is crucial to be ready to provide better care of these patients by knowing that the prognosis is impacted by the infection and not by the respiratory disease, as the virus is here to stay and its capacity to adapt is rather impressive [41].

Limitations: This was a single-center study; therefore, certain aspects cannot be generalized. Second, the sample had mostly good outcomes, but for better prognostic models, more cases with poor outcome are needed. Third, COPD diagnosis could have been underestimated, given that spirometry was not performed during the pandemic period and the disease might have been even more prevalent. The COPD risk class was not assessed; consequently, COPD severity could have an impact on COVID-19 impact and not be detected in our study. We did not assess the relationship between COPD severity and patients' outcomes. This was important, as in Romania all patients with COVID-19 were hospitalized regardless of the COVID-19 severity, so the population was very heterogenous.

5. Conclusions

The factors identified in the current research that were linked to a poor prognosis in patients with COPD and COVID-19 were similar to those linked to a poor prognosis in patients with COVID-19 alone. The severity of COVID-19 affected patient outcomes far more than COPD itself. Although COPD patients may be more at risk for COVID-19 infection, COVID-19 seemed to have an influence on how the disease progressed.

Author Contributions: Conceptualization, N.Ș.M. and D.A.T.; methodology, N.Ș.M. and D.A.T.; validation, N.Ș.M., I.F. and A.E.U.-C.; formal analysis, A.E.U.-C.; investigation, N.Ș.M. and I.F.; resources, N.Ș.M. and D.A.T.; data curation, N.Ș.M. and I.F.; writing—original draft preparation, N.Ș.M., I.F. and A.E.U.-C.; writing—review and editing, D.A.T. and A.E.U.-C.; visualization, N.Ș.M.; supervision, N.Ș.M. and D.A.T.; project administration, D.A.T. All authors have read and agreed to the published version of the manuscript.

Funding: This research received no external funding.

Institutional Review Board Statement: This study was conducted in accordance with the Declaration of Helsinki, and approved by the Hospital Ethics Committee of "Leon Daniello" Clinical Hospital of Pulmonology (nr. 35/25 January 2021).

Informed Consent Statement: Informed consent was obtained from all subjects involved in this study.

Data Availability Statement: The data presented in this study are available on request from the corresponding author.

Conflicts of Interest: The authors declare no conflict of interest.

References

1. Chung, C.C.Y.; Ng, Y.N.C.; Jain, R.; Chung, B.H.Y. A thematic study: Impact of COVID-19 pandemic on rare disease organisations and patients across ten jurisdictions in the Asia Pacific region. *Orphanet J. Rare Dis.* **2021**, *16*, 119. [CrossRef]
2. Limongelli, G.; Iucolano, S.; Monda, E.; Elefante, P.; De Stasio, C.; Lubrano, I.; Caiazza, M.; Mazzella, M.; Fimiani, F.; Galdo, M.; et al. Diagnostic issues faced by a rare disease healthcare network during COVID-19 outbreak: Data from the Campania Rare Disease Registry. *J. Public Health* **2022**, *44*, 586–594. [CrossRef]
3. Higham, A.; Mathioudakis, A.; Vestbo, J.; Singh, D. COVID-19 and COPD: A narrative review of the basic science and clinical outcomes. *Eur. Respir. Rev.* **2020**, *29*, 200199. [CrossRef]
4. Centers for Disease Control and Prevention. *Underlying Medical Conditions Associated with High Risk for Severe COVID-19: Information for Healthcare Providers [Internet]*; Centers for Disease Control and Prevention: Atlanta, GA, USA, 2021; [updated date—9 February 2023]. Available online: https://www.cdc.gov/coronavirus/2019-ncov/hcp/clinical-care/underlyingconditions.html (accessed on 1 March 2022).
5. Centers for Disease Control and Prevention. *Science Brief: Evidence Used to Update the List of Underlying Medical Conditions That Increase a Person's Risk of Severe Illness from COVID-19 [Internet]*; Centers for Disease Control and Prevention: Atlanta, GA, USA, 2021; [updated date 9 February 2023]. Available online: https://www.cdc.gov/coronavirus/2019-ncov/hcp/clinical-care/underlyingconditions.html#anchor_1618433687270 (accessed on 1 March 2022).
6. Centers for Disease Control and Prevention. *Risk for COVID-19 Infection, Hospitalization, and Death by Age Group [Internet]*; Centers for Disease Control and Prevention: Atlanta, GA, USA, 2021; [updated date—25 April 2023]. Available online: https://www.cdc.gov/coronavirus/2019-ncov/covid-data/investigations-discovery/hospitalization-death-by-age.html (accessed on 16 June 2022).
7. McIntosh, K. *COVID-19: Clinical Features [Internet]*; Up to Date: Alphen aan den Rijn, The Netherlands, 2023; [updated date—27 March 2023]; Available online: https://www.uptodate.com/contents/covid-19-clinical-features?search=covid%2019%20risk%20factors&sectionRank=1&usage_type=default&anchor=H2249070035&source=machineLearning&selectedTitle=1~150&display_rank=1#H2249070035 (accessed on 16 January 2022).
8. Guan, W.J.; Liang, W.H.; Shi, Y.; Gan, L.X.; Wang, H.B.; He, J.X.; Zhong, N.S. Chronic Respiratory Diseases and the Outcomes of COVID-19: A Nationwide Retrospective Cohort Study of 39,420 Cases. *J. Allergy Clin. Immunol. Pract.* **2021**, *9*, 2645–2655. [CrossRef]
9. Bloom, C.I.; Drake, T.M.; Docherty, A.B.; Lipworth, B.J.; Johnston, S.L.; Nguyen-Van-Tam, J.S.; Carson, G.; Dunning, J.; Harrison, E.M.; Baillie, J.K.; et al. Risk of adverse outcomes in patients with underlying respiratory conditions admitted to hospital with COVID-19: A national, multicentre prospective cohort study using the ISARIC WHO Clinical Characterisation Protocol UK. *Lancet Respir. Med.* **2021**, *9*, 699–711. [CrossRef]
10. Aveyard, P.; Gao, M.; Lindson, N.; Hartmann-Boyce, J.; Watkinson, P.; Young, D.; Coupland, C.A.; San Tan, P.; Clift, A.K.; Harrison, D.; et al. Association between pre-existing respiratory disease and its treatment, and severe COVID-19: A population cohort study. *Lancet Respir. Med.* **2021**, *9*, 909–923. [CrossRef]
11. Signes-Costa, J.; Nunez-Gil, I.J.; Soriano, J.B.; Arroyo-Espliguero, R.; Eid, C.M.; Romero, R.; Uribarri, A.; Fernandez-Rozas, I.; Aguado, M.G.; Becerra-Muñoz, V.M.; et al. Prevalence and 30-Day Mortality in Hospitalized Patients with COVID-19 and Prior Lung Diseases. *Arch. Bronconeumol.* **2021**, *57*, 13–20. [CrossRef]

12. Schultze, A.; Walker, A.J.; MacKenna, B.; Morton, C.E.; Bhaskaran, K.; Brown, J.P.; Rentsch, C.T.; Williamson, E.; Drysdale, H.; Croker, R.; et al. Risk of COVID-19-related death among patients with chronic obstructive pulmonary disease or asthma prescribed inhaled corticosteroids: An observational cohort study using the OpenSAFELY platform. *Lancet Respir. Med.* **2020**, *8*, 1106–1120. [CrossRef]
13. Liu, S.; Cao, Y.; Du, T.; Zhi, Y. Prevalence of Comorbid Asthma and Related Outcomes in COVID-19: A Systematic Review and Meta-Analysis. *J. Allergy Clin. Immunol. Pract.* **2021**, *9*, 693–701. [CrossRef]
14. Peters, M.C.; Sajuthi, S.; Deford, P.; Christenson, S.; Rios, C.L.; Montgomery, M.T.; Woodruff, P.G.; Mauger, D.T.; Erzurum, S.C.; Johansson, M.W.; et al. COVID-19-related Genes in Sputum Cells in Asthma. Relationship to Demographic Features and Corticosteroids. *Am. J. Respir. Crit. Care Med.* **2020**, *202*, 83–90. [CrossRef]
15. He, Z.F.; Zhong, N.S.; Guan, W.J. Impact of Chronic Respiratory Diseases on the Outcomes of COVID-19. *Arch. Bronconeumol.* **2022**, *58*, 5–7. [CrossRef]
16. Polverino, F.; Kheradmand, F. COVID-19, COPD, and AECOPD: Immunological, Epidemiological, and Clinical Aspects. *Front. Med.* **2021**, *7*, 627278. [CrossRef] [PubMed]
17. Leung, J.M.; Niikura, M.; Yang, C.W.T.; Sin, D.D. COVID-19 and COPD. *Eur. Respir. J.* **2020**, *56*, 2002108. [CrossRef]
18. Richardson, S.; Hirsch, J.S.; Narasimhan, M.; Crawford, J.M.; McGinn, T.; Davidson, K.W.; Barnaby, D.P.; Becker, L.B.; Chelico, J.D.; Cohen, S.L.; et al. Presenting Characteristics, Comorbidities, and Outcomes Among 5700 Patients Hospitalized With COVID-19 in the New York City Area. *JAMA* **2020**, *323*, 2052–2059. [CrossRef]
19. Goyal, P.; Choi, J.J.; Pinheiro, L.C.; Schenck, E.J.; Chen, R.; Jabri, A.; Satlin, M.J.; Campion, T.R., Jr.; Nahid, M.; Ringel, J.B.; et al. Clinical Characteristics of COVID-19 in New York City. *N. Engl. J. Med.* **2020**, *382*, 2372–2374. [CrossRef] [PubMed]
20. Berghella, V.; Hughes, B.L. Classification of Disease Severity [Internet]. Up to Date: Alphen aan den Rijn, The Netherlands, 2023; [updated date—28 April 2023]; Available online: https://www.uptodate.com/contents/covid-19-overview-of-pregnancy-issues?search=covid19%20classification&sectionRank=1&usage_type=default&anchor=H750940065&source=machineLearning&selectedTitle=1~150&display_rank=1#H750940065 (accessed on 16 January 2022).
21. Li, K.; Fang, Y.; Li, W.; Pan, C.; Qin, P.; Zhong, Y.; Liu, X.; Huang, M.; Liao, Y.; Li, S. CT image visual quantitative evaluation and clinical classification of coronavirus disease (COVID-19). *Eur. Radiol.* **2020**, *30*, 4407–4416. [CrossRef]
22. Mihaltan, F.; Ulmean, R.; Nemes, R.; Nedelcu, R. Chronic obstructive pulmonary disease day—A traditional strategy of the Romanian Society of Pneumology. *Pneumologia* **2019**, *68*, 200–201. [CrossRef]
23. Huang, K.; Yang, T.; Xu, J.; Yang, L.; Zhao, J.; Zhang, X.; Bai, C.; Kang, J.; Ran, P.; Shen, H.; et al. Prevalence, risk factors, and management of asthma in China: A national cross-sectional study. *Lancet* **2019**, *394*, 407–418. [CrossRef]
24. Zhang, J.J.; Dong, X.; Cao, Y.Y.; Yuan, Y.D.; Yang, Y.B.; Yan, Y.Q.; Akdis, C.A.; Gao, Y.D. Clinical characteristics of 140 patients infected with SARS-CoV-2 in Wuhan, China. *Allergy* **2020**, *75*, 1730–1741. [CrossRef]
25. Guan, W.J.; Ni, Z.Y.; Hu, Y.; Liang, W.H.; Ou, C.Q.; He, J.X.; Liu, L.; Shan, H.; Lei, C.L.; Hui, D.S.; et al. Clinical Characteristics of Coronavirus Disease 2019 in China. *N. Engl. J. Med.* **2020**, *382*, 1708–1720. [CrossRef]
26. Au Yeung, S.L.; Li, A.M.; He, B.; Kwok, K.O.; Schooling, C.M. Association of smoking, lung function and COPD in COVID-19 risk: A two-step Mendelian randomization study. *Addiction* **2022**, *117*, 2027–2036. [CrossRef]
27. Leung, J.M.; Yang, C.X.; Tam, A.; Shaipanich, T.; Hackett, T.L.; Singhera, G.K.; Dorscheid, D.R.; Sin, D.D. ACE-2 expression in the small airway epithelia of smokers and COPD patients: Implications for COVID-19. *Eur. Respir. J.* **2020**, *55*, 2000688. [CrossRef]
28. Monserrat, J.; Gómez-Lahoz, A.; Ortega, M.A.; Sanz, J.; Muñoz, B.; Arévalo-Serrano, J.; Rodríguez, J.M.; Gasalla, J.M.; Gasulla, Ó.; Arranz, A.; et al. Role of Innate and Adaptive Cytokines in the Survival of COVID-19 Patients. *Int. J. Mol. Sci.* **2022**, *23*, 10344. [CrossRef]
29. Cai, G.; Bossé, Y.; Xiao, F.; Kheradmand, F.; Amos, C.I. Tobacco Smoking Increases the Lung Gene Expression of ACE2, the Receptor of SARS-CoV-2. *Am. J. Respir. Crit. Care Med.* **2020**, *201*, 1557–1559. [CrossRef]
30. Lee, S.C.; Son, K.J.; Han, C.H.; Park, S.C.; Jung, J.Y. Impact of COPD on COVID-19 prognosis: A nationwide population-based study in South Korea. *Sci. Rep.* **2021**, *11*, 3735. [CrossRef]
31. Gomez Antunez, M.; Muino Miguez, A.; Bendala Estrada, A.D.; Maestro de la Calle, G.; Monge Monge, D.; Boixeda, R.; Ena, J.; Mella Perez, C.; Anton Santos, J.M.; Lumbreras Bermejo, C.; et al. Clinical Characteristics and Prognosis of COPD Patients Hospitalized with SARS-CoV-2. *Int. J. Chron. Obstruct. Pulmon. Dis.* **2021**, *15*, 3433–3445. [CrossRef]
32. Bellou, V.; Tzoulaki, I.; van Smeden, M.; Moons, K.G.M.; Evangelou, E.; Belbasis, L. Prognostic factors for adverse outcomes in patients with COVID-19: A field-wide systematic review and meta-analysis. *Eur. Respir. J.* **2022**, *59*, 2002964. [CrossRef]
33. Razek, A.; Fouda, N.; Fahmy, D.; Tanatawy, M.S.; Sultan, A.; Bilal, M.; Zaki, M.; Abdel-Aziz, M.; Sobh, D. Computed tomography of the chest in patients with COVID-19: What do radiologists want to know? *Pol. J. Radiol.* **2021**, *86*, e122–e135. [CrossRef]
34. Hefeda, M.M. CT chest findings in patients infected with COVID-19: Review of literature. *Egypt. J. Radiol. Nucl. Med.* **2020**, *51*, 239. [CrossRef]
35. Okoye, C.; Finamore, P.; Bellelli, G.; Coin, A.; Del Signore, S.; Fumagalli, S.; Gareri, P.; Malara, A.; Mossello, E.; Trevisan, C.; et al. Computed tomography findings and prognosis in older COVID-19 patients. *BMC Geriatr.* **2022**, *22*, 166. [CrossRef]
36. Diamond, M.S.; Kanneganti, T.D. Innate immunity: The first line of defense against SARS-CoV-2. *Nat. Immunol.* **2022**, *23*, 165–176. [CrossRef]

37. Papi, A.; Bellettato, C.M.; Braccioni, F.; Romagnoli, M.; Casolari, P.; Caramori, G.; Fabbri, L.M.; Johnston, S.L. Infections and airway inflammation in chronic obstructive pulmonary disease severe exacerbations. *Am. J. Respir. Crit. Care Med.* **2006**, *173*, 1114–1121. [CrossRef]
38. Bafadhel, M.; McKenna, S.; Terry, S.; Mistry, V.; Reid, C.; Haldar, P.; McCormick, M.; Haldar, K.; Kebadze, T.; Duvoix, A.; et al. Acute exacerbations of chronic obstructive pulmonary disease: Identification of biologic clusters and their biomarkers. *Am. J. Respir. Crit. Care Med.* **2011**, *184*, 662–671. [CrossRef]
39. Sethi, S.; Murphy, T.F. Infection in the pathogenesis and course of chronic obstructive pulmonary disease. *N. Engl. J. Med.* **2008**, *359*, 2355–2365. [CrossRef]
40. Leung, J.M.; Tiew, P.Y.; Mac Aogáin, M.; Budden, K.F.; Yong, V.F.; Thomas, S.S.; Pethe, K.; Hansbro, P.M.; Chotirmall, S.H. The role of acute and chronic respiratory colonization and infections in the pathogenesis of COPD. *Respirology* **2017**, *22*, 634–650. [CrossRef]
41. Ortega, M.A.; García-Montero, C.; Fraile-Martinez, O.; Colet, P.; Baizhaxynova, A.; Mukhtarova, K.; Alvarez-Mon, M.; Kanatova, K.; Asúnsolo, A.; Sarría-Santamera, A. Recapping the Features of SARS-CoV-2 and Its Main Variants: Status and Future Paths. *J. Pers. Med.* **2022**, *12*, 995. [CrossRef]

Disclaimer/Publisher's Note: The statements, opinions and data contained in all publications are solely those of the individual author(s) and contributor(s) and not of MDPI and/or the editor(s). MDPI and/or the editor(s) disclaim responsibility for any injury to people or property resulting from any ideas, methods, instructions or products referred to in the content.

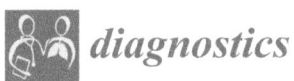

Article

Triiodothyronine and Protein Malnutrition Could Influence Pulse Wave Velocity in Pre-Dialysis Chronic Kidney Disease Patients

Crina Claudia Rusu [1,2], Ina Kacso [1,2], Diana Moldovan [1,2], Alina Potra [1,2], Dacian Tirinescu [1,2], Maria Ticala [1,2], Ancuta M. Rotar [3], Remus Orasan [4], Cristian Budurea [4], Andrada Barar [2], Florin Anton [5], Ana Valea [6], Cosmina Ioana Bondor [7,*] and Madalina Ticolea [2]

1 Department of Nephrology, University of Medicine and Pharmacy "Iuliu Hatieganu" Cluj, 8 Victor Babeș Street, 400012 Cluj-Napoca, Romania
2 Department of Nephrology, County Emergency Clinical Hospital Cluj, 3-5 Clinicilor Street, 400006 Cluj-Napoca, Romania
3 Department of Food Science, Faculty of Food Science and Technology, University of Agricultural Sciences and Veterinary Medicine Cluj-Napoca, Calea Manastur 3-5, 400372 Cluj-Napoca, Romania
4 Nefromed Dialysis Center, 40 Ana Aslan Street, 400528 Cluj-Napoca, Romania
5 Department of Cardiology, University of Medicine and Pharmacy "Iuliu Hatieganu" Cluj, 8 Victor Babeș Street, 400012 Cluj-Napoca, Romania
6 Department of Endocrinology, University of Medicine and Pharmacy "Iuliu Hatieganu" Cluj, 8 Victor Babeș Street, 400012 Cluj-Napoca, Romania
7 Department of Medical Informatics and Biostatistics, University of Medicine and Pharmacy "Iuliu Hatieganu" Cluj, 6 Pasteur Street, 400349 Cluj-Napoca, Romania
* Correspondence: cbondor@umfcluj.ro

Abstract: Cardiovascular diseases (CVD) are the first cause of chronic kidney disease (CKD) mortality. For personalized improved medicine, detecting correctable markers of CVD can be considered a priority. The aim of this study was the evaluation of the impact of nutritional, hormonal and inflammatory markers on brachial-ankle Pulse Wave Velocity (PWV) in pre-dialysis CKD patients. A cross-sectional observational study was conducted on 68 pre-dialysis CKD patients (median age of 69 years, 41.2% with diabetes mellitus, 52.9% male). Laboratory data were collected, including levels of prolactin, triiodothyronine, TGF α, IL-6, and IL-1β. The high values of brachial-ankle PWV were associated with reduced muscle mass ($p = 0.001$, $r = -0.44$), low levels of total cholesterol ($p = 0.04$, $r = -0.26$), triglycerides ($p = 0.03$, $r = -0.31$), triiodothyronine ($p = 0.04$, $r = -0.24$), and prolactin ($p = 0.02$, $r = -0.27$). High PWV was associated with advanced age ($p < 0.001$, $r = 0.19$). In the multivariate analysis, reduced muscle mass ($p = 0.018$), low levels of triiodothyronine ($p = 0.002$), and triglycerides ($p = 0.049$) were significant predictors of PWV, but age ($p < 0.001$) remained an important factor. In conclusion, reduced triiodothyronine together with markers of malnutrition and age were associated with PWV in pre-dialysis CKD patients.

Keywords: pulse wave velocity; chronic kidney disease; malnutrition; inflammation triiodothyronine; prolactin

1. Introduction

High cardiovascular risk in chronic kidney disease (CKD) patients is associated with accelerated atherosclerosis, endothelial dysfunction, and arterial stiffness (AS) and it has major consequences on survival and quality of life. Arterial stiffness is a negative prognostic factor for CKD progression [1] and for associated cardiovascular diseases, contributing to the increase in medical services costs [2–4]. Previous studies have suggested that therapeutic modification of AS can improve cardiovascular mortality in CKD [5,6]. AS was influenced by angiotensin-converting enzyme (ACE) inhibitors/angiotensin II receptor blockers (ARB), vitamin D in the pre-dialysis CKD patients [6,7], and by hypotensive medication combined with the reduction of calcium in the dialysis solution in hemodialysis patients [8]. A relationship between increased AS and declining kidney function was shown [8].

According to experts, the PWV remains a standard parameter for the assessment of AS [9,10]. There are different devices for measuring PWV, based on tonometry, oscillometry, and magnetic resonance [11].

AS is characterized by chronic structural modifications in the arterial wall expressed by elastin fragmentation and media calcification, but molecular changes in the intimal layer may also occur through the atherosclerotic inflammatory process [12,13].

Hyperphosphatemia, the fluctuations of calcium such as hyper and hypocalcemia, hyperparathyroidism, the reduction of alpha Klotho, and the increase in FGF-23 are the main determinants of AS in CKD. Classic cardiovascular risk factors also intervene: hypertension, obesity, dyslipidemia, advanced age (through decreased endothelium nitric oxide availability and increased production of vasoconstrictors), diabetes mellitus (DM), and hyperuricemia [10–12]. In addition, advanced glycation end products (AGEs) that accumulate in CKD activate Nuclear Factor Kappa B, favoring the activation of the vascular inflammatory cascade and promoting the vessel's stiffening by stimulating fibrosis and proliferation of the vascular smooth muscle cells [14,15]. There was also an association of serum glucose concentrations with PWV, independent of the diabetic status [16].

In fact, AS in CKD is based on an enormously increased cardiovascular risk due to, on the one hand, the additional cardiovascular risk factors (oxidative stress, protein malnutrition, alteration of the phospho-calcium balance, etc.) and, on the other hand, due to certain particularities of the classic cardiovascular risk factors such as the appearance of the reverse epidemiology phenomenon [17]. It is well known that malnutrition and inflammation are associated with atherosclerosis (malnutrition inflammation atherosclerosis syndrome) in these patients [18], and it can be a major determinant of vascular stiffness in CKD. There are few data in the literature about the correlation between nutritional markers and PWV in pre-dialysis and dialysis CKD patients. Thus, in a study that evaluated pre-dialysis CKD patients from Korea, it was shown that reduced muscle mass was associated with high brachial-ankle PWV [19]. In addition, another study revealed that hydration status and blood pressure might be major determinants of PWV in hemodialysis patients [20], while in peritoneal dialysis patients a significant association between nutritional markers and PWV was described, suggesting that malnutrition could be the major contributor to vascular dysfunction [21]. It was noted that body mass index (BMI), body fat mass, waist-hip ratio, abdominal circumference, neck circumference, and visceral fat are positively correlated with PWV in the general population [22].

There are also studies that have shown that the hormonal changes occurring in CKD could also influence cardiovascular morbidity and AS. Prolactin is a hormone which is considered as a uremic toxin by some authors. It accumulates with loss of renal function, and it is associated with cardiovascular diseases in the general population and CKD population as well [23]. Hyperprolactinemia is implicated in biological processes such as insulin resistance, metabolic syndrome, inflammation modulation, endothelial dysfunction, and lastly, accelerated atherosclerosis [24,25]. A 27% increased risk of cardiovascular events was observed for each 10 ng/mL prolactin elevation in non-dialysis CKD patients [26].

The presence of subclinical hypothyroidism was also recorded in CKD. It was associated with general mortality in advanced CKD [27]. Low triiodothyronine levels are the most common laboratory finding followed by subclinical hypothyroidism in CKD patients. Hypothyroidism can cause vascular calcification and endothelial damage [28,29].

Currently, it is still not clear how prolactin and triiodothyronine influence cardiovascular diseases in CKD, and if they affect PWV, in fact, what are the most important factors that influence PWV in pre-dialysis CKD patients.

That is why the aim of this study was to evaluate the impact of some inflammatory, nutritional, and hormonal markers on PWV in pre-dialysis CKD patients, and as a second aim in the subgroup of the patients with diabetes.

2. Materials and Methods

2.1. The Participants

We conducted a cross-sectional observational study on a cohort of pre-dialysis CKD patients. The patients were selected from those admitted to the Department of Nephrology, County Clinical Emergency Hospital Cluj, and taken into this study based on the inclusion and exclusion criteria. All patients provided written informed consent. The study methodology was in accordance with institutional and national research ethical standards and with the 1964 Helsinki Declaration and its subsequent amendments.

Inclusion criteria were the following: patients aged $\geq$ 18 years, diagnosed with CKD for at least 6 months, defined according to Kidney Disease: Improving Global. Outcomes (KDIGO) guidelines, with estimated glomerular filtration rate (eGFR) less than 60 mL/min, (predialytic stage), having a stable renal function during 3 months prior to study (change in eGFR < 5 mL/min/1.73 m^2), and no change in medication during the same 3 months.

The exclusion criteria were the following: cancer patients with a life expectancy <6 months, acute inflammatory diseases, terminal neoplasia, hepatitis viral infection, and any other chronic or acute diseases that required changes in treatment during 3 months prior to study.

The patient's clinical data: age, weight, height, systolic blood pressure (SBP), and diastolic blood pressure (DBP), comorbidities (diabetes, hypertension) and the medication data were registered. The diagnosis of hypertension was established on the basis of BP values, namely SBP/DBP $\geq$ 140/90 mmHg as well as on the basis of the use of hypotensive drugs. We calculated pulse pressure (PP) as the difference between the SBP and DBP.

2.2. Evaluation of Anthropometric Parameters

In addition to body mass index (BMI), nutritional status was assessed by bioimpedance using the Body Composition Monitor, a certified device (manufacturer by Fresenius Medical Care, Bad Homburg, Germany) which provided body composition as follows: lean tissue mass (LTM) (kg), and adipose tissue mass (ATM) (kg) [30].

2.3. Laboratory Parameters

Blood samples were collected in the morning after 8 h fasting. Serum electrolytes, albumin, creatinine, lipid profile, inflammatory markers, intact parathormone (iPTH) and the medular response (hemoglobin and white blood cells) were determined. Serum IL-6, IL-1β, TNF-α, prolactin and triiodothyronine were determined by enzyme-linked immunosorbent assay (ELISA) using commercially available kits (R & D System, Minneapolis, MN, USA). The minimum detection limit for TNF-α was 15.6 pg/mL, for IL-6–3.2 pg/mL, for IL-1β–10.2 pg/mL, for prolactin 1.5 ng/mL, and for triiodothyronine < 0.1 ng/mL). Low-density lipoprotein-cholesterol (LDL-cholesterol) was calculated according to the Friedewald formula: LDL cholesterol = total cholesterol-(HDL-cholesterol + triglycerides/5).

2.4. Assessment of Arterial Stiffness

Brachial-ankle PWV was evaluated to assess arterial stiffness with the Mobil-O-Graph NG device (Medexpert Ltd., Budapest, Hungary), based on an oscillometric method. The device gave the augmentation pressure, augmentation index, central SBP, central DBP, and PWV. Brachial BP [31] was initially recorded, then the cuff was automatically re-inflated above DBP for approximately 10 s and brachial pulse waves were recorded with a high-fidelity pressure sensor (MPX5050, Freescale Halbleiter Deutschland GmbH, Muenchen, Germany). Brachial BP was used to calibrate the pulse waveform. Finally, the aortic pulse wave form was reconstructed by the software (HMS version 5.1) using an ARCSolver algorithm [32,33]. The aortic pulse wave was decomposed into forward traveling (incident) and backward traveling (reflected) pulse waves for wave separation analysis. PWV was estimated by mathematical models based on the characteristic impedance and age and assuming a three-element Windkessel model [32,33].

2.5. Statistical Analysis

Data were presented using different statistical measures depending on the nature of the variables. For normally distributed variables the mean ± standard deviation (SD) was reported. For non-normally distributed variables, median (25th–75th percentile) was used. Nominal variables were expressed as absolute and relative frequencies.

To examine the relationships between quantitative variables, either the Spearman or Pearson coefficient of correlation was employed. Spearman coefficient of correlation was used when the relationship was non-linear or when the outliers were present.

In the multivariate linear regression analysis, PWV was considered the dependent variable. Independent variables included those that showed significant correlation in the univariate analysis and those previously identified in relevant literature as influencing PWV levels were considered. However, SBP was excluded from the model due to multicollinearity.

To compare two groups, different statistical tests were employed based on the nature of the variables. The t-test or Mann–Whitney U test for quantitative variables depending on their distribution (normal and non-normal, respectively), while the Chi-square test or Fisher exact test was used for qualitative variables. A p-value less than 0.05 was considered statistically significant.

3. Results

In this study 80 patients were selected, from which six patients were excluded: four with acute infection, one with acute myocardial infarction, and one with malignancy. Another six patients were excluded due to missing data. Finally, 68 patients remained in the study.

3.1. Patients' Characteristics

The demographical, clinical and laboratory patients' characteristics are presented in Table 1. In our group, the median (25th, 75th percentile) age was 69 (62.5, 76) years; 41.2% had diabetes and 52.9% were men.

Table 1. Characteristics of participants.

Parameter	Group (n = 68)
Age (years)	69 (62.5, 76)
Male, n (%)	36 (52.9)
Diabetes mellitus [1], n (%)	28 (41.2)
Hypertension, n (%)	60 (89.6)
SBP (mmHg)	144 (126.5, 162)
DBP (mmHg)	87.07 ± 12.42
PP (mmHg)	58 (45.5, 72.5)
eGFR (mL/min/1.73 m^2)	27 (15, 42)
Body mass index (kg/m^2)	28.6 (26.4, 30.35)
LTM (kg)	38.25 ± 12.16
ATM (kg)	41.74 ± 13.77
Total cholesterol (mg/dL)	177.49 ± 37.45
LDL-cholesterol (mg/dL)	98.73 ± 28.61
HDL-cholesterol (mg/dL)	43.86 ± 12.94
Triglycerides (mg/dL)	125 (91.5, 166)
Fasting glucose (mg/dL)	103 (92, 131)
Calcium (mg/dL)	9.2 (8.64, 9.69)
Phosphorus (mg/dL)	3.66 (3.14, 4.56)
iPTH (pg/mL)	108.85 (84.85, 227.35)
Alkaline phosphatase (UI/L)	80 (72, 96.5)
Hemoglobin (g/dL)	12.46 ± 2.22
Serum albumin (g/L)	3.89 ± 0.49
hs-C reactive protein (mg/dL)	0.47 (0.23, 1.19)
White blood cells (no./mm^3)	7625 (6340, 9050)

Table 1. *Cont.*

Parameter	Group (*n* = 68)
TNF-α (pg/mL)	4.4 (2.94, 6.8)
IL-6 (pg/mL)	2.44 (1.7, 3.55)
IL-1β (pg/mL)	7.06 (6.45, 12.99)
Prolactin (ng/mL)	4.83 (3.1, 7.76)
Triiodothyronine (ng/mL)	1.2 (0.9, 1.3)
Brachial-ankle PWV (m/s)	10.55 ± 2.17
ACEI/ARB, n (%)	29 (42.6)

[1] data about 66 patients. Arithmetic mean ± standard deviation; *n*—number of people; no.—number of cell; SBP—systolic blood pressure; DBP—diastolic blood pressure; PP—pulse pressure; eGFR—estimated glomerular filtration rate; LTM—lean tissue mass; ATM—adipose tissue mass; LDL—low-density lipoprotein; HDL—high-density lipoprotein; iPTH—intact parathormone; PWV—pulse wave velocity; ACEI—angiotensin-converting enzyme inhibitors; ARB—angiotensin II receptor blockers.

3.2. Determinants of Brachial-Ankle PWV

In the analysis of correlations, it was observed that high values of brachial-ankle PWV were associated with reduced values of muscle mass ($p = 0.001$, r = −0.45), low levels of total cholesterol ($p = 0.042$, r = −0.26), triglycerides ($p = 0.023$, r = −0.34) and, respectively, low levels of the hormonal engage: triiodothyronine ($p = 0.04$, r = −0.25) (Figure 1) and prolactin ($p = 0.026$, r = −0.27) (Figure 2). Additionally, increasing brachial-ankle PWV was directly associated with high values of SBP ($p < 0.001$, r = 0.56), PP ($p < 0.001$, r = 0.57) and advanced age ($p < 0.001$, r = 0.92), all of these findings are described in Table 2 listed below.

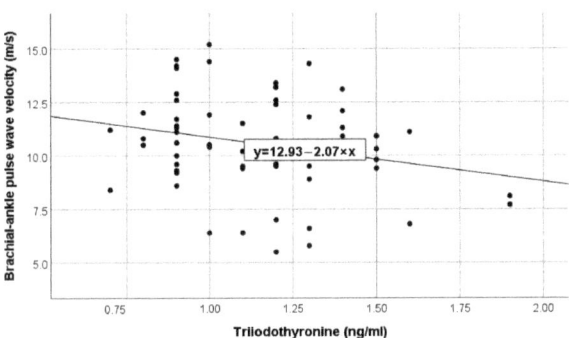

Figure 1. Negative linear correlation between PWV and triiodothyronine in the total group.

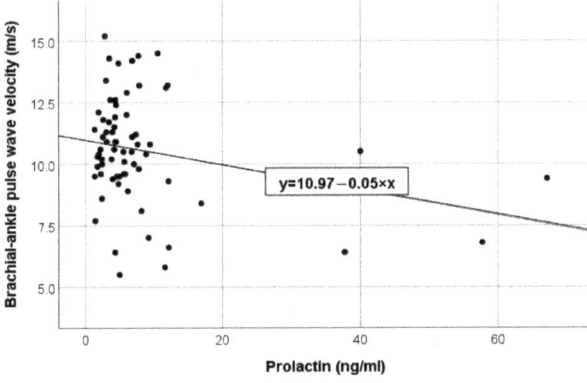

Figure 2. Negative linear correlation between PWV and prolactin in the total group.

Table 2. The brachial-ankle PWV correlation in the group.

Parameters	r—Coefficient of Correlation	p
Age (years)	0.92	<0.001
SBP (mmHg)	0.56	<0.001
PP (mmHg)	0.57	<0.001
Lean tissue mass (kg)	−0.45	0.001
Prolactin (ng/mL)	−0.27	0.026
Triiodothyronine (ng/mL)	−0.25	0.040
Total Cholesterol (mg/dL)	−0.26	0.042
Triglycerides (mg/dL)	−0.34	0.023

SBP—systolic blood pressure, PP—pulse pressure.

In the multivariate analysis it was noted that muscle mass ($p = 0.019$) and triiodothyronine ($p = 0.014$), PP ($p = 0.013$), and triglycerides ($p = 0.024$), respectively, remained with a significant impact on brachial-ankle PWV, but its strongest determinant was age ($p < 0.001$).

3.3. Analysis of the Subgroups

Diabetic vs. non-diabetic patients were analyzed (Table 3). In the DM subgroup there were significantly higher values of SBP ($p = 0.010$) and PP ($p = 0.009$) identified, significantly higher ATM ($p = 0.032$), and significantly higher IL-1β levels ($p = 0.015$).

Table 3. Comparisons between diabetes vs. non-diabetes groups ($n = 66$).

Parameter	Non-Diabetes Subgroup ($n = 38$)	Diabetes Subgroup ($n = 28$)	p
Age (years)	68.5 (61, 76)	68 (62.5, 76)	0.689
Male, n (%)	17 (45.9)	13 (46.4)	0.969
Hypertension, n (%)	34 (89.5)	24 (88.9)	0.940
SBP (mmHg)	138 (121, 156)	150.5 (138.5, 172)	0.010
DBP (mmHg)	82 (76, 98)	89 (80, 97.5)	0.508
PP (mmHg)	49.5 (41, 68)	63 (52, 74)	0.009
eGFR (mL/min/1.73 m^2)	26 (19, 38)	27.85 (12.5, 47)	0.910
BMI (kg/m^2)	28.45 (25.5, 29.9)	29.5 (27.1, 31.55)	0.109
LTM (kg)	38.35 ± 12	38.13 ± 12.63	0.948
ATM (kg)	38.27 ± 12.19	46.22 ± 14.62	0.032
Total cholesterol (mg/dL)	185.97 ± 36.06	168.62 ± 36.58	0.072
Triglycerides (mg/dL)	130 (94, 159.5)	124 (85.5, 175.5)	0.961
Calcium (mg/dL)	9.34 (8.67, 9.76)	9.17 (8.78, 9.47)	0.410
Phosphorus (mg/dL)	3.63 (3.13, 4.41)	3.7 (3.3, 5.22)	0.425
TNF-α (pg/mL)	4.6 (3.11, 6.03)	4.02 (2.69, 8.3)	0.678
IL-6 (pg/mL)	2.44 (1.7, 3.27)	2.2 (1.6, 4.36)	0.830
IL-1β (pg/mL)	6.86 (6.38, 9.96)	9.54 (6.79, 19.35)	0.015
Prolactin (ng/mL)	4.98 (3.07, 8.16)	4.66 (3.91, 7.24)	0.912
Triiodothyronine (ng/mL)	1.2 (0.9, 1.3)	1.1 (0.9, 1.35)	0.568
Brachial-ankle PWV (m/s)	10.14 ± 2.42	10.94 ± 1.58	0.135

Arithmetic mean ± standard deviation; SBP—systolic blood pressure; DBP—diastolic blood pressure; PP—pulse pressure; eGFR—estimated glomerular filtration rate; LTM—lean tissue mass; ATM—adipose tissue mass; PWV—pulse wave velocity.

In the DM subgroup, brachial-ankle PWV was directly correlated with inflammatory markers (TNF alpha $p = 0.012$, r = 0.46; IL-6 $p = 0.034$, r = 0.40), age ($p < 0.001$, r = 0.39) and serum phosphorus ($p = 0.012$, r = 0.39), but not with the eGFR (Table 4).

In the multivariate analysis the parameters which were correlated significantly with brachial-ankle PWV were included in our study, and it was noted that only age ($p < 0.001$) remained statistically significantly associated with PWV.

Table 4. The brachial-ankle PWV correlation in the subgroup of patients with DM.

Parameters	r—Coefficient of Correlation	p
Age (years)	0.89	<0.001
Phosphorus (mg/dL)	−0.51	0.014
eGFR (mL/min/1.73 m^2)	0.11	0.593
TNF-α (pg/mL)	0.47	0.012
IL-6 (pg/mL)	0.40	0.034

eGFR—estimated glomerular filtration rate.

4. Discussion

Age was the strongest determinant of arterial stiffness in the studied group, even though triiodothyronine and prolactin values were also correlated with brachial-ankle PWV. Similar data were published from the CRIC study, in which the worsening of AS with age, the reduction of eGFR, and the increase in PP in CKD were noted [34]. Additionally, in our study, strong correlations of PWV with SBP and PP values were obtained. It is known that hypertension, diabetes mellitus, and CKD are the major determinants of the loss of elasticity and reduced compliance of the vascular wall and, consecutively, increased arterial stiffness. Impaired collagen-elastin ratio, calcification of blood vessels, endothelial dysfunction, increased intima media-thickness, and genetic determinants can produce arterial wall remodeling [35]. All these factors have a prevalence that increases with age.

In addition, it is known that malnutrition is among the risk factors for atherosclerosis and, implicitly, for the increase in AS in CKD. In our study, we remarked that reduced values of muscle mass, therefore protein malnutrition, were associated with the increase of AS. In the longitudinal analysis, in the CRIC study, serum albumin concentration, which is another marker reflecting the protein nutritional status, was predictive of changes in PWV over time [34]. In addition, Harada et al. [36] observed that malnutrition in CKD was a factor associated with vascular calcifications and, consecutively, arterial stiffness, while Cordeiro, in a study, emphasized that another parameter reflecting the nutritional status, the abdominal fat, was associated with coronary artery calcification in non-dialysis dependent CKD patients [37] and then stiffening. In addition, secondary to the reverse epidemiology phenomenon of cardiovascular risk factors in CKD, we noticed that reduced values of lipid markers were associated with increased PWA, not with cardiovascular protection. Therefore, low values of total cholesterol and triglycerides may show a poor nutritional status in this population group.

Regarding the low values of T3 in CKD, they can express a deficit of thyroid function, known in this group of patients, most of the time subclinical (without having a thyroid disease as a substrate) and this could be associated with increased cardiovascular risk. Low values of T3 were associated with AS in our study, consistent with other studies in which FT3, was inversely associated with arterial stiffness in CKD patients [38]. In fact, Klotho synthesis seems to be influenced by the thyroid hormone level [39], and Klotho has a vascular protective effect by reducing vascular calcification. Therefore, the alteration of thyroid hormones in CKD may increase vascular calcifications by reducing the protective effects of Klotho [38]. In addition, overt hypothyroidism has been associated with altered vascular function and altered endothelial-dependent vasodilation [40], partly because of the lack of vasodilatory effect of triiodothyronine (subsequent vasodilation was reported when triiodothyronine increases the NO production by endothelial and smooth muscle cells) [41–43]. An increase in central arterial stiffness may be due the overt hypothyroidism as previous studies have shown.

Prolactine was reported to be correlated with PWV. Carrero et al. observed increased prolactin levels in subjects with endothelial dysfunction/stiffness and which further increased the risk of cardiovascular events and mortality [26]. The increase in prolactinoma in CKD is determined by the reduction of its metabolism, by the increased secretion of PRL in the uremic state and by the reduced availability of dopamine in the brain. Secondary to the decrease in dopaminergic activity, there can be an increase in the release of norepinephrine with a negative result on the endothelial function and other organs, favoring myocardial hypertrophy, hypertension, and other cardiovascular diseases [44]. On the other hand, prolactin retention can inhibit the production of gonadotropic hormone, and consequently induce a testosterone deficiency in male patients with CKD, and through this mechanism, atherosclerosis. Prolactin retention was indeed linked to increased intima–media thickness, atherosclerotic plaque occurrence, systemic inflammation, and cardiovascular risk [45,46].

As evidence in our study, not the high values, but the low values of prolactin, a polypeptide hormone, were associated with the increase in PWA and we consider this type of association as an effect of the protein malnutrition present in the patients enrolled in the study. Moreover, in the study by Haring et al., they noted the association of low prolactin values with increased left ventricular mass, these changes only affecting males [47], without finding a clear explanation. Prolactin has 23 kDa and can induce angiogenesis. After proteolytic cleavage, a 5.6–18 kDa, isoform of prolactin, called vasoinhibins, appears with antiangiogenic properties [48]. Thus, the balance between prolactin and vasoinhibins regulates vascular functions [49].

In diabetic patients, PWV is higher than in the general population and promotes an increase in general and cardiovascular mortality [50]. If a diabetic patient has CKD, s/he has also all specific CKD cardiovascular risk factors and PWV increases additionally, with the impact being more significant. In the present study, the analysis of the subgroup of diabetic patients highlighted several aspects. First, age was also the strongest determinant of PWA values. Second, we did not identify significant differences between PWV in diabetics vs. non-diabetics, although we identified several cardiovascular risk markers that were significantly modified in the DM group. Thus, IL-1β (an inflammatory marker) was significantly higher as well as SBP, PP, and adipose tissue mass (expressed by ATM). Third, other inflammatory markers, TNF alpha, and IL-6, as well as phosphorus, a marker of mineral and bone metabolism, were found among the factors significantly associated with the PWA value in the subgroup with DM.

Other studies also reported that inflammatory markers such as fibrinogen and IL-10 were independently associated with PWV [34,51]. Moreover, it is known that micro-inflammation is present in CKD from the early stages and that there is a link between inflammation and atherosclerosis regarding malnutrition (malnutrition inflammation atherosclerosis syndrome). Several possible pathophysiological pathways can explain the association between chronic inflammation and arterial wall disease [14]. Initially, the circulation of inflammatory mediators favors leukocyte migration into the arterial wall [52]. Then, macrophages' activation by different factors amplifies the inflammatory reaction. This inflammatory cascade then alters the endothelium's function that interacts and conditions the remodeling of the tunica media, further along with changing the artery's mechanical properties [53]. Moreover, endothelial cells decrease the usual production of nitric oxide (NO) and increase endothelin (E1), favoring arterial stiffness.

Regarding the connection between phosphorus and AS as noted in our study, it is probably via vascular calcification. In fact, CKD alters hormonal processes that regulate phosphate levels (intestinal absorption, renal excretion by remaining nephrons, bone metabolism modulated by vitamin D, fetuin-A, Klotho, and fibroblast growth factor 23 (FGF-23); all these processes mentioned favoring hyperphosphatemia [54]. Excessive levels of phosphorous and calcium are endogenous minerals capable of stimulating the phenotypic transformation of vascular smooth muscle cells into osteoblast-like cells [55]. Experimental studies indicate that arterial medial calcification-related vascular alterations develop in the early stages of CKD [56].

All these processes initiated in pre-dialysis stages of CKD explain the significant cardiovascular changes detected in dialysis CKD patients [57].

In conclusion, in pre-dialysis CKD patients, age is the strongest determinant of PWV even among diabetic patients. Reduced triiodothyronine and prolactin values are associated with arterial stiffness, while also being markers of malnutrition. Inflammatory markers and hyperphosphatemia influenced PWV in diabetic patients. No variations of PWV were recorded with eGFR or determined by the DM presence. Therefore, we speculate that if we detect and treat the inflammatory syndrome, respectively the malnutrition, the triiodothyronine, and prolactin levels, probably the value of PWV can be influenced. We believe that knowing the factors that influence PWV as a marker of AS, can help to administer a personalized treatment.

The study has some limitations, the first being the relatively small number of included patients, which makes additional studies necessary in order to validate the correlations and associations between PWV and the level of triiodothyronine, prolactin, and inflammatory markers with nutritional status. Secondly, due to the nature of our cross-sectional data, this study was limited in what we can infer about the causality of the results. Thirdly, by design it was an observational study and the conclusions need to be confirmed in the future, possibly by larger prospective studies.

Author Contributions: Conceptualization, C.C.R. and I.K.; Data curation, C.I.B.; Formal analysis, A.P., A.B. and C.I.B.; Investigation, C.B.; Methodology, C.C.R., D.M. and C.I.B.; Project administration, C.C.R.; Resources, C.C.R.; Software, D.T., A.B. and C.I.B.; Supervision, C.C.R. and I.K.; Validation, C.C.R. and F.A.; Visualization, M.T. (Maria Ticala), R.O., C.B., A.V. and M.T. (Madalina Ticolea); Writing—original draft, C.C.R.; Writing—review and editing, C.C.R., M.T. (Maria Ticala), A.M.R., C.I.B. and M.T. (Madalina Ticolea). All authors have read and agreed to the published version of the manuscript.

Funding: This study was funded by the Grant CNCSIS for young research teams, Project No. PN-II-RU-TE-2014-4-1819.

Institutional Review Board Statement: The study was conducted in accordance with the Declaration of Helsinki, and approved by the Ethics Committee of "Iuliu Hatieganu" University of Medicine and Pharmacy Cluj-Napoca 348/26.09.2017.

Informed Consent Statement: Informed consent was obtained from all subjects involved in the study.

Data Availability Statement: Not applicable.

Conflicts of Interest: The authors declare no conflict of interest.

References

1. Kim, H.; Yoo, T.H.; Choi, K.H.; Oh, K.; Lee, J.; Kim, S.W.; Kim, T.H.; Sung, S.; Han, S.H. Baseline cardiovascular characteristics of adult patients with chronic kidney disease from the KoreaN Cohort Study for Outcomes in Patients with Chronic Kidney Disease (KNOW-CKD). *J. Kor. Med. Sci.* **2017**, *32*, 231–239. [CrossRef] [PubMed]
2. Briet, M.; Collin, C.; Karras, A.; Laurent, S.; Bozec, E.; Jacquot, C.; Stengel, B.; Houillier, P.; Froissart, M.; Boutouyrie, P.; et al. Arterial remodeling associates with CKD progression. *J. Am. Soc. Nephrol.* **2011**, *22*, 967–974. [CrossRef] [PubMed]
3. Hannan, M.; Ansari, S.; Meza, N.; Anderson, A.H.; Srivastava, A.; Waikar, S.; Charleston, J.; Weir, M.R.; Taliercio, J.; Horwitz, E.; et al. CRIC Study Investigators; Chronic Renal Insufficiency Cohort (CRIC) Study Investigators. Risk Factors for CKD Progression Overview of Findings from the CRIC Study. *Clin. J. Americ Soc. Nephrol.* **2021**, *16*, 648–659. [CrossRef] [PubMed]
4. Tripepi, G.; Agharazii, M.; Pannier, B.; D'Arrigo, G.; Mallamaci, F.; Zoccali, C.; London, G. Pulse wave velocity and prognosis in end-stage kidney disease. *Hypertension* **2018**, *71*, 1126–1132. [CrossRef]
5. Toussaint, N.D.; Kerr, P.G. Vascular calcification and arterial stiffness in chronic kidney disease: Implications and management. *Nephrology* **2007**, *12*, 500–509. [CrossRef]
6. Kumar, V.; Yadav, A.K.; Lal, A.; Kumar, V.; Singhal, M.; Billot, L.; Gupta, K.L.; Banerjee, D.; Jha, V.J. Randomized Trial of Vitamin D Supplementation on Vascular Function in CKD. *Am. Soc. Nephrol.* **2017**, *28*, 3100–3108. [CrossRef]
7. Frimodt-Møller, M.; Kamper, A.L.; Strandgaard, S.; Kreiner, S.; Nielsen, A.H. Beneficial effects on arterial stiffness and pulse-wave reflection of combined enalapril and candesartan in chronic kidney disease—A randomized trial. *PLoS ONE* **2012**, *7*, e41757. [CrossRef]
8. LeBoeuf, A.; Mac-Way, F.; Utescu, M.S.; de Serres, S.A.; Douville, P.; Desmeules, S.; Lebel, M.; Agharazii, M. Impact of dialysate calcium concentration on the progression of aortic stiffness in patients on haemodialysis. *Nephrol. Dial. Transplant.* **2011**, *26*, 3695–3701. [CrossRef]
9. Townsend, R.R.; Wilkinson, I.B.; Schiffrin, E.L.; Avolio, A.P.; Chirinos, J.A.; Cockcroft, J.R.; Heffernan, K.S.; Lakatta, E.G.; McEniery, C.M.; Mitchell, G.F.; et al. Recommendations for improving and standardizing vascular research on arterial stiffness: A scientific statement from the American Heart Association. *Hypertension* **2015**, *66*, 698–722. [CrossRef]

10. Laurent, S.; Cockcroft, J.; van Bortel, L.; Boutouyrie, P.; Giannattasio, C.; Hayoz, D.; Pannier, B.; Vlachopoulos, C.; Wilkinson, I.; Struijker-Boudier, H. Expert consensus document on arterial stiffness: Methodological issues and clinical applications. *Eur. Heart J.* 2006, *27*, 2588–2605. [CrossRef]
11. Townsed, R.R. Arterial stiffness: Recomendations and standarization. *Pulse* 2017, *4* (Suppl. S1), 3–7. [CrossRef]
12. Lioufas, N.; Hawley, C.M.; Cameron, J.D.; Toussaint, N.D. Chronic Kidney Disease and Pulse Wave Velocity: A Narrative Review. *Int. J. Hypertens.* 2019, *2019*, 9189362. [CrossRef]
13. Yao, J.; Dong, Z.; Wang, Q.; Li, Z.; Zhang, W.; Lin, W.; Luo, Y.; Li, H.; Guo, X.; Zhang, L.; et al. Clinical Factors Associated with Arterial Stiffness in Chronic Kidney Disease. *J. Clin. Med.* 2023, *12*, 1077. [CrossRef]
14. Drechsler, M.; Megens, R.T.A.; van Zandvoort, M.; Weber, C.; Soehnlein, O. Hyperlipidemia-triggered neutrophylia promotes early atherosclerosis. *Circulation* 2010, *122*, 1837–1845. [CrossRef]
15. Inserra, F.; Forcada, P.; Castellaro, A.; Castellaro, C. Chronic Kidney Disease and Arterial Stiffness: A Two-Way Path. *Front. Med.* 2021, *8*, 765924. [CrossRef]
16. Raymond, R.; Townsend, M.D. Arterial Stiffness in CKD: A Review of Findings from the CRIC Study. *Am. J. Kidney Dis.* 2019, *73*, 240–247. [CrossRef]
17. Stevens, P.E.; Levin, A. Kidney Disease: Improving Global Outcomes Chronic Kidney Disease Guideline Development Work Group Members. Evaluation and management of chronic kidney disease: Synopsis of the Kidney Disease: Improving Global Outcomes 2012 clinical practice guideline. *Ann. Intern. Med.* 2013, *158*, 825–830. [CrossRef]
18. Wu, H.C.; Lee, L.C.; Wang, W.J. Associations among Serum Beta 2 Microglobulin, Malnutrition, Inflammation, and Advanced Cardiovascular Event in Patients with Chronic Kidney Disease. *J. Clin. Lab. Anal.* 2017, *31*, e22056. [CrossRef]
19. Hyun, Y.Y.; Kim, H.; Sung, S.; Kim, S.W.; Chae, D.W.; Kim, Y.; Choi, K.H.; Ahn, C.; Lee, K. Association between Urine Creatinine Excretion and Arterial Stiffness in Chronic Kidney Disease: Data from the KNOW-CKD Study. *Kidney Blood Press Res.* 2016, *41*, 527–534. [CrossRef]
20. Czyżewski, Ł.; Wyzgał, J.; Czyżewska, E.; Sierdziński, J.; Szarpak, Ł. Contribution of volume overload to the arterial stiffness of hemodialysis patients. *Ren. Fail.* 2017, *39*, 333–339. [CrossRef]
21. Gu, Y.; Cheng, L.T.; Chen, H.M.; Sun, X.Y.; Tang, L.J.; Guo, L.J.; Axelsson, J.; Wang, T. Strong association between nutritional markers and arterial stiffness in continuous ambulatory peritoneal dialysis patients. *Blood Purif.* 2008, *26*, 340–346. [CrossRef] [PubMed]
22. Sobhani, S.; Vakili, S.; Javid Jam, D.; Aryan, R.; Khadem-Rezaiyan, M.; Eslami, S.; Alinezhad-Namaghi, M. Relationship between anthropometric indices and arterial stiffness: Insights from an epidemiologic study. *Obes. Sci. Pract.* 2022, *8*, 494–499. [CrossRef] [PubMed]
23. Dourado, M.; Cavalcanti, F.; Vilar, L.; Cantilino, A. Relationship between Prolactin, Chronic Kidney Disease, and Cardiovascular Risk. *Int. J. Endocrinol.* 2020, *2020*, 9524839. [CrossRef] [PubMed]
24. Ignacak, A.; Kasztelnik, M.; Sliwa, T.; Korbut, R.A.; Rajda, K.; Guzik, T.J. Prolactin—Not only lactotrophin. *J. Physiol. Pharmacol.* 2012, *63*, 435–443. [PubMed]
25. Tzanakis, N.D.; Gregerson, K.A. Prolactin actions. *J. Molecul Endocrinol.* 2013, *52*, 95–106. [CrossRef]
26. Carrero, J.J.; Kyriazis, J.; Sonmez, A.; Tzanakis, I.; Qureshi, A.R.; Stenvinkel, P.; Saglam, M.; Stylianou, K.; Yaman, H.; Taslipinar, A.; et al. Prolactin levels, endothelial dysfunction, and the risk of cardiovascular events and mortality in patients with CKD. *Clin. J. Am. Soc. Nephrol.* 2012, *7*, 207–215. [CrossRef]
27. Rhee, C.M.; Alexander, E.K.; Bhan, I.; Brunelli, S.M. Hypothyroidism and mortality among dialysis patients. *Clin. J. Am. Soc. Nephrol.* 2013, *8*, 593–601. [CrossRef]
28. Rhee, C.M.; Brent, G.A.; Kovesdy, C.P.; Soldin, O.P.; Nguyen, D.; Budoff, M.J.; Brunelli, S.M.; Kalantar-Zadeh, K. Thyroid functional disease: An under-recognized cardiovascular risk factor in kidney disease patients. *Nephrol. Dial. Transplant.* 2015, *30*, 724–737. [CrossRef]
29. Liu, T.; Guan, Y.; Li, J.; Mao, H.; Zhan, Y. Thyroid dysfunction and cardiovascular events in patients with chronic kidney disease: A protocol of systematic review and meta-analysis. *Medicine* 2020, *99*, e23218. [CrossRef]
30. Onofriescu, M.; Mardare, N.G.; Segall, L.; Voroneanu, L.; Cuşai, C.; Hogaş, S.; Ardeleanu, S.; Nistor, I.; Prisadă, O.V.; Sascău, R.; et al. Randomized trial of bioelectrical impedance analysis versus clinical criteria for guiding ultrafiltration in hemodialysis patients: Effects on blood pressure, hydration status, and arterial stiffness. *Int. Urol. Nephrol.* 2012, *44*, 583–591. [CrossRef]
31. Sarafidis, P.A.; Lazaridis, A.A.; Imprialos, K.P.; Georgianos, P.I.; Avranas, K.A.; Protogerou, A.D.; Doumas, M.N.; Athyros, V.G.; Karagiannis, A.I. A comparison study of brachial blood pressure recorded with Spacelabs 90217A and Mobil-O-Graph NG devices under static and ambulatory conditions. *J Hum Hypertens* 2016, *30*, 742–749. [CrossRef]
32. Karpetas, A.; Sarafidis, P.A.; Georgianos, P.I.; Protogerou, A.; Vakianis, P.; Koutroumpas, G.; Raptis, V.; Stamatiadis, D.N.; Syrganis, C.; Liakopoulos, V.; et al. Ambulatory recording of wave reflections and arterial stiffness during intra- and interdialytic periods in patients treated with dialysis. *Clin. J. Am. Soc. Nephrol.* 2015, *10*, 630–638. [CrossRef]
33. Weber, T.; Wassertheurer, S.; Rammer, M.; Maurer, E.; Hametner, B.; Mayer, C.C.; Kropf, J.; Eber, B. Validation of a brachial cuff-based method for estimating central systolic blood pressure. *Hypertension* 2011, *58*, 825–832. [CrossRef]
34. Townsend, R.R.; Hyre Anderson, A.; Chirinos, J.A.; Feldman, H.I.; Grunwald, J.E.; Nessel, L.; Roy, J.; Weir, M.R.; Wright, J.T.; Bansal, N.; et al. Association of Pulse Wave Velocity with Chronic Kidney Disease Progression and Mortality. *Hypertension* 2018, *71*, 1101–1107. [CrossRef]

35. Castelli, R.; Gidaro, A.; Casu, G.; Merella, P.; Profili, N.I.; Donadoni, M.; Maioli, M.; Delitala, A.P. Aging of the Arterial System. *Int. J. Mol. Sci.* **2023**, *24*, 6910. [CrossRef]
36. Harada, K.; Suzuki, S.; Ishii, H.; Hirayama, K.; Aoki, T.; Shibata, Y.; Negishi, Y.; Sumi, T.; Kawashima, K.; Kunimura, A.; et al. Nutrition Status Predicts Severity of Vascular Calcification in Non-Dialyzed Chronic Kidney Disease. *Circ. J.* **2017**, *81*, 316–321. [CrossRef]
37. Cordeiro, A.C.; Qureshi, A.R.; Lindholm, B.; Amparo, F.C.; Tito-Paladino-Filho, A.; Perini, M.; Lourenço, F.S.; Pinto, I.M.; Amodeo, C.; Carrero, J.J. Visceral fat and coronary artery calcification in patients with chronic kidney disease. *Nephrol. Dial. Transplant.* **2013**, *28* (Suppl. 4), iv152–iv159. [CrossRef]
38. Meuwese, C.L.; Olauson, H.; Qureshi, A.R.; Ripsweden, J.; Barany, P.; Vermeer, C.; Drummen, N.; Stenvinkel, P. Associations between Thyroid Hormones, Calcification Inhibitor Levels and Vascular Calcification in End-Stage Renal Disease. *PLoS ONE* **2015**, *10*, e0132353. [CrossRef]
39. Mizuno, I.; Takahashi, Y.; Okimura, Y.; Kaji, H.; Chihara, K. Upregulation of the klotho gene expression by thyroid hormone and during adipose differentiation in 3T3-L1 adipocytes. *Life Sci.* **2001**, *68*, 2917–2923. [CrossRef]
40. Lekakis, J.; Papamichael, C.; Alevizaki, M.; Piperingos, G.; Marafelia, P.; Mantzos, J.; Stamatelopoulos, S.; Koutras, D.A. Flow-mediated, endothelium-dependent vasodilation is impaired in subjects with hypothyroidism, borderline hypothyroidism, and high-normal serum thyrotropin (TSH) values. *Thyroid* **1997**, *7*, 411–414. [CrossRef]
41. Owen, P.J.; Sabit, R.; Lazarus, J.H. Thyroid disease and vascular function. *Thyroid* **2007**, *17*, 519–524. [CrossRef] [PubMed]
42. Hiroi, Y.; Kim, H.H.; Ying, H.; Furuya, F.; Huang, Z.; Simoncini, T.; Noma, K.; Ueki, K.; Nguyen, N.-H.; Scanlan, T.S.; et al. Rapid nongenomic actions of thyroid hormone. *Proc. Natl. Acad. Sci. USA* **2006**, *103*, 14104–14109. [CrossRef] [PubMed]
43. Carrillo-Sepulveda, M.A.; Ceravolo, G.S.; Fortes, Z.B.; Carvalho, M.H.; Tostes, R.C.; Laurindo, F.R.; Clinton Webb, R.; Barreto-Chaves, M.L.M. Thyroid hormone stimulates NO production via activation of the PI3K/Akt pathway in vascular myocytes. *Cardiovasc. Res.* **2010**, *85*, 560–570. [CrossRef] [PubMed]
44. McKenna, T.M.; Woolf, P.D. Prolactin metabolic clearance and resistance to dopaminergic suppression in acute uremia. *Endocrinology* **1985**, *116*, 2003–2007. [CrossRef] [PubMed]
45. Kyriazis, J.; Tzanakis, I.; Stylianou, K.; Katsipi, I.; Moisiadis, D.; Papadaki, A.; Mavroeidi, V.; Kagia, S.; Karkavitsas, N.; Daphnis, E. Low serum testosterone, arterial stiffness and mortality in male haemodialysis patients. *Nephrol. Dial. Transplant.* **2011**, *26*, 2971–2977. [CrossRef]
46. Gungor, O.; Kircelli, F.; Carrero, J.J.; Asci, G.; Toz, H.; Tatar, E.; Hur, E.; Sever, M.S.; Arinsoy, T.; Ok, E. Endogenous testosterone and mortality in male hemodialysis patients: Is it the result of aging? *Clin. J. Am. Soc. Nephrol.* **2010**, *5*, 2018–2023. [CrossRef]
47. Haring, R.; Völzke, H.; Vasan, R.S.; Felix, S.B.; Nauck, M.; Dörr, M.; Wallaschofski, H. Sex-specific associations of serum prolactin concentrations with cardiac remodeling: Longitudi-nal results from the study of health Pomerania (SHIP). *Atherosclerosis* **2012**, *221*, 570–576. [CrossRef]
48. Morohoshi, K.; Mochinaga, R.; Watanabe, T.; Nakajima, R.; Harigaya, T. 16 kDa vasoinhibin binds to integrin alpha5 beta1 on endothelial cells to induce apoptosis. *Endocr. Connect.* **2018**, *7*, 630–636. [CrossRef]
49. Ma, Z.; Mao, C.; Jia, Y.; Fu, Y.; Kong, W. Extracellular matrix dynamics in vascular remodeling. *Am. J. Physiol. Cell Physiol.* **2020**, *319*, C481–C499. [CrossRef]
50. Kim, J.M.; Kim, S.S.; Kim, I.J.; Kim, J.H.; Kim, B.H.; Kim, M.K.; Lee, S.H.; Lee, C.W.; Kim, M.C.; Ahn, J.H.; et al. Arterial stiffness is an independent predictor for risk of mortality in patients with type 2 diabetes mellitus: The REBOUND study. *Cardiovasc. Diabetol.* **2020**, *19*, 143. [CrossRef]
51. London, G.M. Arterial Stiffness in Chronic Kidney Disease and End-Stage Renal Disease. *Blood Purif.* **2018**, *45*, 154–158. [CrossRef]
52. Aznaouridis, K.A.; Stefanadis, C.I. Inflammation and arterial function. *Artery Res.* **2007**, *1*, 32–38. [CrossRef]
53. Yildiz, M. Arterial distensibility in chronic inflammatory rheumatic disorders. *Open Cardiovasc. Med. J.* **2010**, *4*, 83–88. [CrossRef]
54. Kuro-O, M. Phosphate as a pathogen of arteriosclerosis and aging. *J. Atheroscler. Thromb.* **2021**, *28*, 203–213. [CrossRef]
55. Giachelli, C.M.; Jono, S.; Shioi, A.; Nishizawa, Y.; Mori, K.; Morii, H. Vascular calcification and inorganic phosphate. *Am. J. Kidney Dis.* **2001**, *38*, S34–S37. [CrossRef]
56. Van den Bergh, G.; Opdebeeck, B.; Neutel, C.; Guns, P.J.; de Meyer, G.; D'Haese, P.; Verhulst, A. Towards a better understanding of arterial calcification disease progression in CKD: Investigation of early pathological alterations. *Nephrol. Dial. Transplant.* **2023**, *38*, 1127–1138. [CrossRef]
57. Arcari, L.; Ciavarella, G.M.; Altieri, S.; Limite, L.R.; Russo, D.; Luciani, M.; de Biase, L.; Mené, P.; Volpe, M. Longitudinal changes of left and right cardiac structure and function in patients with end-stage renal disease on replacement therapy. *Eur. J. Intern. Med.* **2020**, *78*, 95–100. [CrossRef]

Disclaimer/Publisher's Note: The statements, opinions and data contained in all publications are solely those of the individual author(s) and contributor(s) and not of MDPI and/or the editor(s). MDPI and/or the editor(s) disclaim responsibility for any injury to people or property resulting from any ideas, methods, instructions or products referred to in the content.

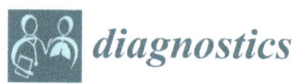

Article

Identifying Optical Coherence Tomography Markers for Multiple Sclerosis Diagnosis and Management

Larisa Cujba [1], Cristina Stan [2], Ovidiu Samoila [2,*], Tudor Drugan [3], Ancuta Benedec (Cutas) [3,*] and Cristina Nicula [2]

[1] Medical Doctoral School, University of Oradea, 410087 Oradea, Romania
[2] Department of Ophthalmology, Faculty of Medicine, "Iuliu Hatieganu" University of Medicine and Pharmacy, 400006 Cluj-Napoca, Romania
[3] Department of Medical Informatics and Biostatistics, "Iuliu Hațieganu" University of Medicine and Pharmacy, 400012 Cluj-Napoca, Romania
* Correspondence: iovidius@yahoo.com (O.S.); cutas.ancuta@umfcluj.ro (A.B.)

Abstract: Background: Multiple sclerosis (MS) is a common neurological disease affecting the optic nerve, directly or indirectly, through transsynaptic axonal degeneration along the visual pathway. New ophthalmological tools, arguably the most important being optical coherence tomography (OCT), could prove paramount in redefining MS diagnoses and shaping their follow-up protocols, even when the optic nerve is not involved. Methods: A prospective clinical study was conducted. In total, 158 eyes from patients previously diagnosed with relapsing remitting MS (RRMS)—with or without optic neuritis (ON), clinically isolated syndrome (CIS) with or without ON, and healthy controls were included. Each patient underwent an ophthalmologic exam and OCT evaluation for both eyes (a posterior pole analysis (PPA) and the optic nerve head radial circle protocol (ONH-RC)). Results: The macular retinal thickness (the 4×4, respectively, 2×2 grid) and thickness of the peripapillary retinal nerve fiber layer (pRNFL) were investigated. Various layers of the retina were also compared. Our study observed significant pRNFL thinning in the RRMS eyes compared to the control group, the pRNFL atrophy being more severe in the RRMS-ON eyes than the RRMS-NON eyes. In the ON group, the macular analysis showed statistically significant changes in the RRMS-ON eyes when compared only to the CIS-ON eyes, regarding decreases in the inner plexiform layer (IPL) thickness and inner nuclear layer (INL) on the central 2×2 macular grid. The neurodegenerative process affected both the inner retina and pRNFL, with clinical damage appearing for the latter in the following order: CIS-NON, CIS-ON, RRMS-NON, and RRMS-ON. In the presence of optic neuritis, SMRR patients presented an increase in their outer retina thickness compared to CIS patients. Conclusions: To differentiate the MS patients from the CIS patients, in the absence of optic neuritis, OCT Posterior Pole Analysis could be a useful tool when using a central 2×2 sectors macular grid. Retinal changes in MS seem to start from the fovea and spread to the posterior pole. Finally, MS could lead to alterations in both the inner and outer retina, along with pRNFL.

Keywords: multiple sclerosis; neurodegeneration; clinically isolated syndrome; optical coherence tomography; retinal fiber layers; ganglion cell layer; posterior pole analysis; macular retinal segmentation

Citation: Cujba, L.; Stan, C.; Samoila, O.; Drugan, T.; Benedec, A.; Nicula, C. Identifying Optical Coherence Tomography Markers for Multiple Sclerosis Diagnosis and Management. *Diagnostics* **2023**, *13*, 2077. https://doi.org/10.3390/diagnostics13122077

Academic Editor: Tomasz Litwin

Received: 8 May 2023
Revised: 1 June 2023
Accepted: 9 June 2023
Published: 15 June 2023

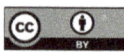

Copyright: © 2023 by the authors. Licensee MDPI, Basel, Switzerland. This article is an open access article distributed under the terms and conditions of the Creative Commons Attribution (CC BY) license (https://creativecommons.org/licenses/by/4.0/).

1. Introduction

Multiple sclerosis (MS) is the most common inflammatory neurological disease of the central nervous system that affects young adults [1,2].

Regarding the pathogenesis of MS, the following processes are involved in the destruction of the myelin sheath: neurodegeneration, neuroinflammation, autoimmune response, excitotoxicity, and gliosis [3].

Considering neurodegeneration, the underlying cause of disability in MS, intensive research has been conducted in order to identify markers able to quantify and track these neuronal changes. The retina offers the opportunity to study the central nervous system, with retinal changes in MS reflecting both focal and global aspects of neurodegeneration and inflammation [4].

The most common subtype of MS is relapsing-remitting MS (RRMS), which comprises 85% of all cases [5].

Clinically isolated syndrome (CIS) is typically the first and earliest clinical manifestation of MS, making patients with this diagnosis vital for research and offering doctors the opportunity to evaluate the earliest signs and quantify the changes in MS [6].

The last revision of the MS diagnostic criteria proposed introducing the optic nerve as the fifth CNS location to quantify the dissemination in time and space of its characteristic lesions, therefore emphasizing the importance of precise evaluations of the optic nerve in refining this diagnostic criteria [7].

Considering The 2017 revisions of the McDonald criteria for the diagnosis of multiple sclerosis: typical CIS-presenting clinical or magnetic resonance imaging (MRI) evidence of dissemination in space of the central nervous system's (CNS) lesions, along with cerebral spinal fluid (CSF)-specific oligoclonal bands, allow for the diagnosis of multiple sclerosis [7].

Visual dysfunction is common in MS, usually occurring after optic neuritis (ON). Less frequently, however, demyelinating lesions can affect the retro-chiasmatic visual pathway [8].

Many MS lesions are asymptomatic, including optic nerve ones. Their early detection would prevent diagnoses at advanced stages of the disease [9]. Identifying subclinical lesions of the visual pathways has become a significant aspect in the evaluation of newly diagnosed cases of MS [10,11].

Optic neuritis is an inflammatory lesion, frequently involving the retrobulbar portion of the optic nerve. It represents the most well-defined clinically isolated syndrome associated with MS [5]. Optic neuritis is the presenting complaint in 20% of multiple sclerosis patients [12]. Furthermore, up to 70% of patients with MS develop an episode of neuritis during the course of the disease [13].

Optical coherence tomography (OCT) is a fast, inexpensive, reproducible, and noninvasive imaging technique. It uses near-infrared light to generate cross-sections or three-dimensional images of the retina [14]. Imaging biomarkers of the retinal structure are important for recognizing and monitoring the inflammation and neurodegeneration in MS. With the advent of spectral domain OCT (SD-OCT), the supervised automatic segmentation of each individual retinal layer is possible. The essential changes observed in those with MS were in the macular ganglion cell-inner plexiform layer (GCIPL) and peripapillary retinal nerve fiber layer (pRNFL) [15]. These two elements are recommended to be used for diagnoses, monitoring, and research. The inflammatory activity of the disease could also be captured by the changes observed in the inner nuclear layer [15].

Considering the difficulties in diagnosing MS, especially in CIS cases, new ophthalmological tools, arguably the most important being OCT, could prove paramount in redefining MS diagnoses and shaping their follow-up protocols, even when the optic nerve is not involved.

Previous studies have demonstrated the phenomenon of transsynaptic axonal degeneration along the visual pathway in MS. We want to identify the OCT markers that are characteristic of MS patients, as well as their patterns, in order to differentiate MS-ON patients from MS-NON patients and MS patients from CIS patients. In this regard, we want to analyze the utility of a less used macular test grid for quantifying the retinal changes in all the layers of the eye in MS patients, in order to develop better diagnosis and monitoring tools for neurodegeneration. Identifying the subclinical activity of this disease with the use of optical coherence tomography is a secondary aim of the study, in order to facilitate earlier diagnoses and the easier surveillance of the global neurodegenerative process in clinical practice.

2. Materials and Methods
2.1. Study Design

The present study is analytical, observational, and monocentric. The selection of the participants was based on selective, convenient sampling, with the data collection being performed prospectively. The subjects gave their informed consent to participate in the study. The study respected the principles of the Declaration of Helsinki and the research protocol was approved by the Ethics Committee of the Iuliu Hațieganu University of Medicine and Pharmacy, Cluj-Napoca (No. 227/22.06.2020), and the Research Ethics Committee of the Faculty of Medicine and Pharmacy, University of Oradea (No. CEFMF/02 of 31.10.2022). The patients were enrolled between November 2021 and March 2022.

2.2. Participants

A total of 170 eyes were evaluated for the study, 158 were included in the final analysis, and 12 eyes were excluded.

We included 54 eyes of healthy subjects, 64 eyes of relapsing-remitting multiple sclerosis (RRMS) patients with prior optic neuritis (RRMS-ON), 26 eyes from RRMS patients without a history of optic neuritis (RRMS-NON), 6 eyes from clinically isolated syndrome (CIS) patients with prior optic neuritis (CIS-ON), and 8 eyes of CIS patients without a history of optic neuritis (CIS-NON). The ON patients were evaluated at least 3 months after an acute episode.

The MS and CIS patients were recruited from the Neurology Department of the Cluj-Napoca Emergency County Hospital. The healthy age- and sex-matched subjects were selected during the same time from the Ophthalmology Department of the same hospital.

The inclusion criteria for this study were: (1). patients assigned by the Specialty Commission for Multiple Sclerosis with a definite diagnosis of multiple sclerosis (RRMS); (2). patients diagnosed with CIS by the neurological department; (3). patients who presented at the clinic at least 3 months after an optic neuritis episode (documentation required); (4). patients able to understand the instructions provided; and (5). patients who gave their written consent to participate in the study

The exclusion criteria were: (1). patients with other ocular or systemic pathologies whose consequences overlap with the researched pathology; (2). patients without an acceptable SD-OCT evaluation; (3). a history of posterior pole surgery, cranio-cerebral trauma, cerebral vascular accidents, meningitis, encephalitis, or brain tumors; and (4). patients with mental health issues and those without temporal and spatial orientation.

2.3. Clinical and Paraclinical Assessment

Each subject was evaluated by the same team of ophthalmologists recording the following data: best-corrected visual acuity (BCVA) (measured with the Snellen scale), anterior and posterior pole biomicroscopy evaluation, aplanotonometry (Goldman, New York, NY, USA), visual field 30-2 (Humphrey Field Analyzer, Carl Zeiss Meditec, Dublin, CA, USA), and OCT measurements (Spectralis, Heidelberg Engineering GmbH, Heidelberg, Germany). ONH-RC and posterior pole analyses were used. Personal data were collected, such as: age, gender, level of education, the clinical form of MS, the ophthalmological onset of the disease, the number of years since receiving the diagnosis, the presence or absence of optic neuritis episodes, the presence or absence of MS-specific treatment upon entering the study, and EDSS score. All the RRMS and CIS patients had undergone a brain MRI with contrast within 3 months prior to entering the study.

2.4. The Methodology of OCT Measurements

The OCT measurements were performed on both eyes of each participant by a single technician who used the same Spectral Domain OCT device (Spectralis, Heidelberg Engineering GmbH, Heidelberg, Germany), which has a built-in real-time eye-tracking system that records the movements of eyeballs and generates feedback to the scan mechanism to stabilize the scan position.

The scans of both the optic nerve and macular region were recorded using ONH-RC and posterior pole analysis protocols. The global and sector thickness of the pRNFL, as well as the macular thickness (a central grid of 2×2 and 4×4 central sectors) on the 7 individually targeted layers: the macular retinal nerve fiber layer (mRNFL), ganglion cell layer

(GCL), inner plexiform layer (IPL), inner nuclear layer (INL), outer plexiform layer (OPL), outer nuclear layer (ONL), retinal pigment epithelium (RPE), and total macular thickness (TMT), were compared between the groups. Figure 1 summarizes all the retinal layers.

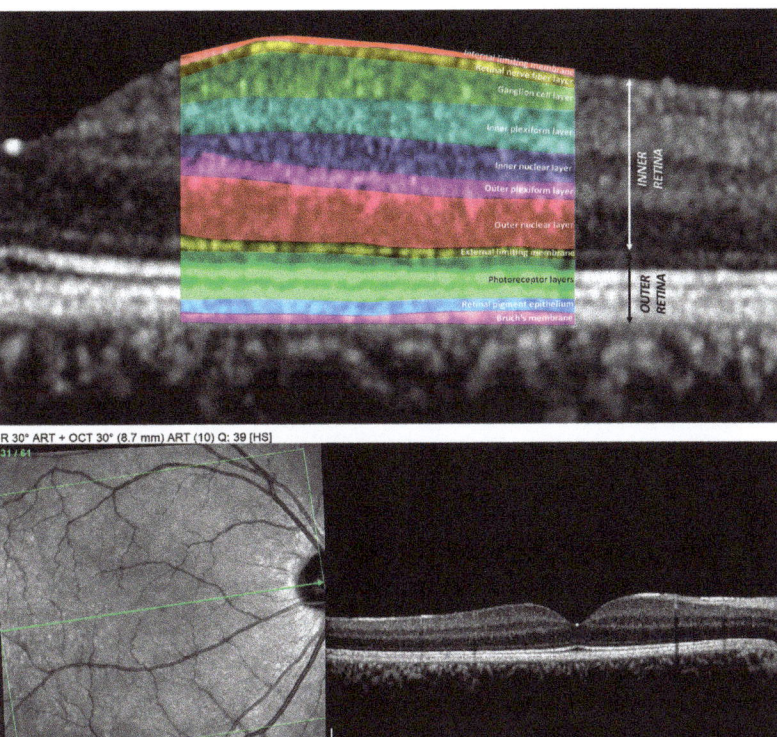

Figure 1. Cross-section images of the macula obtained using SD-OCT. Upper image represents the magnified view of the retinal layers as follows: internal limiting membrane (IML), mRNFL, GCL, IPL, INL, OPL, ONL, external limiting membrane (ELM), photoreceptors layers (PR), RPE, and Bruch membrane (BM). The image bellow: on the left: "En face" OCT scan of the macula (green line showing the level of the scan through the center of the fovea), on the right: cross-section of the macula corresponding to a healthy control.

The pRNFL analysis was performed by scanning a 3.5 mm circumferential area centered on the optic nerve head, resulting in a pie chart (Figure 2) divided into 7 sectors (G—global average, TS—temporal superior, T—temporal, TI—temporal inferior, NI—nasal inferior, N—nasal, and NS—nasal superior) that recorded the pRNFL's mean thickness value in microns for each quadrant.

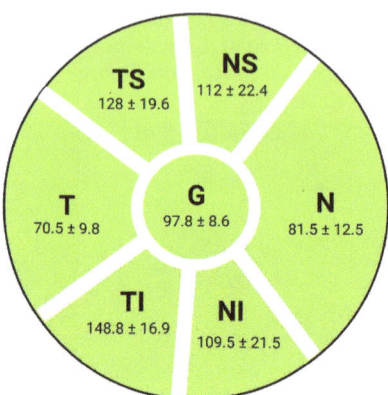

Figure 2. OCT diagram of optic nerve head sectors measurements (right eye) and correspondent RNFL thickness values (μm) from normative database [16]: G—global average, TS—temporal superior, T—temporal, TI—temporal inferior, NI—nasal inferior, N—nasal, and NS—nasal superior.

The analysis of the macular retina was carried out using the posterior pole analysis protocol of Heidelberg SD-OCT, which uses the APS (Anatomic Positioning System) system to adjust the acquisitions to the unique axis of each eye (FoBMOC, fovea-to-Bruch's membrane opening center). This aspect allows for an elimination of the variability in the results from the recording sectors, accurately ensuring the repeatability of the measurements on clearly defined sectors. Thus, 61 horizontal scan lines (1024 A-scans/line), parallel to the central reference line, were recorded. The scan area used 64 sectors, in the form of an 8 × 8 (3° × 3°) cube, but only the central 2 × 2 and 4 × 4 grids were used and analyzed in our study. The 16 sectors were numbered as in Figure 3, using their divisions into temporal, nasal, superior, and inferior, depending on the position relative to the fovea. The values in micrometers of each sector of the 4 and 16 central macular sectors were recorded and analyzed at the level of: the total macular retinal thickness, inner and outer retinal thickness, and thickness of each individual retinal layer, as mentioned above.

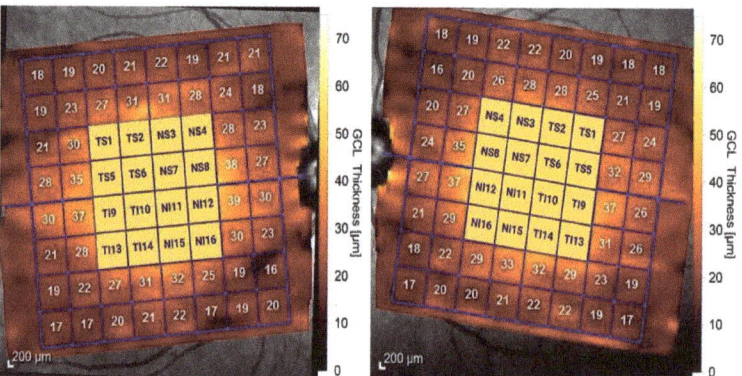

Figure 3. SD-OCT macular scan using posterior pole analysis. We analyzed the 16 central sectors numbered from 1 to 16, divided into nasal sectors (NS3, NS4, NS7, NS8, NI11, NI12, NI15, and NI16) and temporal sectors (TS1, TS2, TS5, TS6, TI9, TI10, TI13, and TI14). Superior sectors were from 1–8 and inferior sectors were from 9–16.

2.5. Statistical Analysis

The data collection and graphical representations were performed in Microsoft Excel 2019. For the statistical analysis, IBM SPSS v24 was used. The normality was verified using the Shapiro–Wilk test and, according to its values for the group comparations, we used means and standard deviations. The Student *t* test was performed for the two groups' comparisons, together with the Levene test for the homogeneity of the variances. For multiple sample comparisons, ANOVA testing was performed, and for a post hoc analysis, a Bonferroni correction was used. The mean difference was considered significant at the 0.05 level.

3. Results

A total of 158 eyes were evaluated as follows: 64 eyes of RRMS-NON patients, 26 eyes of RRMS-ON patients, 8 eyes of CIS-NON patients, 6 eyes of CIS-ON patients, and 54 eyes of healthy controls. The age and sex distributions are documented in Table 1.

Table 1. Age and sex distribution.

		CTRL	CIS-NON	CIS-ON	RRMS-NON	RRMS-ON
Sex	F	42	7	5	47	21
	M	12	1	1	17	5
	Mean Age	31.85	30.88	33.83	37.64	30.35

3.1. Peripapillary RNFL Changes in MS

Table 2 summarizes the average thickness of the peripapillary nerve fiber layer (pRNFL) on each individual sector for each group of participants. Figure 4 serves as a visual representation of the pRNFL thickness variation.

Table 2. Descriptive statistics of group analysis of pRNFL thickness (μm) on each sector.

	CTRL		CIS-NON		CIS-ON		RRMS-NON		RRMS-ON	
	Mean	SD	Mean	SD	Mean	SD	Mean	SD	Mean	SD
NS	120.11	24.96	99.25	24.11	118.17	24.11	109.00	23.20	98.88	18.47
TS	133.30	18.66	139.13	17.75	127.17	17.75	121.19	21.95	111.92	26.94
N	86.35	12.88	81.75	7.36	85.83	7.36	78.02	13.18	71.42	12.31
T	71.93	9.63	70.88	10.93	62.67	10.93	61.45	13.39	52.15	13.73
G	103.83	8.62	100.75	9.09	100.17	9.09	93.05	12.39	83.88	12.60
NI	125.39	18.49	127.38	16.15	129.00	16.15	111.98	25.29	102.54	23.17
TI	154.70	20.07	157.13	22.78	150.67	22.78	141.00	22.38	127.35	24.97

CTRL—healthy controls; CIS-NON—clinically isolated syndrome without ON history; CIS-ON—clinically isolated syndrome with optic neuritis (ON); RRMS-NON—relapsing remitting multiple sclerosis without ON history; and RRMS-ON—relapsing remitting multiple sclerosis with history of optic neuritis. G—global average, TS—temporal superior, T—temporal, TI—temporal inferior, NI—nasal inferior, N—nasal, NS—nasal superior; and pRNFL—peripapillary nerve fiber layer.

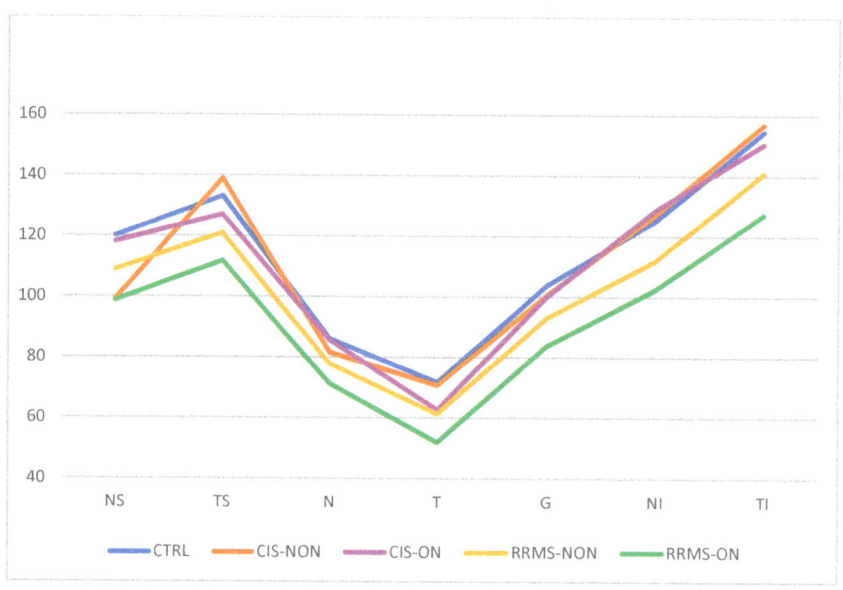

Figure 4. OCT thickness (μm) variation on each pRNFL sector of each group. CTRL—healthy controls; CIS-NON—clinically isolated syndrome without ON history; CIS-ON—clinically isolated syndrome with optic neuritis (ON); RRMS-NON—relapsing remitting multiple sclerosis without ON history; and RRMS-ON—relapsing remitting multiple sclerosis with history of optic neuritis. G—global average, TS—temporal superior, T—temporal, TI—temporal inferior, NI—nasal inferior, N—nasal, NS—nasal superior; and pRNFL—peripapillary nerve fiber layer.

Among the RRMS-NON patients, a statistically significant thinning of the pRNFL was observed in all the quadrants compared to the control group ($p < 0.05$). Among the CIS-NON patients, no significant statistical differences were identified in the pRNFL analysis compared to the control group (Table 3), as was the case for RRMS-NON eyes compared to CIS-NON eyes.

Table 3. The variation in pRNFL thickness (μm) on each sector compared to healthy controls group.

	NS	TS	N	G	T	NI	TI
CIS-NON	−20.86	5.83	−4.60	−3.08	−1.05	1.99	2.42
CIS-ON	−1.94	−6.13	−0.52	−3.67	−9.26	3.61	−4.04
RRMS-NON	−11.11 *	−12.11 *	−8.34 *	−10.79 *	−10.47 *	−13.40 *	−13.70 *
RRMS-ON	−21.23 *	−21.37 *	−14.93 *	−19.95 *	−19.77 *	−22.85 *	−27.36 *

* significant statistical differences, $p < 0.05$; CIS-NON, clinically isolated syndrome without ON history; CIS-ON, clinically isolated syndrome with optic neuritis (ON); RRMS-NON, relapsing remitting multiple sclerosis without ON history; and RRMS-ON, relapsing remitting multiple sclerosis with history of optic neuritis.

Comparing the RRMS-ON and CIS-ON eyes, we observed a statistically significant difference between the pRNFL thicknesses in five of the seven measured sectors: NS ($p = 0.037$), N ($p = 0.01$), G ($p = 0.006$), NI ($p = 0.013$), and TI ($p = 0.045$).

Among the CIS patients, the pRNFL analysis showed that there were no statistically significant differences between those with or without a history of optic neuritis.

Comparing the RRMS patient groups (with and without optic neuritis), a statistically significant difference in the pRNFL thinning in the RRMS-ON patients was noted in the following sectors: G ($p = 0.002$), T ($p = 0.004$), TI ($p = 0.013$), and N ($p = 0.31$).

3.2. Macular Thickness Changes in MS

A statistical analysis of the values of the central macular grid of the 4 × 4 and 2 × 2 sectors was performed on each macular layer separately and on the results that provided global indicators such as inner retina, outer retina, and total macular thickness (Tables 4 and 5, Figures 5 and 6).

Table 4. Descriptive statistics of the distribution of the mean values (μm) on the 4 × 4 central macular grid (16 sectors) of each retinal layer.

	CTRL		CIS-NON		CIS-ON		RRMS-NON		RRMS-ON	
	4 × 4 Sectors		4 × 4 Sectors		4 × 4 Sectors		4 × 4 Sectors		4 × 4 Sectors	
	Mean	SD	Mean	SD	Mean	SD	Mean	SD	Mean	SD
mRNFL	24.027	2.343	25.164	1.538	21.427	1.971	22.633	2.592	20.565	2.145
GCL	47.816	2.578	46.164	3.192	40.000	5.085	41.142	6.205	35.315	6.358
IPL	38.182	2.251	37.657	2.522	34.073	3.143	34.919	4.949	31.185	3.584
INL	38.371	2.761	38.711	2.726	39.990	1.931	38.403	2.156	38.505	2.936
OPL	29.113	2.068	28.617	1.926	29.698	4.017	29.216	2.281	29.890	2.492
ONL	70.149	6.128	70.602	6.211	72.709	5.170	70.422	6.971	71.608	6.795
EPR	13.948	1.102	14.047	1.095	13.927	0.749	14.765	1.792	13.927	0.749
Inner Retina	246.603	11.584	247.016	8.100	247.016	8.100	226.382	14.068	238.188	10.118
Outer Retina	80.408	6.183	79.438	1.923	79.438	1.923	81.253	1.674	79.219	3.083
TMT	327.959	12.124	326.430	7.608	326.430	7.608	308.730	12.978	318.302	11.275

CIS-ON, clinically isolated syndrome with prior optic neuritis (ON); RRMS-ON, relapsing remitting multiple sclerosis with prior optic neuritis; CTRL, control group; CIS-NON, clinically isolated syndrome without ON history; and RRMS-NON, relapsing remitting multiple sclerosis without ON history. mRNFL = macular nerve fiber layer; GCL = ganglion cell layer; IPL = inner plexiform layer; INL = inner nuclear layer; OPL = outer plexiform layer; ONL = outer nuclear layer; RPE = retinal pigment epithelium; and TMT = total macular thickness.

Table 5. Descriptive statistics of the distribution of the mean values (μm) on the 2 × 2 OCT central macular grid of each retinal layer.

	CTRL		CIS-NON		CIS-ON		RRMS-NON		RRMS-ON	
	2 × 2 Central Grid		2 × 2 Central Grid		2 × 2 Central Grid		2 × 2 Central Grid		2 × 2 Central Grid	
	Mean	SD	Mean	SD	Mean	SD	Mean	SD	Mean	SD
mRNFL	15.431	1.115	16.094	0.743	15.167	0.785	15.215	0.903	14.462	1.254
GCL	39.000	4.300	40.500	3.703	29.792	6.454	31.492	6.485	25.163	6.355
IPL	34.663	3.422	35.969	2.750	31.042	3.610	30.551	4.039	26.837	3.752
INL	33.306	3.830	35.094	3.119	33.417	1.821	32.361	3.344	30.800	2.896
OPL	29.846	2.947	29.031	2.466	29.000	5.736	29.195	3.655	29.558	3.106
ONL	79.830	7.519	80.750	8.169	83.833	7.627	80.944	8.107	83.029	6.859
EPR	15.838	1.231	15.688	1.534	14.750	0.880	15.586	1.449	15.990	1.419
Inner Retina	230.731	14.363	237.344	6.463	222.167	9.497	219.953	14.056	209.990	13.025
Outer Retina	84.019	2.529	83.375	2.722	82.833	2.910	84.195	3.283	85.087	1.512
TMT	317.234	14.780	305.125	7.325	295.960	11.667	295.960	14.940	295.960	13.994

CIS-ON, clinically isolated syndrome with optic neuritis (ON); RRMS-ON, relapsing remitting multiple sclerosis with history of optic neuritis; CTRL, control group; CIS-NON, clinically isolated syndrome without ON history; and RRMS-NON, relapsing remitting multiple sclerosis without ON history. mRNFL = macular nerve fiber layer; GCL = ganglion cell layer; IPL = inner plexiform layer; INL = inner nuclear layer; OPL = outer plexiform layer; ONL = outer nuclear layer; RPE = retinal pigment epithelium; and TMT = total macular thickness.

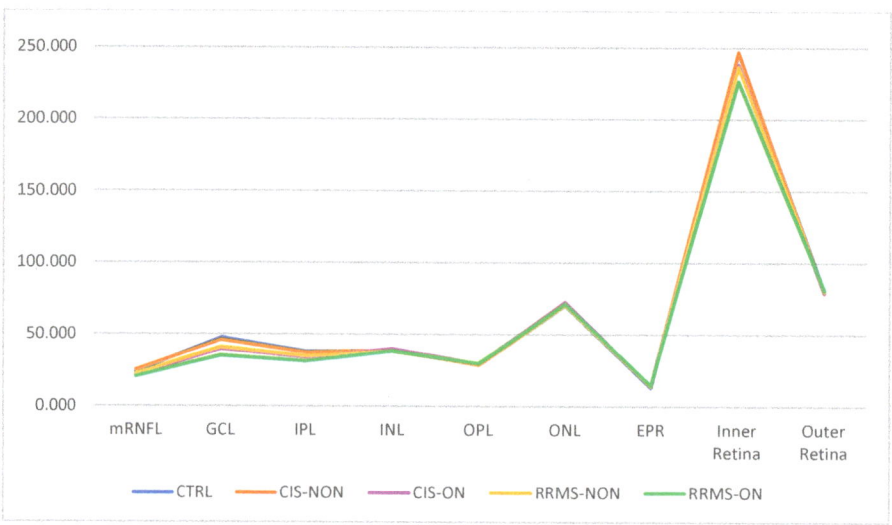

Figure 5. Distribution of the mean values (μm) on the 4 × 4 central macular grid (16 sectors) of each retinal layer.

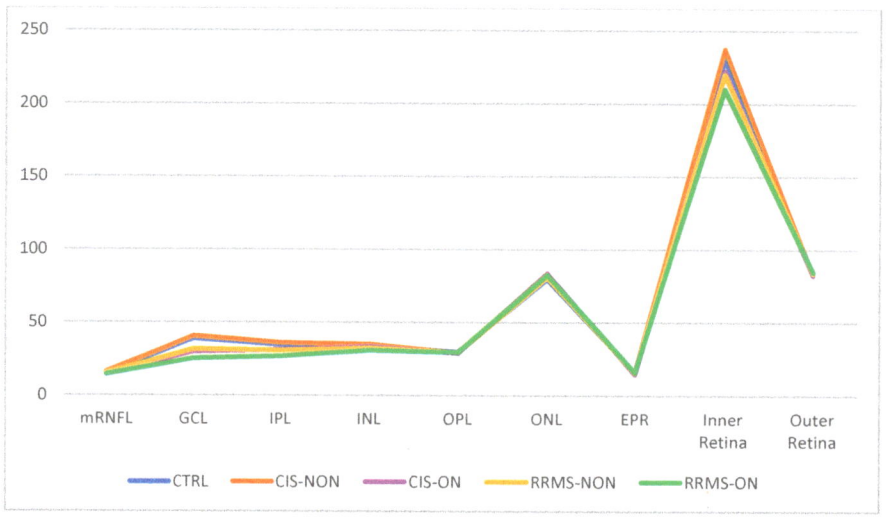

Figure 6. Distribution of the mean values (μm) on the 2 × 2 OCT central macular grid of each retinal layer.

Based on our results, in the macular analysis of the NON group for the central 16 sectors grid, we noticed a significant thinning of the mRNFL ($p = 0.019$), GCL ($p = 0.019$), and IPL ($p < 0.001$) in the RRMS eyes compared to the CTRL eyes and also a thinning of both the mRNFL ($p = 0.007$) and GCL ($p < 0.001$) in the RRMS eyes compared to the CIS eyes. For the four central sectors grid, there was a significant decrease in the thicknesses of the GCL and IPL layers between both the RRMS and CTRL groups ($p = 0.019/p = 0.001$) and RRMS versus CIS group ($p < 0.001$). No other retinal layers showed significant differences between any groups.

Regarding the ON group (RRMS-ON and CIS-ON), no statistically significant difference could be observed for any of the retinal layers in the central 16 sectors grid analysis. For the four central sectors grid analysis, the study revealed a greater thinning in the RRMS-ON eyes for the following layers: IPL ($p = 0.019$) and INL ($p = 0.045$). However, due to the small number of CIS-ON patients (six), no statistical significance could be highlighted.

An analysis of the cumulative INNER and OUTER retinal layers revealed differences both in the patients without ON and those with previous ON. Among the NON group, there was a significant thinning of the four sectors central grid in the INNER retina thickness in the RRMS eyes compared to both the CTRL ($p < 0.001$) and CIS ($p = 0.03$) eyes. For the 16 sectors central grid, the INNER retina was thinner in the RRMS-NON eyes only when compared to the CTRL group ($p = <0.001$). Analyzing the outer retina thickness in the NON group (CTRL, RRMS-NON, and CIS-NON), the results revealed the lack of a statistically significant difference, for both the 4 and 16 sectors central grids.

Among the ON group, analyzing the inner retina thickness values, we observed a thinning in the RRMS-ON group compared to the CIS-ON ($p = 0.004$) group, only for the central four sectors central grid. Analyzing the OUTER retina thickness for the same group, we noticed an increase in the thickness in the RRMS-ON eyes for both the 4 ($p = 0.010$) and 16 ($p = 0.031$) sectors central grids compared to the CIS-ON eyes.

Analyzing the TMT for the four sectors central grid in the NON-group, the results showed a thinning of the TMT in the RRMS-NON group compared to both the CTRL ($p < 0.001$) and CIS-NON ($p = 0.012$) groups. For the 16 sectors central grid, the difference was statistically significant only between the RRMS-NON and CTRL groups ($p = 0.001$) (Figure 7).

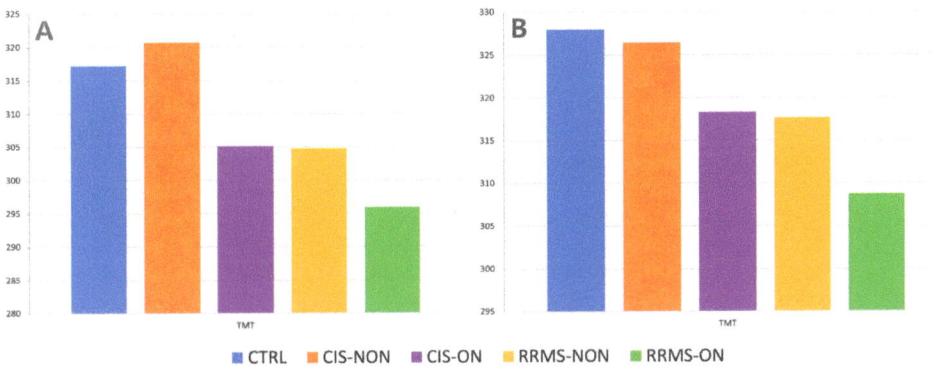

Figure 7. Total macular thickness (TMT) variation on 4 × 4 (**A**), and 2 × 2 (**B**) central macular grid on each group.

Regarding the TMT difference between the RRMS-ON and CIS-ON groups, there was no statistically significant value for any of the studied central macular grids (4 and 16 sectors).

Upon comparing the RRMS-ON and RRMS-NON eyes, in the central 16 sectors grid analysis, we found a greater thinning in the ON eyes for the following layers: mRNFL ($p = 0.001$), GCL ($p < 0.001$), IPL ($p = 0.001$), INNER retina ($p = 0.004$), and TMT ($p = 0.012$), and also a thickening of the OUTER retina ($p = 0.033$). For the four central sectors grid, the thinning was significant in the RRMS-ON eyes in the mRNFL ($p = 0.009$), GCL ($p < 0.001$), IPL ($p = 0.001$), INL ($p = 0.044$), inner retina ($p = 0.003$), and TMT ($p = 0.014$).

Comparing the macular thickness for the central 16 sectors between the CIS-ON and CIS-NON groups, there was a thinning of the mRNFL ($p = 0.002$), GCL ($p = 0.016$), and IPL ($p = 0.035$) in the ON eyes. For the four central sectors, the CIS-ON eyes presented a thinning in the mRNFL ($p = 0.044$), GCL ($p = 0.002$), IPL ($p = 0.013$), inner retina ($p = 0.004$), and TMT ($p = 0.010$) compared to the CIS-NON eyes.

4. Discussion

Today, SD-OCT allows for in vivo quantifications of axonal loss (pRNFL measurements) and neuronal damage (macular thickness assessments) in MS. Even though it has not yet been included in the multiple sclerosis diagnostic criteria, OCT is recommended as a useful diagnostic and monitoring tool for measuring the neurodegeneration in MS [15].

Our study aimed to assess the retinal differences in two concentric macular grids of the posterior pole, analyzing each retinal layer, along with the optic nerve changes in RRMS and CIS patients (with or without prior optic neuritis) in comparison to healthy controls.

The retinal macular area has the highest density of ganglion cells; therefore, OCT analyses of the macula can be an adequate method of quantifying neuronal damage [17]. Additionally, approximately 50% of the ganglion cells are located in the area 4.5 mm from the center of the fovea (approximately 16 degrees) [18]. The 4×4 macular grid analysis approximately covered this area, while the 2×2 covered it only partially.

Anatomically, the GCL, mRNFL, and pRNFL constitute the first units within the visual pathway. Irreversible axonal damage at any level can cause transsynaptic retrograde axonal degeneration, which will lead to an atrophy of the inner retinal structures (RNFL and GCIPL) [15].

Optic neuritis is one of the most frequent manifestations of MS. After an acute episode of optic neuritis, the pRNFL has no immediate change and is substantially decreased only at three months [19]. In this study, we only included patients more than 3 months after an ON event. It seems that pRNFL atrophy ends about 6 months after the onset of optic neuritis, the majority of the loss occurring in the first 3 months [20].

GCIPL analyses are reported to be superior compared to pRNFL measurements in tracking the early atrophy caused by optic neuritis, being less influenced by the axonal swelling following edema and inflammation [15,21]. Additionally, GCIPL atrophy after optic neuritis can be detected earlier than pRNFL atrophy, at 1 month after onset [15]. Moreover, if the optic neuritis episode is extremely severe, the pRNFL will show a floor effect, and only the GCIPL will still be useful as a biomarker of visual pathway neurodegeneration [15].

Consistent with previously reported data [15], our study observed significant pRNFL thinning in the RRMS eyes compared to the control group eyes, with the pRNFL atrophy being more severe in the RRMS-ON eyes than the RRMS-NON eyes.

The normal average thickness of the global pRNFL has been shown to be approximately 100 μm. Following an episode of optic neuritis in MS patients, SD-OCT measurements have confirmed previously published data, recording a pRNFL atrophy of 20.10 μm [15]. Our study results regarding the average thinning of the global pRNFL in RRMS-ON patients recorded a similar value of 19.95. The average global pRNFL thinning in the RRMS-NON eyes was 10.79 μm compared to 7.41 μm reported by Petzold et al. [15].

It is already known that ON in MS has an impact on pRNFL thinning, especially in the temporal sector, where papillomacular bundle nerve fibers appear that are important for central vision [22].

We noticed that the RNFL atrophy in the RRMS eyes (both ON and NON eyes) affected all the pRNFL sectors. There was pronounced pRNFL thinning in the RRMS-ON eyes compared to the RRMS-NON eyes identified in the T, TI, and N sectors.

In the presence of optic neuritis, the RRMS eyes suffered a greater decrease in their pRNFL thickness compared to the CIS eyes. This was observed only for the NS, N, NI, and TI sectors.

We could not identify any change in the pRNFL thickness in the CIS-NON eyes when compared to the control group, except for a decrease in thickness observed in the SN sector, which was probably due to the small number of enrolled CIS-NON patients, presenting an unidentified feature. No statistical difference was noticed in the pRNFL thickness between the CIS-ON and CIS-NON eyes. Our results were consistent with previously reported data [23].

We observed no statistically significant difference between he CIS-ON and CTRL eyes regarding the pRNFL, contrary to what Rzepisnki et al. [23] reported. In our study, due to the small sample of CIS-ON patients, even if there was thinning in the pRNFL, especially in the T sector, it could not have gained statistical significance.

We can also conclude that the pRNFL thinning was significantly influenced by the presence of prior optic neuritis in the RRMS patients, emphasizing its value in proving dissemination in the space of characteristic lesions in the CIS-ON patients, as Rzepinski et al. [23] already stated.

Over time, several studies have shown statistically significant decreases in the pRNFL and GCL thicknesses among RRMS patients, regardless of optic neuritis, compared control groups [24–27].

In their meta-analysis, Petzold et al. [15] reported the atrophy of the GCIPL in both MS-ON and MS-NON eyes compared to controls, the atrophy being more significant in the MS-ON eyes. They also found no changes regarding the ONPL thickness in either MS-ON or MS-NON eyes compared to controls and a minimal increase in its thickness in MSON eyes versus MSNON eyes.

In their study, Martucci et al. [28] created a map of regions of interest in a posterior pole analysis, characterized by statistically significant thinning in MS-NON eyes versus control eyes, with each individual retinal layer showing an irregular damage distribution of the same layers in MS patients. Additionally, in their study, the GCL and IPL damage was more concentrated in the parafoveal area, so we consider it appropriate to analyze the center of posterior pole assessment (comprising our 4×4 macular grid).

In our study, the OCT analysis using a 16-sector macular grid of the retinal layers in RRMS-NON eyes revealed a significant thinning for the mRNFL, GCL, and IPL layers compared those in the CTRL group, but only for the mRNFL and GCL when compared to the CIS-NON eyes. Additionally, in this case, the four central sectors of the PP analysis on the RRMS-NON eyes showed atrophy in both the GCL and IPL when compared to either the CTRL or CIS-NON eyes. The macular 2×2 mRNFL presented no changes, as its thickness was anatomically decreased in the foveal region.

The changes in the macular area of the RRMS-NON and CIS-NON eyes interest the inner retina layers, regarding retinal ganglion cell layer complex (which is the thickest in macular area [15]). When measuring the TMT and inner retina thickness, there was a significant atrophy in the 2×2 and 4×4 central grids of the RRMS-NON eyes compared to the CTRL eyes. Contrary to our results regarding TMT, a recent study [28] reported no statistically significant difference in the average retinal thicknesses between RRMS-NON and control eyes when comparing the entire posterior pole grid (64 sectors) analysis, suggesting that macular 2×2 and 4×4 sector analyses could be more useful for detecting early MS retinal changes. When comparing the RRMS-NON eyes with the CIS-NON eyes, the average values for the TMT and inner retina had a significant decrease only on the 2×2 macular grid. There was no significant alteration in the outer retinas in either the RRMS-NON or CIS-NON eyes when comparing them to each other or to the controls. With respect to the controls, the same finding, regarding the non-alteration in the outer retinas in the MS-NON patients, was ascribable to a sparing of the outer retina from neurodegeneration in the absence of ON [29–31]. Contrary to our findings, Saidha et al. [32] hypothesized the existence of "primary retinal pathology" as a process totally independent of optic nerve damage, based on their results regarding inner and outer retina thinning being mainly in progressive MS-NON eyes.

In other words, we could say that the closer the macular analysis was performed to the foveal area, the greater the discriminating power of the RRMS-NON changes compared to the CIS-NON eyes. A question arises from this: do the retinal changes in MS start in the central macular area?

In the ON group, the macular analysis showed statistically significant changes in the RRMS-ON eyes when compared only to the CIS-ON eyes, with regard to the decrease in the IPL and INL thickness on the central 2×2 macular grid. No changes appeared in the

TMT values on either the 2 × 2 or 4 × 4 macular grid. The inner retina was thinner on the 2 × 2 macular grid of the RRMS-ON patients. Additionally, the outer retina displayed an increase in its thickness on both the 2 × 2 and 4 × 4 macular grids in the RRMS-ON eyes compared to the CIS-ON eyes. Although there have been reports of inner and outer retinal alterations in MS patients, best-corrected vision acuity seems to be mainly influenced by inner retinal changes in the parafoveal area [29].

The RRMS-ON eyes recorded a significant thinning of the mRNFL, GCL, IPL, inner retina, and TMT on both the 2 × 2 and 4 × 4 macular grids compared to the RRMS-NON eyes. They also had a decrease in the INL thickness in the 2 × 2 macular area and an increase in the outer retina for the 4 × 4 macular grid. Thus, based on our results, the presence of optic neuritis seems to produce changes regarding all the retinal layers.

The CIS-ON eyes experienced a significant decrease in their ganglion complex cell layers for both the 2 × 2 and 4 × 4 macular grids and a decrease in the inner retina and TMT for only the 2 × 2 macular grid when comparing them to the CIS-NON eyes.

In their study, Eslami et al. [33] and Rzepinski et al. [23] could not find significant differences in the TMV (total macular volume) in either CIS-ON or CIS-NON eyes when comparing them to healthy controls.

Regardless of a prior optic neuritis episode, macular retinal layer changes in MS predominantly affect the ganglion cell complex of the inner retina (consistent with previously published data [15]).

In our study, the OCT analysis of the macular retinal layers in RRMS patients revealed atrophy changes only in the retinal ganglion cell layer complex (mRNFL, GCL, and IPL), which is the thickest in the macular area, with no thinning of the other retinal layers. Our results were consistent with previously published data [15,34]. However, the atrophy of INL could occur in some MS eyes of patients with a longstanding or progressive disease [35]. Significant correlations were also described between the increase in the INL thickness and the decrease in the RNFL/GCIPL volume. The first mentioned appears as a compensatory mechanism for the changes in the other retinal layers [36].

There are several limitations of this study. First of all, we had a relatively small number of participants, mostly in the CIS group.

Secondly, we used only the central 4 and 16 sectors of the macular area, avoiding any interference with large superior and inferior temporal retinal vessels and focusing our analyses on the macular area, where the greatest density of ganglion cells is. Additionally, we used the macular area changes as a surrogate for the global retinal neurodegeneration in MS, as SD-OCT measurements could not analyze the nasal retina. Finally, the OCT data were collected manually.

5. Conclusions

Posterior pole analyses could be an important assessment tool for monitoring the protocol of neurodegeneration in multiple sclerosis, thus helping to differentiate MS patients from CIS patients, in the absence of optic neuritis, when using a central 2 × 2 sectors macular grid.

Moreover, the fact that the macula is more affected in MS is an argument that the identified changes are specific to MS and not only related to ON.

The neurodegenerative process affects both the inner retina and pRNFL, with clinical damage appearing for the latter in the following order: CIS-NON, CIS-ON, RRMS-NON, and RRMS-ON. In the presence of optic neuritis, SMRR patients could present alterations in their outer retina too.

Author Contributions: Conceptualization, L.C. and C.S.; methodology, C.S. and C.N.; software, T.D. and A.B.; investigation, L.C.; data curation, L.C.; writing—original draft preparation, L.C.; writing—review and editing, O.S. and L.C.; visualization, L.C., C.S. and C.N.; supervision, C.N. and C.S. All authors have read and agreed to the published version of the manuscript.

Funding: This research received no external funding.

Institutional Review Board Statement: The study was conducted in accordance with the Declaration of Helsinki. and approved by the Ethics Committee of the Iuliu Hațieganu University of Medicine and Pharmacy, Cluj-Napoca (No. 227/22.06.2020) and by the Research Ethics Committee of the Faculty of Medicine and Pharmacy, University of Oradea (No. CEFMF/02 of 31.10.2022).

Informed Consent Statement: Informed consent was obtained from all subjects involved in the study.

Data Availability Statement: The data presented in this study are available on request from the corresponding author.

Conflicts of Interest: The authors declare no conflict of interest.

References

1. Williams, A.L. *Multiple Sclerosis Sourcebook: Basic Consumer Health Information about Multiple Sclerosis (MS) and Its Effects on Mobility, Vision, Bladder Function, Speech, Swallowing, and Cognition, Including Facts about Risk Factors, Causes, Diagnostic Procedures, Pain Management, Drug Treatments, and Physical and Occupational Therapies*; Omnigraphics: Detroit, MI, USA, 2019; p. xiii.
2. Wallin, M.T.; Culpepper, W.J.; Nichols, E.; Bhutta, Z.A.; Gebrehiwot, T.T.; Hay, S.I.; Khalil, I.A.; Krohn, K.J.; Liang, X.; Naghavi, M.; et al. Global, regional, and national burden of multiple sclerosis 1990–2016: A systematic analysis for the Global Burden of Disease Study 2016. *Lancet Neurol.* **2019**, *18*, 269–285. [CrossRef]
3. Henstridge, C.M.; Tzioras, M.; Paolicelli, R.C. Glial Contribution to Excitatory and Inhibitory Synapse Loss in Neurodegeneration. *Front. Cell Neurosci.* **2019**, *13*, 63. [CrossRef]
4. Ikuta, F.; Zimmerman, H.M. Distribution of plaques in seventy autopsy cases of multiple sclerosis in the United States. *Neurology* **1976**, *26*, 26–28. [CrossRef] [PubMed]
5. Costello, F. The Afferent Visual Pathway: Designing a Structural-Functional Paradigm of Multiple Sclerosis. *ISRN Neurol.* **2013**, *2013*, 134858. [CrossRef] [PubMed]
6. Efendi, H. Clinically Isolated Syndromes: Clinical Characteristics, Differential Diagnosis, and Management. *Noro Psikiyatr. Arsivi* **2016**, *52*, S1–S11. [CrossRef]
7. Thompson, A.J.; Banwell, B.L.; Barkhof, F.; Carroll, W.M.; Coetzee, T.; Comi, G.; Correale, J.; Fazekas, F.; Filippi, M.; Freedman, M.S.; et al. Diagnosis of multiple sclerosis: 2017 revisions of the McDonald criteria. *Lancet Neurol.* **2018**, *17*, 162–173. [CrossRef] [PubMed]
8. Cordon, B.; Vilades, E.; Orduna, E.; Satue, M.; Perez-Velilla, J.; Sebastian, B.; Polo, V.; Larrosa, J.M.; Pablo, L.E.; Garcia-Martin, E. Angiography with optical coherence tomography as a biomarker in multiple sclerosis. *PLoS ONE* **2020**, *15*, e0243236. [CrossRef] [PubMed]
9. Petzold, A.; Chua, S.Y.L.; Khawaja, A.P.; Keane, P.A.; Khaw, P.T.; Reisman, C.; Dhillon, B.; Strouthidis, N.G.; Foster, P.J.; Patel, P.J.; et al. Retinal asymmetry in multiple sclerosis. *Brain* **2020**, *144*, 224–235. [CrossRef]
10. Galetta, K.M.; Balcer, L.J. Measures of visual pathway structure and function in MS: Clinical usefulness and role for MS trials. *Mult. Scler. Relat. Disord.* **2013**, *2*, 172–182. [CrossRef]
11. Behbehani, R.; Ahmed, S.; Al-Hashel, J.; Rousseff, R.T.; Alroughani, R. Sensitivity of visual evoked potentials and spectral domain optical coherence tomography in early relapsing remitting multiple sclerosis. *Mult. Scler. Relat. Disord.* **2017**, *12*, 15–19. [CrossRef]
12. Costello, F. Vision Disturbances in Multiple Sclerosis. *Semin. Neurol.* **2016**, *36*, 185–195. [CrossRef]
13. Ciapă, M.A.; Șalaru, D.L.; Stătescu, C.; Sascău, R.A.; Bogdănici, C.M. Optic Neuritis in Multiple Sclerosis—A Review of Molecular Mechanisms Involved in the Degenerative Process. *Curr. Issues Mol. Biol.* **2022**, *44*, 3959–3979. [CrossRef] [PubMed]
14. Wicki, C.A.; Hanson, J.V.; Schippling, S. Optical coherence tomography as a means to characterize visual pathway involvement in multiple sclerosis. *Curr. Opin. Neurol.* **2018**, *31*, 662–668. [CrossRef] [PubMed]
15. Petzold, A.; Balcer, L.J.; Calabresi, P.A.; Costello, F.; Frohman, T.C.; Frohman, E.M.; Martinez-Lapiscina, E.H.; Green, A.J.; Kardon, R.; Outteryck, O.; et al. Retinal layer segmentation in multiple sclerosis: A systematic review and meta-analysis. *Lancet Neurol.* **2017**, *16*, 797–812. [CrossRef]
16. *User Manual Software*, Version 6.5, Spectralis Glaucoma Module Premium Edition; Heidelberg Engineering GmbH: Heidelberg, Germany, 2016; p. 78.
17. Zhang, C.; Tatham, A.J.; Weinreb, R.N.; Zangwill, L.M.; Yang, Z.; Zhang, J.Z.; Medeiros, F.A. Relationship between ganglion cell layer thickness and estimated retinal ganglion cell counts in the glaucomatous macula. *Ophthalmology* **2014**, *121*, 2371–2379. [CrossRef]
18. Curcio, C.A.; Allen, K.A. Topography of ganglion cells in human retina. *J. Comp. Neurol.* **1990**, *300*, 5–25. [CrossRef] [PubMed]
19. Henderson, A.P.D.; Altmann, D.R.; Trip, A.S.; Kallis, C.; Jones, S.J.; Schlottmann, P.G.; Garway-Heath, D.F.; Plant, G.T.; Miller, D.H. A serial study of retinal changes following optic neuritis with sample size estimates for acute neuroprotection trials. *Brain* **2010**, *133*, 2592–2602. [CrossRef]
20. Klistorner, A.; Arvind, H.; Garrick, R.; Graham, S.; Paine, M.; Yiannikas, C. Interrelationship of optical coherence tomography and multifocal visual-evoked potentials after optic neuritis. *Investig. Opthalmol. Vis. Sci.* **2010**, *51*, 2770–2777. [CrossRef]
21. Mehmood, A.; Ali, W.; Song, S.; Din, Z.U.; Guo, R.; Shah, W.; Ilahi, I.; Yin, B.; Yan, H.; Zhang, L.; et al. Optical coherence tomography monitoring and diagnosing retinal changes in multiple sclerosis. *Brain Behav.* **2021**, *11*, e2302. [CrossRef]

22. Saidha, S.; Sotirchos, E.S.; Ibrahim, M.A.; Crainiceanu, C.M.; Gelfand, J.M.; Sepah, Y.J.; Ratchford, J.N.; Oh, J.; Seigo, M.A.; Newsome, S.D.; et al. Microcystic macular oedema, thickness of the inner nuclear layer of the retina, and disease characteristics in multiple sclerosis: A retrospective study. *Lancet Neurol.* **2012**, *11*, 963–972. [CrossRef]
23. Rzepiński, Ł.; Kucharczuk, J.; Maciejek, Z.; Grzybowski, A.; Parisi, V. Spectral-Domain Optical Coherence Tomography Assessment in Treatment-Naïve Patients with Clinically Isolated Syndrome and Different Multiple Sclerosis Types: Findings and Relationship with the Disability Status. *J. Clin. Med.* **2021**, *10*, 2892. [CrossRef] [PubMed]
24. Albrecht, P.; Ringelstein, M.; Müller, A.; Keser, N.; Dietlein, T.; Lappas, A.; Foerster, A.; Hartung, H.; Aktas, O.; Methner, A. Degeneration of retinal layers in multiple sclerosis subtypes quantified by optical coherence tomography. *Mult. Scler. J.* **2012**, *18*, 1422–1429. [CrossRef] [PubMed]
25. Syc-Mazurek, S.; Saidha, S.; Newsome, S.D.; Ratchford, J.N.; Levy, M.; Ford, E.; Crainiceanu, C.M.; Durbin, M.K.; Oakley, J.D.; Meyer, S.A.; et al. Optical coherence tomography segmentation reveals ganglion cell layer pathology after optic neuritis. *Brain* **2011**, *135*, 521–533. [CrossRef]
26. Talman, L.S.; Bisker, E.R.; Sackel, D.J.; Long, D.A., Jr.; Galetta, K.M.; Ratchford, J.N.; Lile, D.J.; Farrell, S.K.; Loguidice, M.J.; Remington, G.; et al. Longitudinal study of vision and retinal nerve fiber layer thickness in multiple sclerosis. *Ann. Neurol.* **2010**, *67*, 749–760. [PubMed]
27. Walter, S.D.; Ishikawa, H.; Galetta, K.M.; Sakai, R.E.; Feller, D.J.; Henderson, S.B.; Wilson, J.A.; Maguire, M.G.; Galetta, S.L.; Frohman, E.; et al. Ganglion cell loss in relation to visual disability in multiple sclerosis. *Ophthalmology* **2012**, *119*, 1250–1257. [CrossRef]
28. Martucci, A.; Landi, D.; Cesareo, M.; Di Carlo, E.; Di Mauro, G.; Sorge, R.P.; Albanese, M.; Nicoletti, C.G.; Mataluni, G.; Mercuri, N.B.; et al. Complex Rearrangement of the Entire Retinal Posterior Pole in Patients with Relapsing Remitting Multiple Sclerosis. *J. Clin. Med.* **2021**, *10*, 4693. [CrossRef]
29. Ziccardi, L.; Barbano, L.; Boffa, L.; Albanese, M.; Grzybowski, A.; Centonze, D.; Parisi, V. Morphological Outer Retina Findings in Multiple Sclerosis Patients with or without Optic Neuritis. *Front. Neurol.* **2020**, *11*, 858. [CrossRef]
30. Schneider, E.; Zimmermann, H.; Oberwahrenbrock, T.; Kaufhold, F.; Kadas, E.M.; Petzold, A.; Bilger, F.; Borisow, N.; Jarius, S.; Wildemann, B.; et al. Optical coherence tomography reveals distinct patterns of retinal damage in neuromyelitis optica and multiple sclerosis. *PLoS ONE* **2013**, *8*, e66151. [CrossRef]
31. Balk, L.J.; Tewarie, P.; Killestein, J.; Polman, C.H.; Uitdehaag, B.; Petzold, A. Disease course heterogeneity and OCT in multiple sclerosis. *Mult. Scler. J.* **2014**, *20*, 1198–1206. [CrossRef]
32. Saidha, S.; Syc, S.B.; Ibrahim, M.A.; Eckstein, C.; Warner, C.V.; Farrell, S.K.; Oakley, J.D.; Durbin, M.K.; Meyer, S.A.; Balcer, L.J.; et al. Primary retinal pathology in multiple sclerosis as detected by optical coherence tomography. *Brain* **2011**, *134*, 518–533. [CrossRef]
33. Eslami, F.; Ghiasian, M.; Khanlarzade, E.; Moradi, E. Retinal Nerve Fiber Layer Thickness and Total Macular Volume in Multiple Sclerosis Subtypes and Their Relationship with Severity of Disease, a Cross-Sectional Study. *Eye Brain* **2020**, *12*, 15–23. [CrossRef] [PubMed]
34. Sotirchos, E.S.; Caldito, N.G.; Filippatou, A.; Fitzgerald, K.C.; Murphy, O.C.; Lambe, J.; Nguyen, J.; Button, J.; Ogbuokiri, E.; Crainiceanu, C.M.; et al. Progressive Multiple Sclerosis Is Associated with Faster and Specific Retinal Layer Atrophy. *Ann. Neurol.* **2020**, *87*, 885–896. [CrossRef]
35. Green, A.J.; McQuaid, S.; Hauser, S.L.; Allen, I.V.; Lyness, R. Ocular pathology in multiple sclerosis: Retinal atrophy and inflammation irrespective of disease duration. *Brain* **2010**, *133*, 1591–1601. [CrossRef] [PubMed]
36. Kaushik, M.; Wang, C.Y.; Barnett, M.H.; Garrick, R.; Parratt, J.; Graham, S.L.; Sriram, P.; Yiannikas, C.; Klistorner, A. Inner nuclear layer thickening is inversley proportional to retinal ganglion cell loss in optic neuritis. *PLoS ONE* **2013**, *8*, e78341. [CrossRef] [PubMed]

Disclaimer/Publisher's Note: The statements, opinions and data contained in all publications are solely those of the individual author(s) and contributor(s) and not of MDPI and/or the editor(s). MDPI and/or the editor(s) disclaim responsibility for any injury to people or property resulting from any ideas, methods, instructions or products referred to in the content.

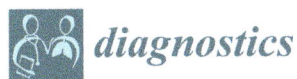

Article

Identification of Histopathological Biomarkers in Fatal Cases of Coronavirus Disease: A Study on Lung Tissue

Ioana-Andreea Gheban-Roșca [1,2], Bogdan-Alexandru Gheban [3,4,*], Bogdan Pop [5,6], Daniela-Cristina Mironescu [7,8], Vasile Costel Siserman [7,8], Elena Mihaela Jianu [4], Tudor Drugan [1] and Sorana D. Bolboacă [1,*]

1. Department of Medical Informatics and Biostatistics, Iuliu Hațieganu University of Medicine and Pharmacy, 400349 Cluj-Napoca, Romania; andreea.gheban-rosca@umfcluj.ro (I.-A.G.-R.); tdrugan@umfcluj.ro (T.D.)
2. Clinical Hospital of Infectious Diseases, 400003 Cluj-Napoca, Romania
3. Rouen University Hospital—Charles-Nicolle, 76000 Rouen, France
4. Department of Histology, Iuliu Hațieganu University of Medicine and Pharmacy, 400347 Cluj-Napoca, Romania; marina.elena@umfcluj.ro
5. The Oncology Institute "Prof. Dr. Ion Chiricuță", 400015 Cluj-Napoca, Romania; bogdan.pop@umfcluj.ro
6. Department of Anatomic Pathology, Iuliu Hațieganu University of Medicine and Pharmacy, 400349 Cluj-Napoca, Romania
7. Institute of Legal Medicine, 400006 Cluj-Napoca, Romania; csiserman@umfcluj.ro (V.C.S.)
8. Department of Forensic Medicine, Iuliu Hațieganu University of Medicine and Pharmacy, 400006 Cluj-Napoca, Romania
* Correspondence: gheban.bogdan@umfcluj.ro (B.-A.G.); sbolboaca@umfcluj.ro (S.D.B.)

Abstract: We aimed to evaluate the primary lung postmortem macro- and microscopic biomarkers and factors associated with diffuse alveolar damage in patients with fatal coronavirus (COVID-19). We retrospectively analyzed lung tissue collected from autopsies performed in Cluj-Napoca, Romania, between April 2020 and April 2021 on patients with severe acute respiratory syndrome coronavirus 2 (SARS-CoV-2). We examined 79 patients with confirmed SARS-CoV-2 infection, ages 34 to 96 years, split into two groups using the cut-off value of 70 years. Arterial hypertension (38%) and type 2 diabetes mellitus (19%) were the most common comorbidities with similar distribution between groups (p-values > 0.14). Macroscopically, bloody exudate was more frequently observed among patients < 70 years (33/36 vs. 29/43, p-value = 0.0091). Diffuse alveolar damage (53.1%) was similarly observed among the evaluated groups (p-value = 0.1354). Histopathological biomarkers of alveolar edema in 83.5% of patients, interstitial pneumonia in 74.7%, and microthrombi in 39.2% of cases were most frequently observed. Half of the evaluated lungs had an Ashcroft score of up to 2 and an alveolar air capacity of up to 12.5%. Bronchopneumonia (11/43 vs. 3/36, p-value = 0.0456) and interstitial edema (9/43 vs. 2/36, p-value = 0.0493) were significantly more frequent in older patients. Age (median: 67.5 vs. 77 years, p-value = 0.023) and infection with the beta variant of the virus (p-value = 0.0071) proved to be significant factors associated with diffuse alveolar damage.

Keywords: histopathology biomarker; severe acute respiratory syndrome coronavirus 2 (SARS-CoV-2); coronavirus disease (COVID-19); autopsy; lung

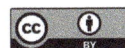

1. Introduction

Severe acute respiratory coronavirus 2 (SARS-CoV-2) is known to produce coronavirus-19 (COVID-19), a pathology classified as a multisystemic disease [1] that primarily affects the lungs [2,3]. Upon entering the host organism, SARS-CoV-2 binds to the angiotensin-converting enzyme-2 (ACE2) receptor on the cell surface, allowing the virus to enter the cell and promote replication. The ACE2 receptors are expressed in several tissues, including the heart, lungs, and kidneys [4,5].

In mild cases of infection, SARS-CoV-2 primarily causes lower respiratory tract infections (LRTIs) and severe pneumonia. In advanced cases, the disease can lead to acute respiratory distress syndrome (ARDS), septic shock, multiple organ dysfunction syndrome

(MODS), and eventually death [6]. Due to the absence of adequate biosafety measures during the initial stages of the pandemic, there were limited histopathological studies conducted, which prevented the medical community from understanding the full extent of the virus's effect on humans [7]. The number of postmortem examination studies is still limited, even though they are an invaluable tool for determining the pathogenesis of any disease, including COVID-19. Furthermore, autopsies can provide additional data to improve clinical care and treatment strategies [8]. Although the virus can cause lesions to other organs and tissues, lung changes are the most severe and will be this study's primary area of focus.

The lung lesions caused by the SARS-CoV-2 virus previously reported in the scientific literature are summarized and briefly presented in Table 1. The table provides a clear overview of the macroscopic and microscopic changes that occur in the lungs due to infection, making it easier to understand the impact of the virus on this vital organ. Despite widespread vaccination campaigns and public health interventions in many countries, the virus continues to spread, leading to illnesses, hospitalizations, and fatalities. New virus variants are emerging, some more transmissible and potentially more resistant to vaccines, making it harder to control the ongoing pandemic [9].

Table 1. Lung pathological findings reported in patients with COVID-19.

Authors	Year *	Country	Age Range (Years)	Sample Size	Macroscopic Findings	Microscopic Findings
Fox et al. [10]	2020	US	44–78	10	(a) Pleurisy; (b) patchy pattern edema; (c) pulmonary infarction	(a) DAD; (b) microthrombi
Roden et al. [11]	2020	US	69–94	8	(a) Consolidation; (b) pleurisy; (c) patchy pattern; (d) fibrosis; (e) pulmonary embolism	(a) DAD; (b) squamous metaplasia; (c) bronchopneumonia; (d) pulmonary embolism
Edler et al. [12]	2020	Germany	52–96	80	(a) Congestion; (b) pleurisy; (c) patchy pattern; (d) tracheobronchitis; (e) bronchopneumonia	(a) DAD; (b) squamous metaplasia; (c) bronchopneumonia; (d) fibrosis
Menter et al. [13]	2020	Switzerland	53–96	21	(a) Severe congestion; (b) consolidation; (c) bronchopneumonia	(a) DAD; (b) capillary stasis; (c) bronchopneumonia; (d) interstitial pneumonia; (e) edema; (f) microthrombi; (g) pulmonary embolism
Carsana et al. [14]	2020	Italy	32–86	38	(a) Congestion; (b) edema; (c) patchy pattern	(a) DAD; (b) capillary stasis; (c) bronchopneumonia; (d) interstitial pneumonia; (e) edema; (f) microthrombi; (g) atypical pneumocytes; (h) fibrosis
Lax et al. [15]	2020	Austria	75–91	11	(a) Congestion; (b) emphysema; (c) pulmonary embolism; (d) pulmonary infarction	(a) DAD; (b) bronchopneumonia; (c) interstitial pneumonia; (d) edema; (e) microthrombi; (f) fibrosis;
Suzuki et al. [16]	2022	Japan	28–96	41	(a) Consolidation; (b) tracheobronchitis; (c) pulmonary embolism	(a) DAD; (b) bronchopneumonia; (c) tracheobronchitis; (d) microthrombi
Viksne et al. [17]	2022	Latvia	22–94	88	No data	(a) DAD; (b) microthrombi; (c) pulmonary embolism; (d) fibrosis

* Year of collected data; DAD = diffuse alveolar damage.

Histopathological findings can accelerate the identification of effective epidemiological and medical strategies to reduce the progression of a pandemic caused by a novel virus with rapid and exponential transmission rates. A higher fatality rate has been reported in older subjects, but histological differences among different age groups were insufficiently documented. Furthermore, limited evidence exists on factors associated with microscopic diffuse alveolar damage. Our study had a two-fold aim: first, to identify the primary lung postmortem macroscopic and microscopic biomarkers observed in patients who died of COVID-19 using standard, special staining, and digital microscopy techniques in relation to age, and second,, to identify and evaluate if there are any factors associated with microscopic diffuse alveolar damage.

2. Materials and Methods

The study followed the Declaration of Helsinki, and its protocol was approved by the Ethics Committee of the Iuliu Hațieganu University of Medicine and Pharmacy Cluj-Napoca (DEP67/14.12.2021) and of the Institute of Legal Medicine, Cluj-Napoca (2406/XII/703/24.03.2022).

2.1. Study Settings and Design

We conducted an observational cohort study. All autopsies performed by forensic pathologists at the Institute of Legal Medicine Cluj-Napoca, Romania, were evaluated on patients who tested positive for SARS-CoV-2 ante- or postmortem between April 2020 and April 2021.

We included in our study only patients with COVID-19 confirmed disease regardless of the comorbidities, to whom an autopsy was performed in our institute in the study timeframe, and the lung tissue blocks were available from both lungs. We excluded patients with uncertain COVID-19 diagnosis from the analysis and those with confirmed COVID-19 disease with autopsy but without lung tissue blocks harvested from both lungs.

Demographic (sex, age, and living environment), epidemiological (symptoms onset, symptomatology duration, and date of death), and clinical (overlapping infections, mechanical ventilation) data were collected retrospectively from forensic reports. Comorbidities (class of body mass index, chronic obstructive pulmonary disease, arterial hypertension, congestive heart failure, myocardial infarction, diabetes mellitus, autoimmune diseases, liver steatosis, hepatitis, cirrhosis, chronic renal disease, malignant tumors, and brain stroke) were documented based on the available clinical data and the morphological observations made during autopsies.

2.2. Histological Processing and Staining

The harvested lung tissues were fixed in 10% neutral buffered formalin, processed, and paraffin embedded. The paraffin block was sectioned at 0.5 μm. Slides were manually stained using hematoxylin and eosin to highlight the cells, nuclei, and trichrome Masson to visualize collagen fibers and evaluate interstitial fibrosis.

Trichrome Masson's special staining implied deparaffinization and rehydration through successive baths of 100%, 95%, and 70% alcohol. The lung tissue was rinsed and then stained in Wiegert's iron hematoxylin for 10 min, rinsed, washed, and stained in Biebrich scarlet-acid fuchsin solution, and washed and differentiated in the phosphomolybdic-phosphotungstic acid solution until the collagen changed color. The lung tissue was dehydrated, cleared in xylene, and mounted on a microscopic slide.

2.3. Microscopic Examination

One independent board-certified pathologist evaluated the lung tissue samples and was blinded to patient characteristics and diagnoses. A Leica DM2500 microscope (Buffalo Grove, IL, USA) was used to examine the H&E slides. The findings were evaluated based on standard histopathological practice [18–20].

The trichrome Masson stained slides were examined as digital whole slide images. The extent of fibrosis in the lung parenchyma was evaluated using the Ashcroft score [21], a semi-quantitative scoring system that assesses the degree of lung fibrosis on histopathological digital slides. The Ashcroft score ranges from 0 to 8, based on the degree of fibrous thickening of the alveolar walls, lung architecture damage, and small fibrous proliferative bundles [21]. Moreover, the number of fibroblastic bundles was manually counted in a 25 cm^2 area of lung tissue.

2.4. Morphometric Analysis

Whole Slide Images were obtained by scanning the physical trichrome Masson's slides using a Pannoramic SCAN 150 by 3DHISTECH (Budapest, Hungary). The average scanning parameters were: 20× magnification, using a Plan-Apochromat objective and a CIS VCC camera with a micrometer/pixel ratio of 0.194475, scan duration of 17 min, calibrated color scheme, 112,640 × 243,200-pixel slide dimension, 9454 scanned fields of view, file size 2.72 GB. Measurement of the percentage of alveolar space was performed using the software SlideViewer by 3DHISTECH (version 2.6, Budapest, Hungary) (SlideViewer, RRID: SCR_017654). Using the plugin "Gradient Map Visualizations" we converted the trichrome Masson microscopic slides into an RGB spectrum (RedGreenBlue) slides where red and green highlighted interstitial and vascular structures and blue highlighted the alveolar space. We took snapshots of the pulmonary section slides and saved them as TIFF.files. Adobe Photoshop CC 2019 (San Jose, CA, USA) (Adobe Photoshop, RRID: SCR_014199) was used to crop and edit the image only to include the lung parenchyma without vascular lumina, which had the same color as alveolar spaces. The digital analysis was performed using the image analysis software ImageJ/Fiji (version 2.13.1, LOCI, University of Wisconsin, Madison, WI, USA) (ImageJ, RRID: SCR_003070) with the RGB Stack option to make a montage and adjust the color threshold of BLUE to 100–250 and analyzed the image by the following measurements: area, area fraction, and limit threshold. The same optical and image parameters, scan settings, and hardware versions were used to evaluate all images. The user defined the area of interest (ROI), and the software retrieved the percentage of free alveolar space from the examined section (Figure 1).

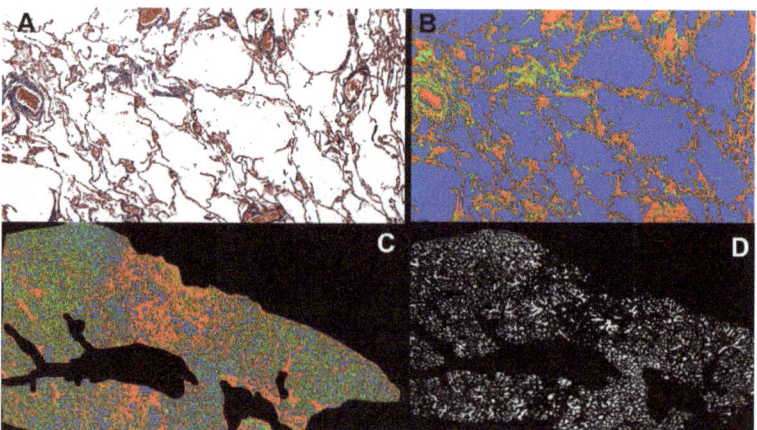

Figure 1. (**A**). Pulmonary parenchyma in Trichrome Masson stain at 20× magnification. (**B**). Red Green Blue (RGB) conversion using the Gradient Map Visualisation tool (SlideViewer by 3DHISTECH) highlights alveolar air space in the blue spectrum. (**C**). Overall view of the pulmonary fragment at 0.5× magnification, in RGB, after cropping vascular spaces using Adobe Photoshop CS9. (**D**). Pulmonary fragment after RGB stacking using ImageJ/Fiji software (version 2.13.1), highlighting only the free alveolar spaces in a white gradient to measure the total air-filled alveolar percentage of entire lung fragment tissue.

2.5. Statistical Analysis

We classified patients as infected with variant alpha (B.1.1.7) or beta (B.1.351, starting from March 2021) according to information available in Global Initiative on Sharing All Influenza Data (GISAID) [22].

We divided the cohort according to age into two groups (<70 years vs. ≥70 years), and we compared demographic, macroscopic, and microscopic characteristics between the two groups.

Shapiro–Wilk test ($p < 0.05$) and Q-Q plots were used to assess the normality of quantitative variables. Continuous data exhibiting non-normal distribution were described as the median and interquartile range (IQR). Categorical variables are summarized as absolute frequencies and percentages. Fisher or Chi-squared tests were applied to test associations in contingency tables based on the appropriate counts of the expected frequency tables. Differences between investigated groups were evaluated with non-parametric tests (Mann–Whitney U test) for continuous variables with non-normal distribution. All tests were two-sided, and the results were considered significant at p-values < 0.05.

Logistic regression was applied to identify factors related to diffuse alveolar damage (DAD) occurrence. Those factors who were associated with DAD at a p-value less than 0.25 in uni-variable models [23] were included in the multivariable regression model using stepwise selection, forward Wald.

Statistical description and analyses were conducted using Simple Interactive Statistical Analysis (SISA by Quantitative Skills, Available Online: https://www.quantitativeskills.com/sisa/ (accessed on 7 March 2023)), IBM SPSS trial version (Armonk, NY, USA) (IBM SPSS Statistics, RRID: SCR_019096), and Microsoft Office Excel 365 (Redmond, WA, USA) (Microsoft Excel, RRID: SCR_016137).

3. Results

3.1. Patients Characteristics

Seventy-nine patients aged between 34 and 96 years old, 36 (45.6%) younger than 70, and 43 (54.4%) older than 70, were evaluated. Among the 79 patients included in the analysis, 51 (64.6%) died in 2020, and 28 (35.4%) died in 2021. Men (median age of 70, IQR = [60 to 79]) were statistically significant younger (Mann–Whitney test: Z statistics = −2.2, p-value = 0.0263) than women (median age of 80, IQR = [68 to 85]). Six patients (7.6%) were under the age of 50, ten patients (12.7%) were between the ages of 50 to 59, and twenty patients (25.3%) were 60 to 69 years old. Most deaths, 51.9% (n = 41), occurred in the hospital setting, followed by 25.3% (n = 20) at home and 13.9% (n = 11) in an ambulance. The place of death could not be determined for one patient. Data regarding days from symptom onset to death was available only for 25 cases and ranged from 1 day to 35 days.

The two investigated groups were similar regarding demographic characteristics, as shown in Table 2.

The number of comorbidities varied from none to nine, without a significant association between the presence of comorbidities (any) and sex ($\chi^2 = 0.1$, p-value = 0.7509). The top three most frequent comorbidities observed in the cohort were: arterial hypertension (38%), type 2 diabetes mellitus (19%), and congestive heart failure (12.7%). A clinical history of myocardial infarction was observed exclusively in patients older than 70. Only one man, 72 years old, had a clinical diagnosis of liver cirrhosis; another man, 46 years old, had chronic renal disease. Fifteen (19%) patients had mechanical ventilation, eleven (25.6%) being in the group older than 70, but the difference did not reach the statistical significance threshold ($\chi^2 = 2.7$, p-value = 0.1024).

Regarding the microbiological results, two patients had positive sputum cultures for *Acinetobacter baumannii*, and another showed the presence of *Aspergillus*. One patient's bronchoalveolar lavage fluid exhibited a mixture of *Acinetobacter baumannii*, *Candida albicans*, and *Pseudomonas aeruginosa*.

Table 2. Demographic and comorbidities characteristics of evaluated patients.

Characteristic	All, n = 79 no. (%)	<70 Years, n = 36 no. (%)	≥70 Years, n = 43 no. (%)	Stat. (p-Value)
Sex				1.2 (0.2721)
Female	20 (25.3)	7 (19.4)	13 (30.2)	
Male	59 (74.7)	29 (80.6)	30 (69.8)	
Living area				0.5 (0.4988)
Urban	54 (68.4)	26 (72.2)	28 (65.1)	
Rural	25 (31.6)	10 (27.8)	15 (34.9)	
Class of BMI				4.4 (0.2220)
underweight	13 (16.5)	3 (8.3)	10 (23.3)	
normal	22 (27.8)	10 (27.8)	12 (27.9)	
obesity grade 1–2	35 (44.3)	17 (47.2)	18 (41.9)	
obesity grade 3	9 (11.4)	6 (16.7)	3 (7)	
Comorbidities				
Arterial hypertension	30 (38)	12 (33.3)	18 (41.9)	0.6 (0.4367)
Type 2 diabetes mellitus	15 (19)	6 (16.7)	9 (20.9)	0.2 (0.6304)
Congestive heart failure	10 (12.7)	4 (11.1)	5 (11.6)	n.a (0.8622)
COPD	7 (8.9)	3 (8.3)	4 (9.3)	n.a (0.8480)
Myocardial infarction	5 (6.3)	0 (0)	5 (11.6)	n.a (0.0381)
Hepatic steatosis	6 (7.6)	2 (5.6)	4 (9.3)	n.a (0.5431)
Malign tumors	7 (8.9)	3 (8.3)	4 (9.3)	n.a (0.8480)
Stroke	6 (7.6)	1 (2.8)	5 (11.6)	n.a (0.1496)

Results are reported as no. (%), where no.= absolute frequency; Stat. is the χ^2 statistics. Statistically significant p-values are highlighted in bold ($p < 0.05$); the remaining values were non-significant. BMI = body mass index; COPD = Chronic obstructive pulmonary disease; n = sample size; n.a. = not applicable, and whenever listed the p-value results are from Fisher's exact test.

3.2. Macroscopic Findings

Upon macroscopic examination, all patients' lungs displayed an increase in consistency, with patchy patterns observed in 63 cases (79.7%) and pulmonary infarctions observed in 39 cases (49.4%). Upon sectioning and palpation, 62 patients (78.5%) exhibited bloody exudate, 58 patients (73.4%) showed edematous exudate, and 17 patients (21.5%) had purulent exudate. Out of the total cases where lung weight measurements were taken (62 cases), the median combined weight of the right and left lungs was 1748 g, ranging between 610 g to 3005 g. The macroscopic findings of the lungs by age group are summarized in Table 3.

Table 3. Macroscopic characteristics of lung tissue by age group.

Characteristic	All, n = 79	<70 Years, n = 36	≥70 Years, n = 43	Stat. (p-Value)
Combined lung weight, g median [Q1 to Q3] {min to max}	1748 [1338 to 2090] {610 to 3005}	1830 [1505 to 2115] {1225 to 2425}	1645 [1235 to 1865] {610 to 3005}	1.5 (0.1276) *
Patchy pattern, no. (%)	63 (79.7)	30 (83.3)	33 (76.7)	0.5 (0.468)
Bloody exudate, no. (%)	62 (78.5)	33 (91.7)	29 (67.4)	6.8 (0.0091)
Edema exudate, no. (%)	58 (73.4)	27 (75)	31 (72.1)	0.1 (0.7708)
Purulent exudate, no. (%)	17 (21.5)	5 (13.9)	12 (27.9)	2.3 (0.1311)
Pulmonary infarction, no. (%)	39 (49.4)	20 (55.6)	19 (44.2)	1 (0.3141)

Results are reported as absolute frequency (percentage) for no. (%); * Mann-Whitney test; Stat. is the χ^2 statistics when the results are reported as no. (%). Q1 = first quartile; Q3 = third quartile; min = minimum; max = maximum.

3.3. Microscopic Findings

Histologically, 42 patients (53.1%) exhibited diffuse alveolar damage (DAD) (Figure 2). Among these patients, twenty-two (27.8%) had DAD in the exudative phase, fifteen (19%) in the organizing phase, and five (6.3%) in the fibrosis phase (Table 4).

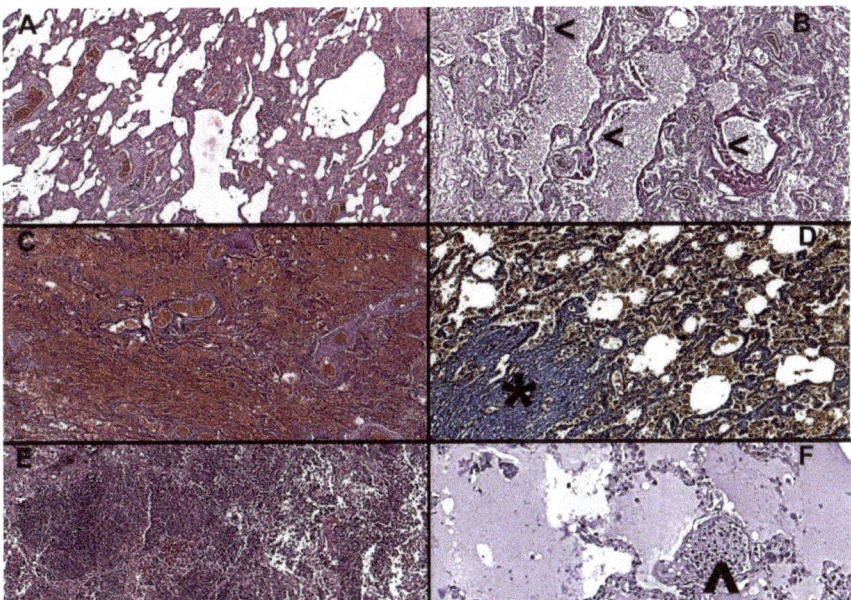

Figure 2. (**A**) Interstitial pneumonia in an 81-year-old male, H&E at 6× magnification, alveolar walls are thickened by inflammatory infiltrate, congestion is marked, and alveolar spaces are deformed. (**B**) Thickened eosinophilic hyaline membranes (<) covering the alveolar walls, indicative of organizing phase diffuse alveolar damage (DAD grade 2) in a 69-year-old male, H&E at 10× magnification. (**C**) Widespread pulmonary infarctions with diffuse hemorrhage in a 77-year-old male, H&E at 5× magnification. (**D**) Increased fibrosis with damage to lung structure and formation of fibrous bands and proliferative nodules (*) in a 60-year-old male, trichrome Masson, at 20× magnification. (**E**) Overlapping bronchopneumonia, with abundant neutrophilic infiltrate within alveolar and bronchial space, in an 87-year-old female, H&E at 10× magnification. (**F**) Recently developed microthrombi, comprised of fibrin and inflammatory cells (^) and alveolar edema in an 84-year-old female, H&E at 20× magnification.

In addition, microthrombi (Table 4) were observed in 31 cases (39.2%), with those aged over 70 years, 18 patients (41.9%), being the most affected group. In 29 patients (36.8%), alveolar epithelial desquamation was observed and graded accordingly. Bronchopneumonia (Table 4) was identified in 14 patients (17.7%), while purulent tracheitis was present in twelve (15.2%). Both bronchopneumonia and tracheobronchitis are defined by the presence of neutrophiles in either bronchial or alveolar spaces. Alveolar edema was observed in 66 cases (83.5%), while interstitial pneumonia (Table 4) was present in 59 patients (74.7%). Interstitial pneumonia is defined by the presence of lymphocytes and plasmocytes in the lung interstitium.

Due to inadequate preanalytical processing, the Ashcroft score was evaluated in 76 patients, highlighting interstitial fibrosis in trichrome Masson (Table 4). A median score of 2, ranging from 1 to 3, was observed, with scores ranging from 0 to 6 in all cases, regardless of age group. Alveolar air capacity was quantified, with a median value of 12.5%, ranging from 7% to 20.1%.

Table 4. Microscopic characteristics of lung tissue by age group.

Characteristic	All, n = 79	<70 Years, n = 36	≥70 Years, n = 43	Stat. (p-Value)
DAD, no. (%)				n.a. (0.1354)
Absent	37 (46.8)	12 (33.3)	25 (58.1)	
Exudative phase	22 (27.8)	13 (36.1)	9 (20.9)	
Organizing phase	15 (19)	9 (25)	6 (14)	
Fibrosis phase	5 (6.3)	2 (5.6)	3 (7)	
Lung congestion, no. (%)				n.a. (0.9935)
Absent	8 (10.1)	4 (11.1)	4 (9.3)	
Slight	22 (27.8)	10 (27.8)	12 (27.9)	
Moderate	29 (36.7)	13 (36.1)	16 (37.2)	
Severe	20 (25.3)	9 (25)	11 (25.6)	
Microthrombi, no. (%)	31 (39.2)	13 (36.1)	18 (41.9)	0.3 (0.6022)
Epithelial desquamation, no. (%)				n.a. (0.8561)
Absent	50 (63.3)	21 (58.3)	29 (67.4)	
Slight	15 (19)	8 (22.2)	7 (16.3)	
Moderate	10 (12.7)	5 (13.9)	5 (11.6)	
Severe	4 (5.1)	2 (5.6)	2 (4.7)	
Bronchopneumonia, no. (%)	14 (17.7)	3 (8.3)	11 (25.6)	4.0 (0.0456)
Tracheobronchitis, no. (%)	12 (15.2)	3 (8.3)	9 (20.9)	2.4 (0.1203)
Alveolar edema, no. (%)	66 (83.5)	31 (86.1)	35 (81.4)	0.3 (0.5734)
Interstitial edema, no. (%)	11 (13.9)	2 (5.6)	9 (20.9)	3.9 (0.0493)
Antrachotic pigment, no. (%)				3.6 (0.1688)
Absent	48 (60.8)	25 (69.4)	23 (53.5)	
Slight	16 (20.3)	4 (11.1)	12 (27.9)	
Moderate	15 (19)	7 (19.4)	8 (18.6)	
Interstitial pneumonia, no. (%)	59 (74.7)	29 (80.6)	30 (69.8)	1.2 (0.2721)
Emphysema, no. (%)	40 (50.6)	17 (47.2)	23 (53.5)	0.3 (0.5790)
Ashcroft Score				−0.4 (0.6692)
Median [Q1 to Q3]	2 [1 to 3]	2 [1 to 3]	2 [1 to 3]	
{min to max}	{0 to 6}	{0 to 6}	{0 to 6}	
Proliferative nodules (no./25 cm^2)				−1.2 (0.2348)
Median [Q1 to Q3]	2 [0 to 3.3]	1 [0 to 3]	2 [0 to 4]	
{min to max}	{0 to 11}	{0 to 7}	{0 to 11}	
Alveolar air capacity				−0.4 (0.6616)
Median [Q1 to Q3]	12.5 [7 to 20.1]	11.4 [6.8 to 21.5]	12.8 [7.9 to 17.1]	
{min to max}	{1 to 50.5}	{1.8 to 50.5}	{1 to 32.5}	

no. (%) stands for no = absolute frequency; Q1 = first quartile; Q3 = third quartile; min = the lowest value; max = the highest value; Stat. is the χ^2 statistics when the results are reported as no. (%), Fisher's exact test when n.a. (not applicable) is displayed, or Z values associated to the Mann-Whitey test otherwise; DAD = diffuse alveolar damage.

3.4. Factors Associated with Diffuse Alveolar Damage

Diffuse alveolar damage (DAD) was present in 42 patients and was more frequently observed in patients infected with beta variant (alpha vs. beta: 30 (46.2%) vs. 12 (85.7%), χ^2 statistics = 7.2, p-value = 0.0071). Patients with DAD were significantly younger than those without DAD (with vs. without 67.5 years—IQR [54.3 to 78.5] vs. 77 years [66 to 82], Mann Whitney test: p-value = 0.023). No significant association was identified between the presence of DAD and sex (women vs. men: 10 (50%) vs. 32 (54.2%), χ^2 statistics = 0.1, p-value = 0.7428), obesity (obesity vs. non-obesity: 27 (61.4%) vs. 15 (42.9%), χ^2 statistics = 2.7, p-value = 0.1015), or mechanical ventilation (with vs. without mechanical ventilation: 9 (60%) vs. 33 (51.6%), χ^2 statistics = 0.3, p-value = 0.5556). Age and variant proved significant risk factors in both uni- and multivariable regression analysis (Table 5).

Table 5. Univariable and multivariable logistic regression model and adjusted OR and associated 95% confidence interval of the presence of DAD.

Variable	Univariable		Multivariable *	
	OR [95%CI]	p-Value	OR [95%CI]	p-Value
Age, years	0.96 [0.92 to 0.99]	0.0204	0.96 [0.92 to 0.99]	0.0190
Obesity	2.12 [0.86 to 5.23]	0.1036		
Variant, alpha = reference	7.00 [1.45 to 33.80]	0.0154	7.59 [1.51 to 38.10]	0.0138

* Hosmer and Lemeshow Test χ^2 = 5.77, p-value = 0.5663; Nagelkerke R2 = 0.219; model with intercept; Model: log (DAD/(1-DAD)) = 3.085–0.046 × ge + 2.027 × Variant (Beta); Percent correct = 62%.

4. Discussion

Our study showed that the top three lung histopathological biomarkers in patients with fatal COVID-19 are alveolar edema, interstitial pneumonia, and microthrombi, with markers of bronchopneumonia and interstitial edema more frequent in older patients (≥70 years). Overall, a low grade of interstitial fibrosis was observed in our cohort, and diffuse alveolar damage (53.1%) was significantly associated with age and beta variant of the virus.

The most frequently observed comorbidities in our cohort were arterial hypertension and type 2 diabetes mellitus. Although our study found similarities in lung histopathological lesions reported in other studies, the incidence and severity of lung lesions, such as DAD, microthrombosis, and interstitial fibrosis, varied. Our study is the first to use the Ashcroft score to quantify interstitial fibrosis, and it found an overall low grade of interstitial fibrosis, which is different from other studies that did not quantify the phenomenon, especially on a microscopic level.

The percentage of free alveolar space in normal lung tissue varies based on factors such as age, smoking history, and environmental exposures, and it ranges from 70–90% depending on the specific location within the lung and the individual's age, with the rest of the space occupied by capillaries, elastic fibers, and other structures [24,25]. Our study is the first to use digital slides and image analysis software to microscopically evaluate the percentage of free alveolar space, which was found to be a median of 12.5%.

Our data showed that most patients died in 2020, while only a small percentage died in 2021. The observed shift in the distribution of COVID-19 fatalities from 2020 to 2021 could be attributed to several factors. Changes in treatment options, such as developing new drugs and therapies, may have reduced the number of deaths [26]. Furthermore, increased vaccination efforts could have contributed to decreased COVID-19 deaths [27]. Other factors, such as the patient's age, underlying comorbidities, and access to medical care, may have also influenced the distribution of deaths between the two years.

Even though most of our participants were men (Table 2), they were statistically significantly younger than women (p-value < 0.03). Jin et al. reported a higher COVID-19 mortality rate in men than in women, even though women are, on average, older than men among COVID-19 patients [28]. Yeap et al. reported that men could be more susceptible to severe COVID-19 disease due to higher levels of testosterone and a higher number of comorbidities, such as hypertension, cardiovascular disease, and diabetes [29]. Our results did not support the association between sex and comorbidities (p-value > 0.70). Another possible explanation is that women have a stronger immune response to viral infections, including SARS-CoV-2, which could help protect them from the severe form of the disease [30]. Women also have higher levels of estrogen, which has been shown to have anti-inflammatory properties that could potentially reduce the severity of COVID-19 symptoms [31]. Overall, more research is needed to fully understand the reasons for the sex differences in COVID-19 mortality and to develop effective strategies for reducing the impact of the disease on both men and women. In our study, the most observed comorbidities were arterial hypertension, diabetes mellitus type 2, and congestive heart failure. This is consistent with previous research that suggests that individuals with preexisting medical conditions and the elderly are more vulnerable to the life-threatening effects of the virus [32].

The findings in our study revealed that all the lungs showed signs of acute lung injury (Tables 3 and 4). One of the common findings in SARS-CoV-2 autopsies is an increased consistency of the lungs, present in all cases in our cohort, similarly reported by other autopsy studies [11]. The average lung weight in human autopsies can vary depending on age, sex, height, weight, and smoking history. Grandmaison et al. reported that adults' average lung weight ranges from 460–800 g per lung, with slight differences based on sex [33]. Increased pulmonary consistency is not a specific or diagnostic feature of COVID-19, as many other lung diseases and conditions can also cause changes in lung density or consistency. In addition, lung weight can vary widely even among healthy individuals, making it difficult to use this measure as a diagnostic tool for lung disease [34]. In our study, the consistency is explained by the lesions associated with ARDS, vascular stasis due to cardiac insufficiency, pulmonary fibrosis, and overlapping bronchopneumonia (Table 4), as described by other histopathological studies of the COVID-19 lung (Table 1) [15,35,36].

In COVID-19, bloody exudate in the lungs can be attributed to a pro coagulative state and microthrombosis [37], causing an inability to drain the blood flow to the heart and systemic circulation, thus leading to a bloody exudate to be found when sectioning the lungs. Ranucci et al. found that COVID-19 patients with ARDS exhibited a procoagulant pattern characterized by elevated levels of D-dimer, fibrinogen, and factor VIII, among other markers suggesting that this procoagulant state may contribute to the development of thrombotic complications in these patients [37]. In our study group, bloody exudate was found more frequently in younger patients (Table 3).

Bronchopneumonia and tracheobronchitis (Table 4) were present in less than 20% of the cases. The two findings can result from bacterial superinfection in patients with SARS-CoV-2 rather than a direct result of the virus-induced lung tissue damage. SARS-CoV-2 primarily targets the respiratory tract and causes lung lesions that predispose to secondary bacterial infections, exacerbating respiratory symptoms and leading to bronchopneumonia and purulent tracheobronchitis. Studies have shown that bacterial superinfection can occur in many patients with COVID-19, particularly those requiring hospitalization or having other underlying health conditions [38,39]. The mechanisms underlying this process are not fully understood but may involve the direct infection of lung cells and the activation of immune responses contributing to tissue damage. Overall, while bacterial superinfection can contribute to the development of bronchopneumonia and purulent tracheobronchitis in patients with SARS-CoV-2, the direct effects of the virus on lung tissue cannot be ruled out, and further research is needed to understand the mechanisms involved.

Interstitial pneumonia is a common finding in severe COVID-19 cases. It is characterized by inflammation and scarring of the tissue between the air sacs in the lungs. Our study identified the presence of interstitial pneumonia (Table 4) in 74.7% of cases, which was similar, albeit higher, to the study conducted by Huang et al., which reported an incidence of 64% [40].

Pulmonary interstitial fibrosis (PIF) is a condition characterized by the scarring of the lung tissue, which can impair lung function; the extent of interstitial fibrosis in COVID-19 patients is still poorly understood and remains an active area of research. Several studies have reported the development of PIF in patients with COVID-19, especially those with severe disease or who require mechanical ventilation [41,42]. In a cohort of 174 COVID-19 patients who underwent chest computed tomography (CT) scans, 25% had evidence of interstitial lung changes, including ground-glass opacities, consolidation, and reticulation, characteristic of PIF [43]. Another study published in European Radiology 2020 reported that PIF was present in 22.4% of COVID-19 patients who required mechanical ventilation [44].

In our research, we have found a degree of interstitial fibrosis (Table 4) in most cases and have used the Ashcroft score [21] to evaluate the extent, as well as counting the number of proliferative fibroblastic nodules present in 25 cm^2 of lung tissue. The Ashcroft score is commonly used to quantify microscopic interstitial lung fibrosis [21]. Barton et al. examined the post-mortem lung tissue of six patients who died of COVID-19 and reported diffuse alveolar damage and PIF in all cases, with varying degrees of severity [45]. Barton et al. noted that PIF suggests that COVID-19 can cause lung fibrosis, which may contribute to the long-term respiratory complications seen in some COVID-19 survivors [45]. However, the long-term extent of PIF in COVID-19 patients and its impact on lung function and overall health outcomes are still unclear, and further research is needed to understand the relationship between SARS-CoV-2 and PIF and its long-term implications.

We found that half of our patients had DAD (Table 4), lower than reported in a multi-institutional autopsy study conducted in Italy and New York City, where DAD was present in 87% of cases [46]. In our analysis, DAD was more frequently observed in patients infected with the beta variant of the virus than the alpha variant. Moreover, patients with DAD were significantly younger than those without DAD. However, it is important to note that this is a cross-sectional analysis, and the causal relationships between the viral variant, age, and DAD cannot be established based on this study design alone.

The presence of microthrombi (Table 4) was lower in our study, with only 39.2% of patients showing microthrombi compared to 84% in the aforementioned study [46]. Similar findings were reported in other studies from northern Italy, where DAD was present in all cases. Despite the same strain of the virus being present in our region, the reason for this discrepancy is not yet fully understood [14].

In our study, the free alveolar space percentage (Table 4) values were below the normal limits, emphasizing that the lesions induced by COVID-19 severely impact the amount of free alveolar space. Imagistic-based studies suggest the same observations. Fox et al. found that COVID-19 lungs had a marked reduction in the volume of the free alveolar space, which was filled with cellular debris, fibrin, and hyaline membranes [10]. Furthermore, COVID-19 patients had a significant reduction in the volume of the free alveolar space compared to healthy controls, and the degree of reduction in the free alveolar space is positively correlated with disease severity [43]. Different staining methods and image analysis algorithms may yield slightly different results. Therefore, it is essential to interpret histological data in the context of the specific method used to obtain it. Histopathological lesions can provide a more detailed understanding of the severity and extent of SARS-CoV-2 infection.

In our study group, various pathological features, including DAD, microthrombosis, emboli, infarctions, edema, bacterial infection, fibrosis, and interstitial pneumonia, indicate that they likely contribute to the reduction of free alveolar space and compromise respiratory function, leading to death. Therefore, our study implicates these pathological features as potential causes of respiratory insufficiency and subsequent mortality in COVID-19 patients.

Histopathological analysis of autopsy cases can help improve the accuracy of diagnosis, particularly in cases where other diagnostic methods are inconclusive or unavailable, helping clinicians to provide appropriate care and reduce the risk of transmission to others. Autopsy analysis can also provide insights into the long-term effects of SARS-CoV-2 infection, including potential damage to organs and tissues, information that can be used to develop long-term patient monitoring and treatment plans.

Our research stands out in the scientific community due to its unique position as one of the few autopsy-based studies on a substantial number of cases, which supports its originality and scientific value. By conducting autopsies soon after death, we obtained high-quality tissue samples, ensuring an accurate assessment of histopathological biomarkers in fatal cases of coronavirus disease. The scarcity of autopsy studies in this context adds significant value, providing crucial insights into the pathological manifestations and underlying mechanisms of lung involvement. Moreover, including a large case number strengthens the robustness and generalizability of our findings. By employing digital analysis of high-quality tissue samples, we have further enhanced the reliability and validity of our histopathological assessments, leading to more accurate and meaningful conclusions.

These factors collectively contribute to the novel histopathological insights that our research provides.

Limitations of the Study

The study's retrospective design limited the availability of clinical documentation (e.g., smoking status, alcohol consumption, weight) for patients who died outside hospitals, which may have impacted the accuracy of the data collected. Some tissue fragments could not be evaluated due to inadequate preanalytical processing, including special staining, which may have resulted in incomplete data. The specific variants of SARS-CoV-2 present in the patients included in the study could not be evaluated for each patient because it was not currently determined, which may have limited the conclusions that can be drawn regarding the virus's impact on the study population. Long-term evaluation of virus-associated histopathological changes could not be evaluated because patients in our cohort did not survive for more than two weeks after the initial COVID-19 infection.

Author Contributions: Conceptualization, I.-A.G.-R. and B.-A.G.; methodology, I.-A.G.-R., B.-A.G. and S.D.B.; software, B.-A.G. and B.P.; validation, S.D.B., T.D., E.M.J. and B.P.; formal analysis, B.-A.G. and S.D.B.; investigation, D.-C.M., V.C.S. and I.-A.G.-R.; resources, I.-A.G.-R. and B.-A.G.; data curation, I.-A.G.-R. and S.D.B.; writing—original draft preparation, I.-A.G.-R.; writing—review and editing, I.-A.G.-R., S.D.B., B.-A.G., B.P., T.D., E.M.J., D.-C.M. and V.C.S.; visualization, I.-A.G.-R.; supervision, S.D.B., T.D., E.M.J. and B.P.; project administration, I.-A.G.-R. and S.D.B. This paper is part of the author's Ph.D. thesis, coordinated by senior author S.D.B. All authors have read and agreed to the published version of the manuscript.

Funding: This research was funded by the Iuliu Hațieganu University of Medicine and Pharmacy Cluj-Napoca grant number PCD 881/43, 12.01.2022.

Institutional Review Board Statement: The study was conducted in accordance with the Declaration of Helsinki, and its protocol was approved by the Ethics Committee of the Iuliu Hațieganu University of Medicine and Pharmacy Cluj-Napoca (DEP67/14.12.2021) and of the Institute of Legal Medicine Cluj-Napoca (2406/XII/703/24.03.2022).

Informed Consent Statement: Patient consent was waived due to this being a retrospective study on autopsy cases. The patients that died in the hospital before exits had signed a formal consent on having their biological materials used for studies as part of a university hospital.

Data Availability Statement: Data are contained within the article.

Acknowledgments: The special staining was performed by histotechnicians M. Benyi and B. Uifălean of the Pathology Department of Children's Emergency Clinical Hospital, Cluj-Napoca, Romania, and histotechnician S. Bara of the Emergency Clinical County Hospital, Cluj-Napoca, Romania.

Conflicts of Interest: The authors declare no conflict of interest.

References

1. Temgoua, M.N.; Endomba, F.T.; Nkeck, J.R.; Kenfack, G.U.; Tochie, J.N.; Essouma, M. Coronavirus Disease 2019 (COVID-19) as a Multi-Systemic Disease and its Impact in Low- and Middle-Income Countries (LMICs). *SN Compr. Clin. Med.* **2020**, *2*, 1377–1387. [CrossRef] [PubMed]
2. Naming the Coronavirus Disease (COVID-19) and the Virus That Causes It. Available online: https://www.who.int/emergencies/diseases/novel-coronavirus-2019/technical-guidance/naming-the-coronavirus-disease-(covid-2019)-and-the-virus-that-causesit#:~:text=Human%20disease%20preparedness%20and%20response,virus%20on%2011%20February%202020 (accessed on 7 March 2023).
3. Solomon, M.; Liang, C. Human coronaviruses: The emergence of SARS-CoV-2 and management of COVID-19. *Virus Res.* **2022**, *319*, 198882. [CrossRef] [PubMed]
4. Beyerstedt, S.; Casaro, E.B.; Rangel, É.B. COVID-19: Angiotensin-converting enzyme 2 (ACE2) expression and tissue susceptibility to SARS-CoV-2 infection. *Eur. J. Clin. Microbiol. Infect Dis.* **2021**, *40*, 905–919. [CrossRef] [PubMed]
5. Abdelrahman, Z.; Li, M.; Wang, X. Comparative Review of SARS-CoV-2, SARS-CoV, MERS-CoV, and Influenza A Respiratory Viruses. *Front. Immunol.* **2020**, *11*, 552909. [CrossRef] [PubMed]
6. Rahman, S.; Montero, M.T.V.; Rowe, K.; Kirton, R.; Kunik, F., Jr. Epidemiology, pathogenesis, clinical presentations, diagnosis and treatment of COVID-19: A review of current evidence. *Expert. Rev. Clin. Pharmacol.* **2021**, *14*, 601–621. [CrossRef]

7. Borczuk, A.C. Pulmonary pathology of COVID-19: A review of autopsy studies. *Curr. Opin. Pulm. Med.* **2021**, *27*, 184–192. [CrossRef]
8. Baj, J.; Ciesielka, M.; Buszewicz, G.; Maciejewski, R.; Budzyńska, B.; Listos, P.; Teresiński, G. COVID-19 in the autopsy room-requirements, safety, recommendations, and pathological findings. *Forensic. Sci. Med. Pathol.* **2021**, *17*, 101–113. [CrossRef]
9. Pagani, I.; Ghezzi, S.; Alberti, S.; Poli, G.; Vicenzi, E. Origin and evolution of SARS-CoV-2. *Eur. Phys. J. Plus* **2023**, *138*, 157. [CrossRef]
10. Fox, S.E.; Akmatbekov, A.; Harbert, J.L.; Li, G.; Quincy Brown, J.; Vander Heide, R.S. Pulmonary and cardiac pathology in African American patients with COVID-19: An autopsy series from New Orleans. *Lancet Respir. Med.* **2020**, *8*, 681–686. [CrossRef]
11. Roden, A.C.; Bois, M.C.; Johnson, T.F.; Aubry, M.C.; Alexander, M.P.; Hagen, C.E.; Lin, P.T.; Quinton, R.A.; Maleszewski, J.J.; Boland, J.M. The Spectrum of Histopathologic Findings in Lungs of Patients With Fatal Coronavirus Disease 2019 (COVID-19) Infection. *Arch. Pathol. Lab. Med.* **2021**, *145*, 11–21. [CrossRef]
12. Edler, C.; Schröder, A.S.; Aepfelbacher, M.; Fitzek, A.; Heinemann, A.; Heinrich, F.; Klein, A.; Langenwalder, F.; Lütgehetmann, M.; Meißner, K.; et al. Dying with SARS-CoV-2 infection-an autopsy study of the first consecutive 80 cases in Hamburg, Germany. *Int. J. Leg. Med.* **2020**, *134*, 1275–1284. [CrossRef] [PubMed]
13. Menter, T.; Haslbauer, J.D.; Nienhold, R.; Savic, S.; Hopfer, H.; Deigendesch, N.; Frank, S.; Turek, D.; Willi, N.; Pargger, H.; et al. Postmortem examination of COVID-19 patients reveals diffuse alveolar damage with severe capillary congestion and variegated findings in lungs and other organs suggesting vascular dysfunction. *Histopathology* **2020**, *77*, 198–209. [CrossRef] [PubMed]
14. Carsana, L.; Sonzogni, A.; Nasr, A.; Rossi, R.S.; Pellegrinelli, A.; Zerbi, P.; Rech, R.; Colombo, R.; Antinori, S.; Corbellino, M.; et al. Pulmonary post-mortem findings in a series of COVID-19 cases from northern Italy: A two-centre descriptive study. *Lancet Infect Dis.* **2020**, *20*, 1135–1140. [CrossRef]
15. Lax, S.F.; Skok, K.; Zechner, P.; Kessler, H.H.; Kaufmann, N.; Koelblinger, C.; Vander, K.; Bargfrieder, U.; Trauner, M. Pulmonary Arterial Thrombosis in COVID-19 With Fatal Outcome: Results From a Prospective, Single-Center, Clinicopathologic Case Series. *Ann. Intern. Med.* **2020**, *173*, 350–361. [CrossRef]
16. Suzuki, H.; Muramatsu, H.; Hayashi, K. Causes of death of forensic autopsy cases tested positive for COVID-19 in Tokyo Metropolis. *Japan. Leg. Med.* **2023**, *62*, 102222. [CrossRef] [PubMed]
17. Viksne, V.; Strumfa, I.; Sperga, M.; Ziemelis, J.; Abolins, J. Pathological Changes in the Lungs of Patients with a Lethal COVID-19 Clinical Course. *Diagnostics* **2022**, *12*, 2808. [CrossRef]
18. Nur Urer, H.; Ersoy, G.; Yılmazbayhan, E.D. Diffuse alveolar damage of the lungs in forensic autopsies: Assessment of histopathological stages and causes of death. *Sci. World J.* **2012**, *2012*, 657316. [CrossRef]
19. Panchabhai, T.S.; Farver, C.; Highland, K.B. Lymphocytic Interstitial Pneumonia. *Clin. Chest Med.* **2016**, *37*, 463–474. [CrossRef]
20. Corrin, B.; Nicholson, A. *Pathology of the Lungs*, 3rd ed.; Churchill Livingstone Elsevier: London, UK, 2011; pp. 1–39.
21. Ashcroft, T.; Simpson, J.M.; Timbrell, V. Simple method of estimating the severity of pulmonary fibrosis on a numerical scale. *J. Clin. Pathol.* **1988**, *41*, 467–470. [CrossRef]
22. Tracking of hCoV-19 Variants. Available online: https://gisaid.org/hcov19-variants/ (accessed on 7 March 2023).
23. Bendel, R.B.; Afifi, A.A. Comparison of stopping rules in forward regression. *J. Am. Stat. Assoc.* **1977**, *72*, 46–53. [CrossRef]
24. Crapo, J.D.; Morris, A.H.; Gardner, R.M. Reference spirometric values using techniques and equipment that meet ATS recommendations. *Am. Rev. Respir. Dis.* **1981**, *123*, 659–664. [CrossRef] [PubMed]
25. Weibel, E.R. Lung morphometry: The link between structure and function. *Cell Tissue Res.* **2017**, *367*, 413–426. [CrossRef] [PubMed]
26. Niknam, Z.; Jafari, A.; Golchin, A.; Danesh Pouya, F.; Nemati, M.; Rezaei-Tavirani, M.; Rasmi, Y. Potential therapeutic options for COVID-19: An update on current evidence. *Eur. J. Med. Res.* **2022**, *27*, 6. [CrossRef] [PubMed]
27. Huang, C.; Yang, L.; Pan, J.; Xu, X.; Peng, R. Correlation between vaccine coverage and the COVID-19 pandemic throughout the world: Based on real-world data. *J. Med. Virol.* **2022**, *94*, 2181–2187. [CrossRef] [PubMed]
28. Jin, J.M.; Bai, P.; He, W.; Wu, F.; Liu, X.F.; Han, D.M.; Liu, S.; Yang, J.K. Gender Differences in Patients With COVID-19: Focus on Severity and Mortality. *Front. Public Health* **2020**, *8*, 152. [CrossRef]
29. Yeap, B.B.; Marriott, R.J.; Manning, L.; Dwivedi, G.; Hankey, G.J.; Wu, F.C.W.; Nicholson, J.K.; Murray, K. Higher premorbid serum testosterone predicts COVID-19-related mortality risk in men. *Eur. J. Endocrinol.* **2022**, *187*, 159–170. [CrossRef]
30. Viveiros, A.; Rasmuson, J.; Vu, J.; Mulvagh, S.L.; Yip, C.Y.Y.; Norris, C.M.; Oudit, G.Y. Sex differences in COVID-19: Candidate pathways, genetics of ACE2 and sex hormones. *Am. J. Physiol. Heart Circ. Physiol.* **2021**, *320*, H296–H304. [CrossRef]
31. Lemes, R.M.R.; Costa, A.J.; Bartolomeo, C.S.; Bassani, T.B.; Nishino, M.S.; Pereira, G.J.D.S.; Smaili, S.S.; Maciel, R.M.B.; Braconi, C.T.; da Cruz, E.F.; et al. 17β-estradiol reduces SARS-CoV-2 infection in vitro. *Physiol. Rep.* **2021**, *9*, e14707. [CrossRef]
32. Chen, N.; Zhou, M.; Dong, X.; Qu, J.; Gong, F.; Han, Y.; Qiu, Y.; Wang, J.; Liu, Y.; Wei, Y.; et al. Epidemiological and clinical characteristics of 99 cases of 2019 novel coronavirus pneumonia in Wuhan, China: A descriptive study. *Lancet* **2020**, *395*, 507–513. [CrossRef]
33. Grandmaison, G.L.; Clairand, I.; Durigon, M. Organ weight in 684 adult autopsies: New tables for a Caucasoid population. *Forensic. Sci. Int.* **2001**, *119*, 149–154. [CrossRef]
34. Matoba, K.; Hyodoh, H.; Murakami, M.; Saito, A.; Matoba, T.; Ishida, L.; Fujita, E.; Yamase, M.; Jin, S. Estimating normal lung weight measurement using postmortem CT in forensic cases. *Leg. Med.* **2017**, *29*, 77–81. [CrossRef] [PubMed]

35. Calabrese, F.; Pezzuto, F.; Fortarezza, F.; Hofman, P.; Kern, I.; Panizo, A.; von der Thüsen, J.; Timofeev, S.; Gorkiewicz, G.; Lunardi, F. Pulmonary pathology and COVID-19: Lessons from autopsy. The experience of European Pulmonary Pathologists. *Virchows Arch.* **2020**, *477*, 359–372. [CrossRef]
36. Valdebenito, S.; Bessis, S.; Annane, D.; Lorin de la Grandmaison, G.; Cramer-Bordé, E.; Prideaux, B.; Eugenin, E.A.; Bomsel, M. COVID-19 Lung Pathogenesis in SARS-CoV-2 Autopsy Cases. *Front. Immunol.* **2021**, *12*, 735922. [CrossRef] [PubMed]
37. Ranucci, M.; Ballotta, A.; Di Dedda, U.; Baryshnikova, E.; Dei Poli, M.; Resta, M.; Falco, M.; Albano, G.; Menicanti, L. The procoagulant pattern of patients with COVID-19 acute respiratory distress syndrome. *J. Thromb. Haemost.* **2020**, *18*, 1747–1751. [CrossRef]
38. Ebner, J.; Van den Nest, M.; Bouvier-Azula, L.; Füszl, A.; Gabler, C.; Willinger, B.; Diab-Elschahawi, M.; Presterl, E. Routine Surveillance of Healthcare-Associated Infections Misses a Significant Proportion of Invasive Aspergillosis in Patients with Severe COVID-19. *J. Fungi* **2022**, *8*, 273. [CrossRef] [PubMed]
39. Kurra, N.; Woodard, P.I.; Gandrakota, N.; Gandhi, H.; Polisetty, S.R.; Ang, S.P.; Patel, K.P.; Chitimalla, V.; Ali Baig, M.M.; Samudrala, G. Opportunistic Infections in COVID-19: A Systematic Review and Meta-Analysis. *Cureus* **2022**, *14*, e23687. [CrossRef] [PubMed]
40. Huang, C.; Wang, Y.; Li, X.; Ren, L.; Zhao, J.; Hu, Y.; Zhang, L.; Fan, G.; Xu, J.; Gu, X.; et al. Clinical features of patients infected with 2019 novel coronavirus in Wuhan, China. *Lancet* **2020**, *395*, 497–506. [CrossRef]
41. Trias-Sabrià, P.; Dorca Duch, E.; Molina-Molina, M.; Aso, S.; Díez-Ferrer, M.; Marín Muñiz, A.; Bordas-Martínez, J.; Sabater, J.; Luburich, P.; Del Rio, B.; et al. Radio-Histological Correlation of Lung Features in Severe COVID-19 Through CT-Scan and Lung Ultrasound Evaluation. *Front. Med.* **2022**, *9*, 820661. [CrossRef]
42. George, P.M.; Wells, A.U.; Jenkins, R.G. Pulmonary fibrosis and COVID-19: The potential role for antifibrotic therapy. *Lancet Respir. Med.* **2020**, *8*, 807–815. [CrossRef]
43. Francone, M.; Iafrate, F.; Masci, G.M.; Coco, S.; Cilia, F.; Manganaro, L.; Panebianco, V.; Andreoli, C.; Colaiacomo, M.C.; Zingaropoli, M.A.; et al. Chest CT score in COVID-19 patients: Correlation with disease severity and short-term prognosis. *Eur. Radiol.* **2020**, *30*, 6808–6817. [CrossRef]
44. Pan, F.; Ye, T.; Sun, P.; Gui, S.; Liang, B.; Li, L.; Zheng, D.; Wang, J.; Hesketh, R.L.; Yang, L.; et al. Time Course of Lung Changes at Chest CT during Recovery from Coronavirus Disease 2019 (COVID-19). *Radiology* **2020**, *295*, 715–721. [CrossRef] [PubMed]
45. Barton, L.M.; Duval, E.J.; Stroberg, E.; Ghosh, S.; Mukhopadhyay, S. COVID-19 Autopsies, Oklahoma, USA. *Am. J. Clin. Pathol.* **2020**, *153*, 725–733. [CrossRef] [PubMed]
46. Borczuk, A.C.; Salvatore, S.P.; Seshan, S.V.; Patel, S.S.; Bussel, J.B.; Mostyka, M.; Elsoukkary, S.; He, B.; Del Vecchio, C.; Fortarezza, F.; et al. COVID-19 pulmonary pathology: A multi-institutional autopsy cohort from Italy and New York City. *Mod. Pathol.* **2020**, *33*, 2156–2168. [CrossRef] [PubMed]

Disclaimer/Publisher's Note: The statements, opinions and data contained in all publications are solely those of the individual author(s) and contributor(s) and not of MDPI and/or the editor(s). MDPI and/or the editor(s) disclaim responsibility for any injury to people or property resulting from any ideas, methods, instructions or products referred to in the content.

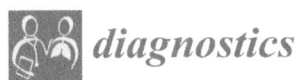

Review

Salivary Biomarkers of Anti-Epileptic Drugs: A Narrative Review

Ioana-Andreea Chiș [1], Vlad Andrei [1], Alexandrina Muntean [2,*], Marioara Moldovan [3], Anca Ștefania Mesaroș [4], Mircea Cristian Dudescu [5] and Aranka Ilea [1]

1. Department of Oral Rehabilitation, Faculty of Dentistry, University of Medicine and Pharmacy "Iuliu Hațieganu", 400012 Cluj-Napoca, Romania; chis.ioana.andreea@elearn.umfcluj.ro (I.-A.C.); vlad.andrei@elearn.umfcluj.ro (V.A.); aranka.ilea@umfcluj.ro (A.I.)
2. Department of Paediatric Dentistry, Faculty of Dentistry, University of Medicine and Pharmacy "Iuliu Hațieganu", 400012 Cluj-Napoca, Romania
3. Department of Polymer Composites, Institute of Chemistry "Raluca Ripan", University Babes-Bolyai, 400294 Cluj-Napoca, Romania; mmarioara2004@yahoo.com
4. Department of Dental Propaedutics and Aesthetics, University of Medicine and Pharmacy "Iuliu Hațieganu", 400012 Cluj-Napoca, Romania; mesaros.anca@umfcluj.ro
5. Department of Mechanical Engineering, Faculty of Automotive, Mechatronics and Mechanical Engineering, Technical University of Cluj-Napoca, 400641 Cluj-Napoca, Romania; mircea.dudescu@rezi.utcluj.ro
* Correspondence: alexandrina.muntean@umfcluj.ro

Abstract: Saliva is a biofluid that reflects general health and that can be collected in order to evaluate and determine various pathologies and treatments. Biomarker analysis through saliva sampling is an emerging method of accurately screening and diagnosing diseases. Anti-epileptic drugs (AEDs) are prescribed generally in seizure treatment. The dose–response relationship of AEDs is influenced by numerous factors and varies from patient to patient, hence the need for the careful supervision of drug intake. The therapeutic drug monitoring (TDM) of AEDs was traditionally performed through repeated blood withdrawals. Saliva sampling in order to determine and monitor AEDs is a novel, fast, low-cost and non-invasive approach. This narrative review focuses on the characteristics of various AEDs and the possibility of determining active plasma concentrations from saliva samples. Additionally, this study aims to highlight the significant correlations between AED blood, urine and oral fluid levels and the applicability of saliva TDM for AEDs. The study also focuses on emphasizing the applicability of saliva sampling for epileptic patients.

Keywords: saliva; biomarkers; anti-epileptic drugs; therapeutic drug monitoring; seizure; epilepsy

1. Introduction

A biomarker can be defined as a "characteristic that is measured and evaluated as an indicator of normal biological processes, pathogenic processes, or responses to an exposure or intervention, including therapeutic interventions" [1,2]. Biomarkers are objective indicators that serve a variety of purposes, from screening and diagnosing conditions to monitoring the effects of treatments or even the progression and prognosis of a disease [1,3].

Most of these biomarkers are assessed through various types of human biological sampling, such as serum, plasma, urine, sputum, etc., depending on the types of investigations required [4]. Blood sampling is usually invasive and anxiety-inducing for patients, with a need for a more restrictive clinical setting. Moreover, there is a limited number of samples that can be collected, and associated difficulties in obtaining those samples from the pediatric and geriatric populations. For that reason, there is a lot of ongoing research regarding the use of other biological matrices for medical investigation purposes, especially for those patients whose clinical status is difficult to assess [1,4].

Saliva biomarker analysis is an emerging field that is attracting an increased interest, being noninvasive and requiring no medical personnel to perform it. Moreover, the fact that it can be performed repeatedly represents the basis of an effective approach in large-scale

Citation: Chiș, I.-A.; Andrei, V.; Muntean, A.; Moldovan, M.; Mesaroș, A.Ș.; Dudescu, M.C.; Ilea, A. Salivary Biomarkers of Anti-Epileptic Drugs: A Narrative Review. Diagnostics 2023, 13, 1962. https://doi.org/10.3390/diagnostics13111962

Academic Editor: Sang Kun Lee

Received: 25 April 2023
Revised: 30 May 2023
Accepted: 2 June 2023
Published: 4 June 2023

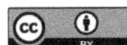

Copyright: © 2023 by the authors. Licensee MDPI, Basel, Switzerland. This article is an open access article distributed under the terms and conditions of the Creative Commons Attribution (CC BY) license (https://creativecommons.org/licenses/by/4.0/).

screening [1]. The hundreds of substances in saliva composition help to detect diseases, provide evidence of exposure to harmful substances and assess overall health status [5].

Saliva composition is influenced by factors such as age, gender, diet, drug intake, level of hygiene, type of stimulus and even the circadian rhythm [5–7]. The production of oral fluid can also be quantitatively and qualitatively modified by numerous physiological and pathological conditions [8]. As a result, saliva samples are variable and unstable, with a composition that varies greatly both intra- and inter-individually [5]. Moreover, all its complex biochemical and physical chemical properties make research into saliva more difficult [5].

Saliva primarily consists of water (99.5%), along with proteins (0.3%) and inorganic and trace substances (0.2%) [5,7,8]. Glycoproteins, enzymes (e.g., α-amylase), immunoglobulins and antimicrobial peptides are some of the protein constituents, whilst the inorganic component consists of electrolytes (e.g., sodium, potassium, chloride, bicarbonate) [5,9,10].

The drug's pH, the degree of protein binding, and its molecular weight, spatial configuration and lipid solubility are among the numerous factors that can influence the passage of drugs from blood to saliva [1,8]. Saliva pH values oscillate between 6 and 7, with more alkaline values exhibited when the secretion is increased [5,7]. The blood and oral fluid's pH influence the passage of drugs from blood to saliva. A more acidic pH of a drug leads to an enhanced drug diffusion. Therefore, acidic drugs are generally present in lower concentrations in oral fluid than blood, whilst alkaline drugs are present at higher concentrations [1,11,12]. On top of that, the substance's acid dissociation constant (the pK_a) is a very important factor that determines the potential utility of saliva therapeutic drug monitoring (TDM) for many drugs [1,8]. The pK_a is a parameter that characterizes a chemical compound's ionization equilibria in relation to the compound's acid–base properties [13]. All the above-mentioned factors influence the passage and, consecutively, the rapport of the blood: saliva drug concentrations.

The objectives of this narrative review are to assess the numerous characteristics of various AEDs and the methods of determining their plasma/serum levels from saliva samples. Additionally, this study aims to highlight the significant correlations between AED blood, urine and oral fluid levels and the applicability of saliva TDM for AEDs. The selected studies focus on AED and TDM from plasma/serum and saliva samples from epileptic patients, from healthy subjects and from in vitro artificially enhanced biofluids. The study also focuses on emphasizing the applicability, the ease and the importance of saliva sampling for epileptic patients.

2. Materials and Methods

A thorough electronic literature search was conducted in MEDLINE through PubMed, Web of Science, the Cochrane Library and Google Scholar. The terms used in this process were: anti-epileptic drugs OR anti-epileptics OR acetazolamide OR benzodiazepines OR adinazolam OR alprazolam OR bromazepam OR climazolam OR clobazam OR clonazepam OR clorazepate OR diazepam OR estazolam OR flumazenil OR flunitrazepam OR flurazepam OR halazepam OR loprazolam OR lorazepam OR lormetazepam OR midazolam OR nimetazepam OR nitrazepam OR oxazepam OR prazepam OR temazepam OR triazolam OR brivaracetam OR carbamazepine OR eslicarbazepine acetate OR ethosuximide OR felbamate OR gabapentin OR lacosamide OR lamotrigine OR levetiracetam OR oxcarbazepine OR perampanel OR phenobarbital OR phenytoin OR pregabalin OR primidone OR rufinamide OR topiramate OR valproic acid AND saliva OR oral fluid OR salivary biomarker.

The inclusion criteria were as follows: any study that described the determination of any of the aforementioned AEDs through sampled or enhanced oral fluid. Commentaries, opinion articles, editorials and conference abstracts were excluded.

After removing duplicates, the titles and abstracts of the articles were read and then, if the studies fit the criteria, the full text was examined and a decision was made regarding study inclusion in this review.

3. Anti-Epileptic Drugs

Anti-epileptic drugs (AEDs) are structurally and functionally diverse drugs prescribed in a number of conditions such as epilepsy, neuropathic pain, mania, anxiety or spasticity. AEDs have clinically relevant differences, leaving the choice of the prescribed drug to be purely empirical [14].

TDM has the optimization of a patient's clinical outcome as an objective, identifying the initial response to a medication and the need for any adjustments [15,16]. TDM supports the management of patients' medication regimens with the aid of measured drug concentrations [15].

Predicting an optimum dose of an AED for a particular patient is an impossible task. Although there are well-defined reference ranges established for most AEDs, the individual differences and the severity of epilepsy make it impossible to accurately pinpoint an optimal dosage [15,16]. In some patients, dosages below the target range can manage seizures well, whilst other patients can require and tolerate drug concentrations in excess of the range [17]. Moreover, seizures occur at irregular intervals, with the clinical symptoms of epilepsy and the signs of toxicity not always being detectable. Since anticonvulsivant therapy is long term, determining if and what AEDs are causing more harm than good is essential. All these aspects, plus the fact that there are no direct laboratory markers for clinical efficacy or for drug toxicity, make it difficult to ascertain if a prescribed dose will be sufficient to control seizures in the long term. Since the correlation between AED serum concentrations and the clinical effects is superior to the correlation between dose and effect, measuring drug concentrations is often the most effective way to guide treatment [15,16].

For most AEDs, saliva reflects the free (pharmacologically active) serum concentrations [15]. Only the fraction of the drug that is unbound from serum proteins is available to diffuse from the vascular system and accumulate in tissues, and to be available for interaction with therapeutic targets. Therefore, the extent of serum binding can have significant effects on the pharmacodynamic properties of a compound, as well. It is, however, important to wait for the drug to reach an equilibrium between the saliva and the blood levels. This equilibrium varies from one person to another and from one drug to another [15,16]. Aman et al. suggest performing regular salivary TDM correlated with neurological assessments, in order to avoid toxic drug concentrations [18].

There are, however, factors that influence the interpretation of the saliva sample, such as the patient's use of concomitant drugs, how the sample was collected, stored and/or analyzed, and the timing of the sample collection in relation to the last orally administered dose [1,16].

Anti-epileptic medication should ideally be introduced slowly, with doses gradually increasing depending on symptoms. The AED should be titrated upwards to the maximum tolerated dose only if seizures still continue to occur. Any type of change in therapy should be made one at a time, gradually, in order to avoid toxicity. Saliva TDM can help with any dose increase in order to predict/avoid toxicity, as side effects are often insidious and might go unrecognized. If the patient has no benefit from a maximum tolerated dose of a drug, the treatment should be switched to an alternative first-line drug [19]. When switching medications (even though the drugs are considered bio-equivalent to the branded product), there may be differences in the drug's bioavailability and, therefore, in the clinical status of the patient, causing potential breakthrough seizures. The determination of AED concentrations is a good practice before and after switching a patient's medication, in order to ascertain both drugs' bioavailability [17].

In clinical practice, about 30% of patients are pharmacoresistant, which can cause high rates of disability, morbidity or mortality [20,21]. During epileptic seizures, using saliva monitoring, drug oscillations can be assessed and concentrations can be correlated with therapeutic profiles, thus avoiding toxicity [20].

In children, dose requirements are less predictable than for adults, being constantly subjected to change—in these cases, TDM is a must for patient management. Since plasma sampling may present difficulties in children, saliva TDM can be particularly helpful. In pregnant women, due to all the metabolic changes, the pharmacokinetics of many AEDs are altered, causing plasma concentrations to more or less significantly decline. Saliva samples reflect the non-protein-bound quantity of AED in plasma, therefore making frequent TDM in pregnant women easier. In the elderly, the plasma concentration is affected by greater pharmacodynamic sensitivity, thus complicating the interpretation of TDM results. Moreover, drug polytherapy is significantly increased in the elderly compared to other age groups, and drug interactions are more likely to occur. Therefore, saliva monitoring fulfills the need for a rapid method for TDM [17].

When it comes to patients with co-morbidities and co-pathologies, possible drug–drug interactions can result in either an increase or a decrease in plasma AED concentrations. Moreover, the absorption, distribution, elimination and protein binding of AEDs can be seriously affected, resulting in either signs of toxicity or with patient experiencing breakthrough seizures. Therefore, the rapid and correct measurement of AED concentrations is essential [22]. In patients with hepatic disease, the elimination of AEDs can be significantly altered, and therefore the prediction of the extent of change in AED clearance can be impossible. Consequently, in these situations, TDM is essential and considered the best practice [17].

4. Salivary Levels of Individual AEDs

4.1. Acetazolamide

Acetazolamide has a pK_a of 7.2, with approximately half of its molecules being charged in blood and oral fluid at a physiological pH. It has a plasma protein binding of 95%, which predicts a poor penetration into oral fluid [16].

Acetazolamide is a drug with no clinically important drug–drug interactions, with a predictable dose-concentration relationship that does not recommend routine TDM [16].

However, two studies by Wallace et al. and Hartley et al. reported saliva as an appropriate source for acetazolamide TDM. The studies were, however, performed on healthy volunteers and the samples were collected within the first hour of administration, which might influence the oral fluid concentrations. A correlation coefficient of $r^2 = 0.99$ and recoveries of more than 87.7% up until 100% were reported [23,24].

4.2. Benzodiazepines

Benzodiazepines act as neural inhibitors, resulting in a slowing of neurotransmission. Commonly used to prevent seizures and to treat anxiety and sleep disorders, their main effects include sedation, hypnosis, tranquilization, decreased anxiety, centrally mediated muscle relaxation and anti-convulsant activity. Among the common side effects, the significant impairment of mental alertness and cognitive performance, as well as amnestic effects, are probably the most notable [25–27].

Some of the most well-known and frequently prescribed benzodiazepines are adinazolam, alprazolam, bromazepam, climazolam, clobazam, clonazepam, clorazepate, diazepam, estazolam, flumazenil, flunitrazepam, flurazepam, halazepam, loprazolam, lorazepam, lormetazepam, midazolam, nimetazepam, nitrazepam, oxazepam, prazepam, temazepam and triazolam [25,26].

Benzodiazepines bind to plasma proteins, having low pK_a values. For that reason, they are generally found in low concentrations in saliva samples, showing a shorter detection time than in blood [28]. Benzodiazepines are known to bind the protein albumin, but mainly on α-glycoprotein. Therefore, due to their consequent low concentration in biofluids, high sensitivity is required for the determination of benzodiazepines in biological samples [27].

Clobazam is prescribed for the treatment of various epilepsies (in generalized seizures, for the adjunctive intermittent treatment of partial seizures and for the management of the non-convulsive status epilepticus) and febrile and alcohol withdrawal seizures [17]. Clobazam and its pharmacologically active metabolite, N-desmethyl clobazam, have a plasma protein binding of 85–90%. The metabolite is present in blood at much higher concentrations than the parent drug [16,17]. One study by Bakke et al. used cut-off limits primarily selected based on the sensitivities of the used analytical methods [29]. There have been reports of clobazam's excessive accumulation correlated with toxicity in patients. Nevertheless, clobazam and N-desmethyl clobazam can be monitored in saliva samples—moreover, the salivary concentrations are highly correlated with serum concentrations ($r^2 = 0.93$ and $r^2 = 0.90$) [15–17,30,31].

Clonazepam is used for the treatment of various seizure types, in Lennox–Gastaut syndrome and in the management of status epilepticus. It is as yet unknown whether clonazepam is secreted into saliva [16]. The elimination of clonazepam is associated with individual differences and variability in the dose-to-plasma concentration relationship [17]. Hart et al. analyzed saliva samples spiked with clonazepam—the samples that were stored overnight at room temperature had drug concentrations 76% lower compared to samples that were analyzed immediately. These findings suggest the fact that clonazepam is unstable in saliva [32]. Moore et al. reported a correlation coefficient of $r^2 = 0.9991$ for clonazepam, after oral fluid was fortified with several benzodiazepines at the concentration of 10 ng/mL [33]. Bakke et al. reported that clonazepam is part of the benzodiazepines he found to be less detected in oral fluid compared to blood [29]. Desharnais et al., in a recent study published in 2020, used a Quantisal® device to collect saliva samples and, using incubation with a precipitation solvent, determined 7-aminoclonazepam in oral fluid samples, but without quantifying its concentration. The authors stated a recovery < 80% for 55 out of the 97 analyzed compounds [34]. Using HPLC, Uddin et al. reported a correlation coefficient of $r^2 = 0.999$ for clonazepam in saliva samples [27]. Using an LC-MS/MS method, Concheiro et al. also reported a correlation coefficient of above 0.99 for several tested drugs (including benzodiazepines and, consequently, clonazepam) [35]. Øiestad et al., using the same method, reported a correlation coefficient of $r^2 = 0.993$ for clonazepam [36]. Using long-column fast gas chromatography/electron impact mass spectrometry (GC/EI-MS), Gunnar et al. quantitated 30 different drugs of abuse from 250 µL of oral fluid, thus determining clonazepam with a 72.8% recovery and with a 0.992 correlation coefficient [37].

Diazepam, while being licensed as a skeletal muscle relaxant, an anxiolytic and a sedative and analgesic, is targeted for the management of febrile convulsions and of status epilepticus. Diazepam is metabolized in the liver to its pharmacologically active metabolite, N-desmethyldiazepam (nordiazepam), with both further metabolized to temazepam and, respectively, oxazepam. N-desmethyldiazepam accumulates in plasma to higher concentrations than diazepam, being responsible for most of the clinical effect. Many patients tend to develop tolerance to the anti-seizure effects of diazepam. Therefore, there are differences between patients when it comes to the dose-to-plasma concentration relationship, as well as the plasma concentration to clinical effect relationship. Both diazepam and N-desmethyldiazepam distribute into saliva, the concentrations reflecting their non-protein bound plasma concentration [17]. Hallstrom et al., in a study published in 1980, reported a correlation coefficient of $r^2 = 0.89$ between salivary and plasma diazepam and $r^2 = 0.81$ between salivary and plasma nordiazepam [38]. Moore et al. reported a correlation coefficient of $r^2 = 0.9996$ for diazepam in oral fluid samples [33]. Gunnar et al. reported a correlation coefficient of $r^2 = 1.000$ for diazepam, with a 63.3% recovery [37]. Bakke et al. reported that diazepam was more often detected in blood samples than in oral fluid [29]. Vindenes et al. stated that benzodiazepines were most commonly detected in urine rather than oral fluid, but, however, N-desmethyldiazepam was substantially more detected in oral fluid samples, with a sensitivity of 95%. This study mentioned cut-off values for all of the screened and confirmed 32 most commonly abused drugs [22]. Gjerde et al. reported correlation coefficients of $r^2 = 0.61$ for diazepam and $r^2 = 0.95$ for nordiazepam, with low oral fluid/blood ratios of 0.036 for diazepam, and, respectively, 0.027 for nordiazepam. This study also mentioned cut-off concentrations for all the 17 tested drugs [39]. Christodoulides et al., using a chip-based Programmable Bio-Nano-Chip platform and LC-MS/MS, detected diazepam from oral fluid samples in approximately 10 min [40].

Midazolam is a short-acting benzodiazepine prescribed as a hypnotic, anesthetic or for the treatment of status epilepticus or generalized seizures. Link et al. reported in their study a liquid chromatography/electrospray ionization tandem mass spectrometry method that was successfully applied to midazolam and its metabolites (1-hydroxymidazolam and 4-hydroxymidazolam). In both oral fluid and plasma, the method showed a good sensitivity in determining midazolam and its metabolites [41]. In another ulteriorly published study, Link et al. noted that the concentrations of midazolam and its metabolites were much lower in saliva than in plasma, although there was a significant linear correlation between midazolam levels in both matrices. The authors also concluded that oral fluid sampling is a good way of determining midazolam and its hydroxy-metabolites, although, because of their low concentrations, sensitive methods are to be used [42]. Using a triple quadrupole LC-MS-MS system, Moore et al. reported a mean recovery of 81.48% of midazolam from oral fluid samples [32]. Using long-column fast gas chromatography/electron impact mass spectrometry (GC/EI-MS), Gunnar et al. determined midazolam with a 73.1% recovery and with an $r^2 = 0.997$ correlation coefficient by using CG/EI-MS [37]. Donzelli et al. simultaneously determined six probe drugs through phenotyping CYP isoforms (human cytochrome P450 enzymes) [43]. These isoforms are involved in the metabolism of many xenobiotics and are responsible for the oxidative metabolism of approximately 50–90% of commonly used drugs [43,44]. The authors have concluded that for midazolam, when a higher dose of 7.5 mg is administered, saliva has a usefulness for non-invasive phenotyping of CYP3A4. Moreover, due to its short plasma half-life, midazolam cannot be reliably determined at timepoints later than 4 h [43].

Benzodiazepines are detectable in oral fluid, but, for the most part, at lower concentrations in urine [45,46]. Moore et al. used the Quantisal® collection device, quantified using solid-phase extraction for analyzing benzodiazepines in oral fluid, and detected them with the use of liquid chromatography with tandem mass spectrometric detection. The authors simultaneously quantified a total of 14 benzodiazepines, with a percentage recovery from 81.4% (the lowest) to 90.17% (the highest), reporting intraday precision assays of 2.8–7.29% [32]. Desharnais et al. also used the Quantisal® collection device. Samples were prepared with an organic precipitation solvent in order to boost drug recovery and the stability of benzodiazepines, and then analyzed with LC-MS/MS [34]. Valen et al. used Intercept® oral fluid sampling kits, but admitted that better recoveries and fewer matrix effects were observed for some substances when Quantisal® kits were used. The authors reported extraction recoveries between 58% and 76% for most tested drugs and recoveries between 23% and 33% for three 7-amino benzodiazepines metabolites [47]. Uddin et al. developed an HPLC method with diode array detection (DAD), in order to determine six benzodiazepines and two metabolites in plasma, urine and saliva samples. The mean recoveries reported for plasma, urine and saliva were 96.0–108.2%, 94.3–107.1% and 97.0–107.0% in within-day assays [27]. Bakke et al. reported, using ultra high-performance liquid chromatography-tandem mass spectrometry (UHPLC-MS-MS) on blood and oral fluid samples, that oxazepam was detected more frequently in oral fluid compared to blood (100% versus 34%). Alprazolam and nitrazepam were detected more frequently in blood compared to oral fluid (100% compared to 69.1% and, respectively, 93.5% compared to 51.6%) [28]. Pil and Verstraete reported that during the "Rosita 2" study, where 10 devices for roadside drug testing for oral fluid were evaluated and over 2000 tests were performed on over 2000 people, sensitivity for benzodiazepines varied between 33% and 69%. For benzodiazepines, in oral fluid samples, the mean sensitivity, specificity and accuracy were reportedly 74.4%, 84.2% and 79.2%, while for whole blood samples these mean percentages were 66.7%, 87.0% and, respectively, 74.4% [48]. Inscore et al., in their published study, developed a new patented method that allowed the detection of five different drugs at 1 ppm in oral fluid in less than 10 min. The method used surface-enhanced Raman spectroscopy (SERS), using gold- and silver-doped sol-gels immobilized in the glass capillaries. The electronegative gold and the electropositive silver's purpose was to attract differently charged chemical groups [49].

4.3. Brivaracetam

Brivaracetam is a novel member of the racetam family of anticonvulsants, prescribed as an adjunctive therapy in partial-onset seizures of epileptic patients [17,50]. It has a wide interindividual variability in the rate of elimination, having a weak plasma protein binding of 35% [17,51]. Brivaracetam plasma concentrations decrease when carbamazepine, phenobarbital, rifampin or phenytoin are administered. Therefore, monitoring plasma concentrations is indicated for evaluating a possible toxicity and for ascertaining possible clinical interactions [17]. Brivaracetam is a small, non-ionizable molecule, with a diffusing capacity from plasma to saliva. It distributes into saliva, the concentrations reflecting the non-protein bound concentration in plasma [17,50].

Rolan et al. reported that oral fluid is a suitable analytic matrix for brivaracetam, with the saliva concentrations being highly correlated to plasma concentrations ($r^2 = 0.97$), with a slope (standard error) similar to the protein-unbound fraction of brivaracetam [50].

4.4. Carbamazepine

Carbamazepine is a first-line drug in the treatment of partial and primary or secondarily generalized seizures. It is also prescribed for treating trigeminal neuralgia and bipolar disorder. Its pharmacologically active metabolite is carbamazepine-epoxide, which accumulates in plasma [17].

Carbamazepine metabolism can be affected by numerous AEDs to increase its blood concentration (clobazam, stiripentol) or decrease it (felbamate, oxcarbazepine, phenobarbital, phenytoin, primidone, rufinamide) [17,52]. Simultaneously taking carbamazepine and lamotrigine may increase the prospect of neurotoxic side effects [53]. Carbamazepine metabolism can also be affected by many non-epilepsy drugs to increase its blood concentration (such as clarithromycin, ciprofloxacin, erythromycin, fluconazole, metronidazole, miconazole, etc.) or decrease it (such as rifampicin, risperidone, etc.). Other drugs can increase carbamazepine–epoxide concentrations and may cause toxicity, such as brivaracetam, valproic acid, zonisamide, etc. [17,52].

Although it is stated that saliva stimulation before probing can affect the drug's pH and, therefore, its determined concentration, for carbamazepine it seems that salivary stimulation, the pH of saliva or the volume of fluid produced have no influence on its determined concentration. Stimulating salivation, besides enabling sampling in dehydrated or comatose patients, does not alter carbamazepine concentrations in saliva [36,37,54–57]. Carbamazepine and carbamazepine–epoxide are 70–75% and, respectively, 50–60% bound to plasma proteins [16,17,51,58]. Therefore, the salivary concentration of both substances is similar to the free concentration of the pharmacologically active, non-protein bound concentration in plasma [15,17]. Usually, carbamazepine-10,11-epoxide is at a steady state of 15–20% of the total carbamazepine concentration for most patients [59]. Considering patient inter-individuality and many drug-to-drug interactions, the TDM of carbamazepine and its metabolite is essential in order to ensure an optimal therapeutic response and to avoid toxicity [17]. Its narrow effective range requires constant monitoring, with repeated blood draws from patients. Therefore, saliva TDM is proposed to non-invasively assess and monitor carbamazepine concentrations [60]. Vasudev et al. reported that the measurement of the unbound concentration of carbamazepine from saliva should induce a better correlation with seizure control [58].

Patrick et al., in their review article, concurred that carbamazepine and carbamazepine–epoxide concentrations in saliva correlate with concentrations in total serum ($r^2 = 0.84$–0.99 and, respectively, $r^2 = 0.76$–0.88) [16]. Dordević et al. used HPLC with UV detection in order to determine carbamazepine from both serum and saliva samples. The authors noted a strong correlation between the two matrices ($r^2 = 0.9481$) [53]. Vasudev et al. studied saliva and blood samples that were centrifuged and analyzed using HPLC. The authors expressed a good linear relationship between the samples from the two matrices, with a correlation coefficient of $r^2 = 0.659$ [58]. Al Za'abi et al. simultaneously quantified carbamazepine in saliva and serum samples using a fluorescence polarization immunoassay with a TDx analyzer. The authors reported a good linear relationship ($r^2 = 0.99$) between the saliva and serum samples, with a 1.02 ± 0.11 mean ratio of carbamazepine salivary to serum-free concentration [61]. Djordjević et al., also using HPLC-UV, analyzed carbamazepine saliva and serum levels in healthy and in acutely poisoned patients. The authors reported lower carbamazepine concentrations in saliva with regard to serum levels when samples from the two matrices were collected at the same time. In patients with acute poisonings, consequent to different ingested doses of carbamazepine, the authors noted high inter-individual variations, with a strong correlation between saliva and serum levels ($r^2 = 0.9117$). In poisonings, due to a saturation of finding proteins and an increase in free serum carbamazepine levels, they also reported an average higher ratio of saliva and serum (0.43) than in the long-term use of therapeutic doses (0.39) [55]. Carona et al., using a novel HPLC technique with DAD, reported a plasma and saliva correlation of $r^2 = 0.8299$ for carbamazepine and of $r^2 = 0.9291$ for carbamazepine-10,11-epoxide [20]. Dziurkowska and Wesolowski, using UHPLC with a DAD, successfully detected carbamazepine and carbamazepine-10,11-epoxide from saliva samples. The method used was reported to have good linearity, reflected by $r^2 > 0.99$ for all the analyzed substances [62]. Carvalho et al. also reported using LC coupled to a diode detector in order to determine carbamazepine and other AEDs from oral fluid, although they determined the drugs from dried saliva spots. A mean recovery for carbamazepine was reported between 40.8 and 45.5%. The authors adapted cards that are commonly applied in dried blood spots sampling to oral fluid sampling and reported a linearity between 0.1 and 10 µg/mL for all AEDs [59]. Dwivedi et al. noted the statistically significant association of carbamazepine levels in serum and saliva, also reporting a positive correlation between the carbamazepine daily dose and the plasma levels [63]. Dziurkowska and Wesolowski tested deproteinization with 1% formic acid solution in acetonitrile, in order to determine carbamazepine and its metabolite from oral fluid. The authors reported a good linearity in the concentration range of 10–5000 ng/mL ($r^2 > 0.999$) and an extraction recovery of over 95% [64]. Chen et al. proposed using SERS as a faster method, which was non-contact, label-free and economic, and does not require professionals in order to determine on-site carbamazepine in oral fluid. The method was based on Au-Ag core–shell nanomaterial substrates that greatly improved the signal of the target molecule and, consequently, increased the detection sensitivity [60]. Capule et al. studied the connection between carbamazepine treatment and Stevens-Johnson syndrome/toxic epidermal necrolysis (SJS/TEN). The authors extracted and analyzed genomic DNA from saliva samples, using a UV–visible spectrophotometer and then genotyping HLA-A alleles by polymerase chain reaction. Despite their small sample size, a significant correlation between HLA-B75 and HLA-B*15:02 alleles and carbamazepine-induced SJS/TEN was reported [65]. Therefore, based on all the aforementioned studies, saliva is a good matrix for carbamazepine TDM.

4.5. Eslicarbazepine Acetate

Eslicarbazepine acetate is a licensed AED used in the adjunctive treatment of partial onset seizures. Its non-licensed uses include the treatment of bipolar disorder, cranial or trigeminal neuralgia, headache and neuropathic pain [17].

Carbamazepine, phenytoin and topiramate enhance eslicarbazepine acetate's elimination and, therefore, decrease its plasma concentrations [17,52]. Eslicarbazepine has linear pharmacokinetics, with protein binding of 30% [16]. Its pharmacologically active metabolite is eslicarbazepine, similar to oxcarbazepine's active metabolite, 10-hydroxycarbazepine, which is secreted into saliva, having a good correlation with plasma levels [15,17]. There were no studies found that quantify eslicarbazepine acetate from saliva samples. Patrick et al. stated in their 2013 review paper that, since eslicarbazepine is the same molecule as 10-hydroxycarbazepine, it can be expected that its saliva transfer will be similar [16].

4.6. Ethosuximide

Ethosuximide is an AED that is prescribed in the monotherapy of absence seizures [17]. It is not protein-bound, and therefore it is distributed into saliva at similar concentrations in plasma, with correlations between the ethosuximide levels of the two matrices ($r^2 = 0.99$). Therefore, for this drug, saliva TDM can be performed [16,17].

4.7. Felbamate

Felbamate is an AED that is prescribed to patients with Lennox–Gastaut syndrome and to those who do not respond well to alternative treatments. Due to the formation of a reactive atropaldehyde metabolite which can cause toxicity in some individuals, felbamate has been correlated with an increased risk of aplastic anemia and hepatotoxicity, which lead to the restriction of its use [16,17]. Carbamazepine and phenytoin enhance felbamate's elimination, decreasing its plasma concentrations. Valproic acid inhibits felbamate's metabolism and gabapentin inhibits felbamate's renal elimination, thus both increasing felbamate's plasma concentration. Felbamate is 48% bound to plasma proteins [17]. To date, saliva TDM for felbamate is still unstudied [16,17].

4.8. Gabapentin

Gabapentin is prescribed in the monotherapy treatment of partial seizures and peripheral neuropathic pain, and as an adjunctive treatment in the epilepsy of adults and children over 6 years of age [16,17]. Gabapentin is not protein bound and not metabolized, its clearance being entirely performed by renal excretion [16,17,66]. Gabapentin is reported to not interact pharmacokinetically with other AED, nor to alter their serum levels [66]. Since gabapentin is not protein bound, salivary levels are assumed to be similar to those in serum [16,66]. Studies have shown that gabapentin is secreted into saliva at lower concentrations than it is found in plasma, but nonetheless with a significant correlation between its levels in the two matrices [16,17,66]. Pujadas et al. successfully determined gabapentin levels in oral fluid using GC-MS and a solid-phase extraction procedure. However, the reported recovery values were 8.2%, 8.8% and 19.7% [54]. Berry et al., using reversed phase HPLC, reported that 5–10% of serum gabapentin concentrations were found in saliva samples, possibly relating that fact to its hydrophilic character. The authors noted that, while there is a linear relationship between gabapentin salivary levels and dosage increments, the saliva TDM of gabapentin is more a means to confirm that the patient has taken the drug rather than for quantifying it for therapeutic monitoring [66].

4.9. Lacosamide

Lacosamide is prescribed in the mono- and adjunctive therapy of partial onset seizures in epilepsy [16,17]. Enzyme-inducing AEDs such as carbamazepine, phenytoin and phenobarbital can decrease plasma lacosamide concentrations by enhancing its elimination [17].

Lacosamide's binding to plasma protein is 14%, with its saliva concentrations reflecting the non-protein bound plasma concentrations [17]. While Carona et al. used the HPLC method to determine AEDs in saliva, they reported a mean recovery of lacosamide of 86.6% ± 7.33 of saliva samples [20]. Greenaway et al. reported, in their study, a correlation coefficient of lacosamide levels between serum free concentrations and saliva concentrations of $r^2 = 0.828$, while Brandt et al. reported a coefficient interval of $r^2 = 0.842$ [67,68]. Cawello et al. reported a ≤10% difference for saliva and total plasma lacosamide concentration ratio [69]. Patrick et al., in their review article, reported a mean saliva/serum lacosamide concentration coefficient interval of $r^2 = 0.84$–0.98, all these findings proving that saliva is a suitable source for investigating lacosamide pharmacokinetics [16].

4.10. Lamotrigine

Lamotrigine is prescribed for the monotherapy treatment of partial and generalized tonic–clonic seizures and also as an adjunctive treatment in seizures and Lennox–Gastaut syndrome. It has other uses in bipolar depression, migraines, neuropathic pain, peripheral neuropathy, psychosis, schizophrenia and trigeminal neuralgia [16,17]. Some of the AEDs that inhibit lamotrigine metabolism and increase its concentrations are felbamate and valproic acid, while carbamazepine, eslicarbazepine acetate, methsuximide, oxcarbazepine, phenobarbital, phenytoin, primidone, retigabine and rufinamide decrease lamotrigine concentrations by inducing its metabolism. Other non-AED pharmacokinetic interactions of lamotrigine include aripiprazole, isoniazid and sertraline, which increase its concentrations, and, respectively, acetaminophen, atazanavir, ethambutol, olanzapine, oral contraceptives, rifampicin and ritonavir, that decrease its blood concentrations [17,52]. Pregnancy can also reduce lamotrigine concentrations [70].

The fact that there are numerous drug–drug pharmacokinetic interactions and, also, that there are large inter-individual differences in dose-to-plasma concentrations, make lamotrigine TDM valuable and necessary [17]. Lamotrigine is 55–66% bound to plasma proteins, with its saliva concentrations reflecting the non-protein bound plasma levels [16,17,51].

Patrick et al. noted that earlier studies reported a high correlation between saliva and serum concentrations of lamotrigine ($r^2 = 0.95$) [16]. Tsiropoulos et al. studied the correlation between lamotrigine concentrations in serum and saliva, while also examining the relationship between the saliva levels and the non-protein bound lamotrigine concentrations in serum. Both stimulated and unstimulated saliva from the same patients were tested, demonstrating a good correlation between lamotrigine serum concentration in both cases (unstimulated and stimulated: $r^2 = 0.85$ and $r^2 = 0.94$, respectively). Saliva lamotrigine concentrations were reported to be in good correlation with the free, non-bound levels [71]. Malone et al. also studied lamotrigine concentrations in both stimulated and unstimulated saliva samples, comparing them to serum samples. The authors reported a mean saliva/serum lamotrigine concentration ratio of 0.49 at a serum lamotrigine concentration of 10 mg/L, with a correlation coefficient of $r^2 = 0.9841$. The authors concluded that, with appropriate timing in sampling, saliva could provide a good alternative for lamotrigine TDM [72]. Incecayir et al. also reported a good lamotrigine saliva/serum correlation of $r^2 = 0.677$, while Mallayasamy et al. and Kuczynska et al. reported values of $r^2 = 0.683$ and, respectively, $r^2 = 0.82$ [70,73,74]. Ryan et al. reported good lamotrigine salivary and serum concentrations ($r^2 = 0.81$–0.84) in both patients under 16 years of age and also adults [75]. Conclusively, saliva TDM is a viable option in monitoring lamotrigine levels.

4.11. Levetiracetam

Levetiracetam is prescribed in the monotherapy treatment of partial seizures, as well as for adjunctive therapy and in primary generalized tonic–clonic seizures associated with idiopathic generalized epilepsy and myoclonic seizures. Carbamazepine, lamotrigine, methsuximide, oxcarbazepine, phenobarbital and phenytoin can lower levetiracetam plasma concentrations by enhancing its metabolism [16,17].

Levetiracetam has an oral bioavailability of 100%, is 3–10% protein bound and is secreted into saliva, the concentrations being highly correlated with those in plasma [16,17,76,77].

Lins et al., in their study, have reported that when performing oral fluid TDM for levetiracetam, the last oral dose is important because administration within two hours of saliva sampling leads to high drug concentrations. The authors recommend saliva TDM for levetiracetam to be performed at least four hours after oral intake [16,78]. Moreover, Grim et al. noted that stimulated saliva samples can result in lower concentration values ($r^2 = 0.87$ stimulated saliva, whereas $r^2 = 0.91$ in unstimulated samples) [76]. Several studies noted a saliva/serum ratio of almost 1/1, matching levetiracetam saliva and serum concentrations ($r^2 = 0.8428$–0.93) [20,77,79]. Grim et al. reported contrasting results: 40% lower levetiracetam concentrations in oral fluid than in serum [76]. The discrepancy is believed to be due to the different sampling and assay procedures [77].

4.12. Oxcarbazepine

Oxcarbazepine is licensed for monotherapy and for the adjunctive treatment of partial seizures, as well as in the treatment of bipolar disorder and trigeminal neuralgia [17]. Its metabolite is mono-hydroxycarbazepine (MHD or 10-hydroxycarbazepine or 10-hydroxy-10,11-dihydrocarbazepine), which has a plasma protein binding of 40%, a concentration that predicts good penetration into the oral fluid [16,17]. The AEDs that enhance its metabolism, leading to a 15–35% reduction in MHD plasma levels, are carbamazepine, lacosamide, phenobarbital and phenytoin. However, the AEDs that decrease its plasma concentrations by 11% and 20% are viloxazine and, respectively, verapamil [17].

Oxcarbazepine is pharmacologically active but is often at a very low, undetectable concentrations. Therefore, the levels of its metabolite, MHD, are routinely monitored [17].

Unstimulated oral fluid/serum MHD levels' correlation values range from $r^2 = 0.91$ to 0.96 [16,80,81]. Stimulated saliva flow can cause a decrease in saliva MHD levels, so that saliva MHD approaches the range of unbound MHD concentrations in serum or plasma. However, increasing the oral fluid flow disrupts the normal correlation between saliva and serum MHD concentrations [81]. Therefore, there is a wide variation between the correlation values when stimulated saliva is collected, with values of 0.21–0.68 [16,82–84]. The time of the fluid collection is another aspect of interest. Miles et al. concluded that unstimulated saliva/plasma ratios correlated well in the 8–72 h window after oral oxcarbazepine administration, but not earlier than 8 h. Therefore, the authors report that saliva is a suitable matrix for MHD TDM and recommend that oral fluid collection should be avoided within 8 h of the last orally administered dose [81].

4.13. Perampanel

Perampanel is prescribed in the adjunctive treatment of partial-onset seizures and of primary generalized tonic–clonic seizures in patients with idiopathic generalized epilepsy [17]. Perampanel has potentially significant drug–drug interactions; carbamazepine, oxcarbazepine, phenytoin and topiramate can decrease perampanel plasma concentrations by enhancing its metabolism, whilst ketoconazole can increase perampanel plasma concentrations by inhibiting its metabolism [16,17]. Although perampanel TDM is not routinely recommended, when patients are taking concomitant medications monitoring is suggested, due to the various possible drug interactions [16].

Perampanel is 98% bound to plasma proteins. To date, there are no studies that recommend saliva as a matrix for perampanel TDM [16,17].

4.14. Phenobarbital

Phenobarbital is prescribed in the treatment of all forms of epilepsy, except absence seizures. Other indications include acute convulsive episodes and status epilepticus, Lennox–Gastaut syndrome, myoclonic seizures, neonatal seizures and in the prophylaxis of febrile seizures [17]. Phenobarbital's metabolism is inhibited and plasma concentrations are increased by acetazolamide, felbamate, methsuximide, oxcarbazepine, phenytoin, retigabine, rufinamide, stiripentol, sulthiame, chloramphenicol, propoxyphene and valproic acid. On the other hand, phenobarbital's metabolism is enhanced and plasma concentrations are lowered by dicoumarol, thioridazone and troleandomycin [16,17]. The significant amount of possible drug–drug interactions and variable dose-concentration relationships recommend phenobarbital TDM [16].

Phenobarbital is 48–55% bound to plasma proteins and it distributes into saliva [16,17]. Since approximately 50% of phenobarbital is charged in blood and oral fluid at physiological pH, its penetration in oral fluid is unreliable [16]. Conclusively, in the literature, oral fluid/blood ratios for phenobarbital have been reported to range from $r^2 = 0.20$ to $r^2 = 0.52$ for total phenobarbital, and from $r^2 = 0.63$ to $r^2 = 0.68$ for free phenobarbital. Oral fluid phenobarbital concentrations correlate with blood phenobarbital concentrations at values of $r^2 = 0.64$–0.98 for total phenobarbital and $r^2 = 0.64$–0.99 for free phenobarbital [15,16,63]. Carvalho et al., adapting cards that are commonly applied in dried blood spots to oral fluid samples and using LC coupled to a DAD, determined phenobarbital at $r^2 = 0.998 \pm 0.001$, with a mean recovery of 50.6 ± 6.5 from dried saliva spots [59]. Therefore, saliva sampling is concluded to be a suitable matrix for phenobarbital TDM.

4.15. Phenytoin

Phenytoin is prescribed in the treatment of tonic–clonic seizures and focal seizures, as well as trigeminal neuralgia and seizures that occur during or following severe head injury and/or neurosurgery [17]. Phenytoin is subjected to more drug–drug interactions than any other AED, with a long list of AEDs that can increase its blood concentrations (acetazolamide, clobazam, eslicarbazepine acetate, felbamate, methsuximide, oxcarbazepine, rufinamide, stiripentol, sulthiame and topiramate). Carbamazepine, phenobarbital and valproic acid can either increase or decrease its blood concentrations. Non-epilepsy drugs that can affect phenytoin metabolism are numerous, as well [16,17,52]. Phenytoin is 92% bound to plasma protein, exhibiting non-linear plasma pharmacokinetics that occur at different doses for different patients. Given all these facts, and phenytoin's narrow therapeutic window, TDM is strongly recommended [16,17].

Phenytoin's distribution into saliva reflects the non-protein bound levels in plasma, with correlation coefficients of $r^2 = 0.92$–0.99 for oral fluid/total phenytoin and $r^2 = 0.98$–0.99 for oral fluid/free phenytoin [15–17]. Therefore, mean saliva to blood concentration ratios of total phenytoin vary from 0.09 to 0.13, whilst for free phenytoin the ratios vary from 0.99 to 1.06 [15,16]. Patrick et al., in their review study, noted that there are three main considerations when sampling saliva for phenytoin TDM: the saliva flow rate, the timing of the sampling and concomitant drug use. Apart from the aforementioned possible drug–drug interactions, the authors concluded that unstimulated saliva samples should be collected due to the fact that higher phenytoin concentrations have been found in unstimulated samples. Moreover, the sampling should be performed more than 4 h after the last phenytoin dose was administered in order to avoid any drug residue in the oral fluid that could alter the concentrations [16]. Several other studies confirmed literature values—the correlation of free plasma phenytoin levels (approximately 10% of total plasmatic values) and saliva phenytoin levels was $r^2 = 0.82$–0.998 [59,61].

4.16. Pregabalin

Pregabalin is prescribed in the treatment of partial seizures, in anxiety disorders, panic disorder and for peripheral and central neuropathic pain. Pregabalin is not bound to plasma proteins and it is not metabolized. Gabapentin and phenytoin can decrease pregabalin plasma concentrations. To date, it is not known if pregabalin is secreted into saliva [15,17].

4.17. Primidone

Primidone is prescribed to treat generalized tonic–clonic, Jacksonian, psychomotor and focal seizures, as well as myoclonic jerks, essential tremor and akinetic attacks [17]. Primidone is 33% bound to plasma proteins [19,51]. Acetazolamide, carbamazepine and phenytoin can decrease plasma primidone concentrations, whilst clobazam, ethosuximide and stiripentol can increase those concentrations [17,52]. Primidone produces two pharmacologically active metabolites, phenobarbital and phenyl-ethyl-malondiamide, that are responsible for most of the drugs' actions [17]. Therefore, saliva TDM for both primidone and phenobarbital is recommended, especially since blood primidone concentrations are correlated with saliva concentrations: $r^2 = 0.71$–0.98 [15–17].

4.18. Rufinamide

Rufinamide is prescribed to treat seizures associated with Lennox–Gastaut syndrome, but also to treat partial seizures, epileptic spasms, myoclonic-astatic epilepsy and status epilepticus [17]. Carbamazepine, methsuximide, oxcarbazepine, phenobarbital, phenytoin, primidone and vigabatrin can induce and inhibit rufinamide's metabolism, enhancing its elimination. Valproic acid increases rufinamide's plasma concentrations [17,52,85,86]. Rufinamide is 28% bound to plasma proteins, with the saliva levels reflecting the non-protein bound plasma concentrations [15,17]. Franco et al. determined a correlation coefficient between saliva and plasma of $r^2 = 0.78$, while stating that the rufinamide concentrations in saliva were moderately lower than those in plasma, with a mean saliva to plasma ratio of 0.7 ± 0.2 [85]. Mazzucchelli et al. reported a mean saliva to plasma concentration ratio of 0.66, a value that confirms that salivary rufinamide concentrations reflect the unbound drug concentrations in plasma [87]. Therefore, saliva is a suitable matrix for rufinamide TDM.

4.19. Topiramate

Topiramate is prescribed in the treatment of generalized tonic–clonic seizures and partial seizures, as well as for seizures associated with Lennox–Gastaut syndrome and in migraines [17]. AEDs such as carbamazepine, eslicarbazepine acetate, methsuximide, oxcarbazepine, phenobarbital, phenytoin, primidone and valproic acid lower topiramate plasma concentrations, whilst non-AEDs such as diltiazem, hydrochlorothiazide, lithium, metformin, propranolol, posaconazole and sumatriptan increase topiramate's plasma concentrations [17,52].

Topiramate is 20% bound to plasma proteins and it is secreted into oral fluid, with a prediction for strong correlations between total plasma and saliva levels r^2 = 0.92–0.98 [15,17,51,88]. As previously stated, consideration should be given to the time of the saliva sampling, regarding the last administered dose. Miles et al. collected unstimulated oral fluid samples > 3 h after the patients received their last topiramate dose [88]. Conclusively, saliva TDM is a good option for monitoring topiramate levels, when the time of sampling is being considered.

4.20. Valproic Acid (Valproate)

Valproic acid is prescribed in the treatment of any form of epilepsy in patients of any age, as well as in several seizure disorders (such as febrile seizures, infantile spasms, juvenile myoclonic epilepsy, Lennox–Gastaut syndrome, neonatal seizures, etc.) and non-epilepsy conditions (such as bipolar depression, psychosis or schizophrenia) [17]. Valproate plasma concentration is decreased by AEDs (such as carbamazepine, eslicarbazepine acetate, ethosuximide, lamotrigine, methsuximide, phenobarbital, phenytoin, primidone, tiagabine and topiramate) and by non-AEDs (such as amikacin, cisplatin, diflunisal, doripenem, efavirenz, ertapenem, imipenem, meropenem, methotrexate, naproxen, oral contraceptives, panipenam, rifampicin and ritonavir). On the other hand, valproate's plasma concentration is increased by AEDs such as clobazam, felbamate and stiripentol, and, respectively, by non-AEDs such as bupropion, chlorpromazine, cimetidine, erythromycin, guanfacine, isoniazid, lithium, sertraline and verapamil [17,52].

Valproic acid's protein-bound plasma level is concentration dependent, with variations from 74% to 93% [17,51]. Pastalos et al. suggested that saliva is not a useful matrix for valproic acid TDM due to the fact that the distribution of valproate in saliva is reported to be erratic [15,17]. Patrick et al. also predicted poor and inconsistent valproic acid penetration into saliva [16]. Saliva stimulation does not enhance the recovery of valproate in saliva and it does not improve the correlation between its salivary and serum-free concentrations [61]. Nevertheless, Dwivedi et al. reported a significant correlation (r^2 = 0.36, $p < 0.004$), with a mean ratio of saliva to serum-free concentration of 0.68 ± 1.29% [89]. Another study by Tonic-Ribarska et al. studied the determination of valproic acid from unstimulated saliva samples, reporting a mean recovery of 99.4% with a concentration coefficient for the calibration function for valproate of r^2 = 0.9989 [90]. Al Za'abi et al. also reported a good linear relationship between the salivary and the serum-free valproic acid, with a correlation coefficient of r^2 = 0.70 ($p < 0.04$) [61]. More studies are required in order to make saliva an appropriate matrix for valproic acid TDM.

The data collected in this narrative review are summarized in Table 1. For each AED, the published studies found are noted (with regard to authors, journal and year of publication). For each AED in particular, the biofluid which saliva AED levels were compared to is noted in the "Biofluid 1" column. Additionally, the method of determination of the AED levels from each biofluid and the correlations between the two measurements are noted. The AEDs included in this table are the AEDs that show promise in salivary biomarker detection.

Table 1. Correlations in the determination of salivary levels of individual AEDs.

AED (and Their Metabolites)	Authors	Publication	Year	Biofluid 1	Biofluid 2	Determination Method	Correlation/ Corresponding Results * Between the Biofluids
Acetazolamide	Wallace et al. [23]	J Pharm Sci	1977	Enhanced Plasma	Enhanced Saliva	GLC	0.99
	Hartley et al. [24]	J Chromatogr.	1986	Enhanced Plasma	Enhanced Saliva	HPLC	0.985
Clobazam and N-desmethyl clobazam	Gorodischer et al. [30]	Ther Drug Monit.	1997	Plasma	Saliva	GC	0.9 (clobazam), 0.93 (N-desmethyl clobazam)
	Bardy et al. [31]	Brain Dev.	1991	Serum	Saliva	HPLC and enzyme multiplied immunoassay technique	0.9 (clobazam), 0.93 (N-desmethyl clobazam)
Clonazepam and 7-acetamidoclonazepam	Moore et al. [33]	J Anal Toxicol	2007	Enhanced Artificial Saliva	-	LC-MS/MS	0.9991
	Bakke et al. [29]	J Anal Toxicol.	2019	Blood	Saliva	UHPLC-MS/MS	71% *
	Desharnais et al. [34]	Forensic Sci Int	2020	Enhanced Saliva	-	LC-MS	-
	Uddin et al. [27]	J Sep Sci.	2008	Enhanced Plasma	Enhanced Saliva	HPLC	0.999
	Concheiro et al. [35]	Anal Bioanal Chem	2008	Enhanced Saliva	-	LC-MS	0.99
	Øiestad et al. [36]	Clin Chem	2007	Enhanced Saliva	-	LC-MS	0.993
	Gunnar et al. [37]	J Mass Spectrom JMS	2005	Enhanced Saliva	-	GC-MS	0.992
Diazepam, nordiazepam and o N-desmethyldiazepam, 3-OH-diazepam, temazepam and oxazepam	Hallstrom et al. [38]	Br J Clin Pharmacol	1980	Plasma	Saliva	GC	0.89 (diazepam), 0.81 (nordiazepam)
	Moore et al. [33]	J Anal Toxicol.	2007	Enhanced Artificial Saliva	-	LC-MS/MS	0.9996 (diazepam)
	Gunnar et al. [37]	J Mass Spectrom JMS	2005	Enhanced saliva	-	GC-MS	1.000 (diazepam, 0.999 (temazepam), 0.998 (nordiazepam and oxazepam)
	Bakke et al. [29]	J Anal Toxicol.	2019	Blood	Saliva	UHPLC-MS/MS	96.2% * (diazepam), 100% * (N-desmethyldiazepam), 88.9% * (oxazepam)
	Vindenes et al. [22]	J Anal Toxicol.	2011	Urine	Saliva	LC-MS	89% * (N-desmethyldiazepam), 75% * (3-OH-diazepam), 68% * (oxazepam)
	Gjerde et al. [39]	J Anal Toxicol.	2010	Blood	Saliva	HPLC-MS/MS	0.61 (diazepam), 0.95 (nordiazepam)

Table 1. Cont.

AED (and Their Metabolites)	Authors	Publication	Year	Biofluid 1	Biofluid 2	Determination Method	Correlation/ Corresponding Results * Between the Biofluids
Midazolam and 1-hydroxymidazolam and 4-hydroxymidazolam	Link et al. [41]	Rapid Commun Mass Spectrom	2007	Enhanced Plasma	Enhanced Saliva	LC-MS	0.9991 (midazolam), 0.9978 (1-hydroxymidazolam), 0.9986 (4-hydroxymidazolam)
	Link et al. [42]	Br J Clin Pharmacol.	2008	Plasma	Saliva	LC-MS/MS	0.864 (midazolam)
	Moore et al. [33]	J Anal Toxicol.	2007	Enhanced Artificial Saliva	-	LC-MS/MS	0.996 (midazolam)
	Gunnar et al. [37]	J Anal Toxicol.	2007	Enhanced Artificial Saliva	-	LC-MS/MS	0.997 (midazolam)
	Donzelli et al. [43]	Clin Pharmacokinet.	2014	Plasma	Saliva	HPLC-MS/MS	0.886–0.959 (midazolam)
Brivaracetam	Rolan et al. [50]	Br J Clin Pharmacol.	2008	Plasma	Saliva	LC-MS	0.97
Carbamazepine and carbamazepine-10,11-epoxide	Vasudev et al. [58]	Neurol India	2002	Serum	Saliva	HPLC	0.659
	Dordevic et al. [53]	Vojnosanit Pregl.	2009	Serum	Saliva	HPLC	0.9481
	Al Za'abi et al. [61]	Acta Neurol Belg.	2003	Serum	Saliva	Fluorescence polarization immunoassay	0.99
	Djordjevic et al. [55]	Vojnosanit Pregl.	2012	Serum	Saliva	HPLC-UV	0.9117
	Carona et al. [20]	J Pharm Biomed Anal.	2021	Plasma	Saliva	HPLC	0.8299 (carbamazepine) 0.9291 (carbamazepine-10,11-epoxide)
	Dziurkowska and Wesolowski [62]	Mol Basel Switz.	2019	Saliva	-	UHPLC-MS/MS-DAD	>0.99 (carbamazepine-10,11-epoxide)
	Carvalho et al. [59]	J Anal Toxicol.	2019	Dried Enhanced Saliva Spots	-	HPLC-DAD	0.998
	Dwivedi et al. [63]	Int J Neurosci.	2016	Serum	Saliva	HPLC	0.6614
	Chen et al. [60]	Biomed Opt Express.	2021	Enhanced Saliva	-	SERS	0.9663–0.9753
Ethosuximide	Patrick et al. [16]	Ther Drug Monit.	2013	Blood	Saliva	GC	0.74–0.99
Gabapentin	Pujadas et al. [54]	J Pharm Biomed Anal.	2007	Enhanced Saliva	-	GC-MS	0.9903
	Berry et al. [66]	Seizure	2003	Plasma	Saliva	HPLC	0.9491

Table 1. Cont.

AED (and Their Metabolites)	Authors	Publication	Year	Biofluid 1	Biofluid 2	Determination Method	Correlation/ Corresponding Results * Between the Biofluids
Lacosamide	Carona et al. [20]	J Pharm Biomed Anal.	2021	Plasma	Saliva	HPLC	0.9912
	Greenaway et al. [68]	Epilepsia	2011	Serum	Saliva	HPLC	0.842
	Brandt et al. [67]	Epilepsia	2018	Serum	Saliva	Unstated	0.578–0.671
	Cawello et al. [69]	Epilepsia	2013	Plasma	Saliva	HPLC-MS	0.9496–0.9577
	Patrick et al. [16]	Ther Drug Monit.	2013	Blood	Saliva	HPLC	0.84–0.98
Lamotrigine	Tsiropoulos et al. [71]	Ther Drug Monit.	2000	Serum	Saliva	HPLC	0.85 (unstimulated) 0.94 (stimulated saliva)
	Malone et al. [72]	J Clin Neurosci Off J Neurosurg Soc Australas.	2006	Plasma	Saliva	HPLC	0.9841
	Incecayir et al. [73]	Arzneimittelforschung	2007	Plasma	Saliva	HPLC	0.677
	Mallayasamy et al. [74]	Arzneimittelforschung	2010	Plasma	Saliva	HPLC	0.6832
	Ryan et al. [75]	Pharmacotherapy	2003	Serum	Saliva	HPLC	0.905, 0.940
	Patrick et al. [16]	Ther Drug Monit.	2013	Blood	Saliva	HPLC	0.95
Levetiracetam	Lins et al. [78]	Int J Clin Pharmacol Ther.	2007	Plasma	Saliva	Unstated	0.88
	Grim et al. [76]	Ther Drug Monit.	2003	Serum	Saliva	HPLC	0.87, 0.86
	Carona et al. [20]	J Pharm Biomed Anal.	2021	Plasma	Saliva	HPLC	0.8428
	Mecarelli et al. [77]	Ther Drug Monit.	2007	Serum	Saliva	GC	0.9
	Hamdan et al. [79]	J Anal Methods Chem.	2017	Plasma	Saliva	HPLC	0.9
	Patrick et al. [16]	Ther Drug Monit.	2013	Blood	Saliva	HPLC	0.91 (unstimulated), 0.87 (stimulated saliva)
Oxcarbazepine and mono-hydroxycarbazepine	Li et al. [80]	Ther Drug Monit.	2016	Plasma	Saliva	HPLC	0.908
	Miles et al. [81]	Ther Drug Monit.	2004	Serum	Saliva	HPLC	0.941
	Klitgaard et al. [82]	Eur J Clin Pharmacol.	1986	Plasma	Saliva	Equilibrium dialysis and an ultrafiltration technique	0.75
	Kristensen et al. [84]	Acta Neurol Scand.	1983	Serum	Saliva	HPLC	0.914
	Patrick et al. [16]	Ther Drug Monit.	2013	Blood	Saliva	HPLC	0.91–0.98

Table 1. Cont.

AED (and Their Metabolites)	Authors	Publication	Year	Biofluid 1	Biofluid 2	Determination Method	Correlation/ Corresponding Results * Between the Biofluids
Phenobarbital	Dwivedi et al. [63]	Int J Neurosci.	2016	Serum	Saliva	HPLC	0.4257
	Carvalho et al. [59]	J Anal Toxicol.	2019	Dried Enhanced Saliva Spots	-	HPLC-DAD	0.998
	Patsalos and Berry [15]	Ther Drug Monit.	2013	Blood	Saliva	Unstated	0.91
	Patrick et al. [16]	Ther Drug Monit.	2013	Blood	Saliva	HPLC	0.91–0.94
Phenytoin	Carvalho et al. [59]	J Anal Toxicol.	2019	Dried Enhanced Saliva Spots	-	HPLC-DAD	0.998
	Al Za'abi et al. [61]	Acta Neurol Belg.	2003	Serum	Saliva	Fluorescence polarization immunoassay	0.98
	Patrick et al. [16]	Ther Drug Monit.	2013	Blood	Saliva	HPLC	0.92–0.99
	Patsalos and Berry [15]	Ther Drug Monit.	2013	Blood	Saliva	Unstated	0.85–0.99
Primidone	Patrick et al. [16]	Ther Drug Monit.	2013	Blood	Saliva	HPLC	0.71–0.98
	Patsalos and Berry [15]	Ther Drug Monit.	2013	Blood	Saliva	Unstated	0.71–0.97
Rufinamide	Franco et al. [85]	Epilepsia	2020	Plasma	Saliva	HPLC-UV	0.78
	Mazzucchelli et al. [87]	Anal Bioanal Chem	2011	Plasma	Saliva	HPLC-UV	0.99
Topiramate	Miles et al. [88]	Pediatr Neurol	2003	Serum	Saliva	Fluorescence polarization immunoassay	0.97
	Patsalos and Berry [15]	Ther Drug Monit.	2013	Blood	Saliva	Unstated	0.97
Valproic acid	Al Za'abi et al. [61]	Acta Neurol Belg.	2003	Serum	Saliva	Fluorescence polarization immunoassay	0.7
	Dwivedi et al. [89]	Seizure	2015	Serum	Saliva	HPLC	0.13
	Tonic-Ribarska et al. [90]	Acta Pharm Zagreb Croat.	2012	Saliva	-	HPLC	0.9989

* corresponding results (%) were noted in articles that did not state a correlation coefficient. GC = gas chromatography, GLC = gas–liquid chromatography, HPLC = high-performance liquid chromatography, HPLC-DAD = high-performance liquid chromatography with diode-array detection, HPLC-UV = high-performance liquid chromatography with ultraviolet spectroscopy, LC-MS = liquid chromatography mass-spectrometry, LC-MS/MS = liquid chromatography tandem mass-spectrometry, SERS = surface-enhanced Raman spectroscopy, UHPLC-MS/MS = ultra-high performance liquid chromatography.

5. Discussion

AEDs are numerous and diverse, with different mechanisms of action, and choosing the right anti-epileptic for a patient is based on numerous factors such as the seizure type, the potential for drug interactions and the associated comorbidities. The initial response of a patient to a prescribed AED and the monitoring of the dosages is traditionally performed through blood sampling TDM. This monitoring is important because of the clinically relevant differences that exist among similarly active AEDs. Moreover, their possible interactions can lead to both beneficial and/or undesirable effects [14]. Furthermore, the importance of AED and TDM also comes from the statement that about 30% of patients are refractory or drug resistant to AEDs [20].

Numerous AEDs have great potential to be routinely determined through saliva sampling, especially clobazam, clonazepam, diazepam, midazolam, carbamazepine, gabapentin, lacosamide, lamotrigine, levetiracetam, oxcarbazepine, phenobarbital, phenytoin, primidone, rufinamide, topiramate and valproic acid. Saliva TDM would greatly facilitate AED administration for practitioners through its rapidity, ease and a better avoidance of possible side effects. Future research should be focused in order to study and confirm the correlations between these AEDs' blood and saliva levels. Additionally, more research is needed to create a basis for saliva TDM for all the other generally prescribed AEDs.

There is usually a constant proportion between the non-protein-bound AED concentration and the protein-bound. In some cases, when protein binding is influenced by various pathologies (such as renal or hepatic diseases), the free non-protein bound dictates the therapeutic outcome and serves as a clinical guideline for dose management. Therefore, traditionally, the free pharmacologically active concentrations of the component are measured through blood withdrawals in order to adapt patients' doses [15,17]. The blood withdrawals should be performed at the moment when the AED reaches its plasmatic peak in order to monitor the effects. The AED oral dose might be constant, whilst the plasma levels, however, may be low, which can cause seizures to appear. In these cases, it is essential to perform TDM correctly [91]. Saliva TDM of AEDs can be carried out, however, as an alternative assessment sampling technique, with knowing the precise timing of the drug's blood:saliva equilibrium for each patient [16]. The majority of AEDs, because of their lipophilic properties, cross the blood–brain barrier and can be determined from saliva [16]. Further research is needed in order to determine the right moment for sampling—especially when switching the medications, when multiple AEDs are prescribed or in pharmacologically resistant patients [17,20,21].

With regard to the ideal biofluid with which to compare saliva AEDs levels, further research is needed. Many of the described studies used in vitro enhanced biofluids to establish correlations, while other studies tested AEDs levels in both healthy and epileptic patients. The metabolic response between subjects with epilepsy and healthy subjects under AEDs treatment is different. Another aspect is that, in general, plasma and serum levels are comparable. Serum is the liquid that remains after the blood has clotted, while plasma is the liquid that remains when clotting is prevented with the addition of an anticoagulant. However, the use of said anticoagulant can impact the plasma TDM, and the results may vary from one study to another [92,93]. All these differences between the biofluids require enhancement and a predictability of the TDM process. Saliva TDM is a valid option in order to monitor AEDs levels. Further research regarding better-established protocols is, however, needed.

The comparisons between AEDs levels between saliva and another biofluid (e.g., blood or urine) have not taken into consideration modifications due to pH, biofluid density, composition or due to any other pathologies or concomitant drug intakes (drugs prescribed for pathologies other than epilepsy). Additionally, AED monitoring through saliva is a practice that is gaining popularity due to several advantages. Its ease in collecting and storing even multiple samples at a time and the lack of invasiveness might result in it being the future matrix of choice for AED TDM [1,16,17].

There are a few disadvantages associated with saliva TDM, such as the modifications of the oral fluid flow rate, consistency and collected amounts that vary from one patient to another. Moreover, there are difficulties in saliva sampling in certain populations with xerostomia or with critical illnesses. Other drawbacks include the contamination of saliva samples with food, with various periodontal and dental caries microorganisms and even with blood from periodontal pockets [1,17]. There is also a very short period of time available for drug detection in saliva: about 12–24 h after consumption [35].

The benefits of using saliva as AED TDM, however, outweigh the drawbacks. Therefore, there is an increased demand for further research in order to improve the detection and the surveillance of biomarkers. The techniques for biomarker determination should be low-cost and simple to use and to integrate in healthcare centers. Moreover, further research should also be aimed at the improvement of electrochemical sensors in order to more selectively and concomitantly determine multiple types of biomarkers from oral fluid samples. The saliva TDM of AEDs should be determined correctly, quickly and accurately with a universal test that can correlate the oral fluid drug levels to plasma levels.

Overall, saliva analysis is a promising way to monitor numerous biomarkers, having significant potential to be used when fast, efficient and specific determinations are needed, hence its applicability in the future in emergency rooms or even schools, workplaces or roadside testing with law enforcement officers [1]. As a general future perspective, monitoring salivary biomarkers has great potential in being a selective means of analysis in numerous medical and legal fields.

6. Conclusions

In various pathologies, the TDM of the drugs prescribed as treatment is required so that the doses can be monitored and updated if needed. In several cases, saliva has become, instead of blood or plasma, the matrix of choice for testing. All that being said, there is a need for further research regarding the sensitivity of the qualitative and quantitative determination of saliva biomarkers from oral fluid samples. With the proper adaptations and the right analytical methods, saliva TDM has great potential to be used and perfected—notably in long-term treatments that need constant monitorization and updating.

Author Contributions: Conceptualization, I.-A.C., A.M., M.M., A.Ș.M., M.C.D. and A.I.; methodology, I.-A.C., A.M., M.M., A.Ș.M., M.C.D. and A.I.; software, I.-A.C. and V.A.; validation, I.-A.C., A.M., M.M., A.Ș.M., M.C.D. and A.I.; formal analysis, I.-A.C., A.M., M.M., A.Ș.M., M.C.D. and A.I.; investigation, I.-A.C., A.M., M.M., A.Ș.M., M.C.D. and A.I.; resources, I.-A.C., A.M., M.M., A.Ș.M., M.C.D. and A.I.; data curation, I.-A.C., A.M., M.M., A.Ș.M., M.C.D. and A.I.; writing—original draft preparation, I.-A.C., A.M., M.M., A.Ș.M., M.C.D. and A.I.; writing—review and editing, I.-A.C., A.M., M.M., A.Ș.M., M.C.D. and A.I.; visualization, I.-A.C., A.M., M.M., A.Ș.M., M.C.D. and A.I.; supervision, I.-A.C., A.M., M.M., A.Ș.M., M.C.D. and A.I.; project administration, I.-A.C. and A.I. All authors have read and agreed to the published version of the manuscript.

Funding: The present study was supported by a grant from the Ministry of Research, Innovation and Digitization, CNCS—UEFISCDI, project number PN-III-P4-PCE-2021-1140, within PNCDI III, a financial support for which the authors are thankful.

Institutional Review Board Statement: Not applicable.

Informed Consent Statement: Not applicable.

Data Availability Statement: Not applicable.

Conflicts of Interest: The authors declare no conflict of interest.

References

1. Gug, I.; Tertis, M.; Ilea, A.; Chiș, I.A.; Băbțan, A.M.; Uriciuc, W.A.; Ionel, A.; Feurdean, C.N.; Boșca, A.B.; Cristea, C. Salivary Biomarkers in Toxicology: An Update Narrative. In *Biomarkers in Toxicology*; Biomarkers in Disease: Methods, Discoveries and Applications; Patel, V.B., Preedy, V.R., Rajendram, R., Eds.; Springer International Publishing: Cham, Switzerland, 2022; pp. 1–27. Available online: https://link.springer.com/10.1007/978-3-030-87225-0_70-1 (accessed on 13 January 2023).
2. FDA-NIH Biomarker Working Group. *BEST (Biomarkers, EndpointS, and other Tools) Resource*; Food and Drug Administration (US): Silver Spring, MD, USA, 2016. Available online: http://www.ncbi.nlm.nih.gov/books/NBK326791/ (accessed on 6 March 2023).
3. Califf, R.M. Biomarker definitions and their applications. *Exp. Biol. Med.* **2018**, *243*, 213–221. [CrossRef] [PubMed]
4. Ilea, A.; Andrei, V.; Feurdean, C.; Băbțan, A.M.; Petrescu, N.; Câmpian, R.; Boșca, A.B.; Ciui, B.; Tertiș, M.; Săndulescu, R.; et al. Saliva, a Magic Biofluid Available for Multilevel Assessment and a Mirror of General Health—A Systematic Review. *Biosensors* **2019**, *9*, 27. [CrossRef] [PubMed]
5. Schipper, R.G.; Silletti, E.; Vingerhoeds, M.H. Saliva as research material: Biochemical, physicochemical and practical aspects. *Arch. Oral. Biol.* **2007**, *52*, 1114–1135. [CrossRef] [PubMed]
6. Battino, M.; Ferreiro, M.S.; Gallardo, I.; Newman, H.N.; Bullon, P. The antioxidant capacity of saliva: The antioxidant capacity of saliva. *J. Clin. Periodontol.* **2002**, *29*, 189–194. [CrossRef] [PubMed]

7. Milanowski, M.; Pomastowski, P.; Ligor, T.; Buszewski, B. Saliva—Volatile Biomarkers and Profiles. *Crit. Rev. Anal. Chem.* **2017**, *47*, 251–266. [CrossRef]
8. Gug, I.T.; Tertis, M.; Hosu, O.; Cristea, C. Salivary biomarkers detection: Analytical and immunological methods overview. *TrAC Trends Anal. Chem.* **2019**, *113*, 301–316. [CrossRef]
9. Humphrey, S.P.; Williamson, R.T. A review of saliva: Normal composition, flow, and function. *J. Prosthet. Dent.* **2001**, *85*, 162–169. [CrossRef]
10. De Smet, K.; Contreras, R. Human Antimicrobial Peptides: Defensins, Cathelicidins and Histatins. *Biotechnol. Lett.* **2005**, *27*, 1337–1347. [CrossRef]
11. Grabenauer, M.; Moore, K.N.; Bynum, N.D.; White, R.M.; Mitchell, J.M.; Hayes, E.D.; Flegel, R. Development of a Quantitative LC-MS-MS Assay for Codeine, Morphine, 6-Acetylmorphine, Hydrocodone, Hydromorphone, Oxycodone and Oxymorphone in Neat Oral Fluid. *J. Anal. Toxicol.* **2018**, *42*, 392–399. [CrossRef]
12. Hutchinson, L.; Sinclair, M.; Reid, B.; Burnett, K.; Callan, B. A descriptive systematic review of salivary therapeutic drug monitoring in neonates and infants: Salivary TDM in neonates and infants. *Br. J. Clin. Pharmacol.* **2018**, *84*, 1089–1108. [CrossRef]
13. Nowak, P.; Woźniakiewicz, M.; Kościelniak, P. Application of capillary electrophoresis in determination of acid dissociation constant values. *J. Chromatogr. A* **2015**, *1377*, 1–12. [CrossRef]
14. Howard, P.; Twycross, R.; Shuster, J.; Mihalyo, M.; Rémi, J.; Wilcock, A. Anti-epileptic drugs. *J. Pain Symptom Manag.* **2011**, *42*, 788–804. [CrossRef]
15. Patsalos, P.N.; Berry, D.J. Therapeutic drug monitoring of antiepileptic drugs by use of saliva. *Ther. Drug Monit.* **2013**, *35*, 4–29. [CrossRef]
16. Patrick, M.; Parmiter, S.; Mahmoud, S.H. Feasibility of Using Oral Fluid for Therapeutic Drug Monitoring of Antiepileptic Drugs. *Eur. J. Drug Metab. Pharmacokinet.* **2021**, *46*, 205–223. [CrossRef]
17. Patsalos, P.N.; Spencer, E.P.; Berry, D.J. Therapeutic Drug Monitoring of Antiepileptic Drugs in Epilepsy: A 2018 Update. *Ther. Drug Monit.* **2018**, *40*, 526–548. [CrossRef]
18. Aman, M.G.; Paxton, J.W.; Field, C.J.; Foote, S.E. Prevalence of toxic anticonvulsant drug concentrations in mentally retarded persons with epilepsy. *Am. J. Ment. Defic.* **1986**, *90*, 643–650.
19. Thijs, R.D.; Surges, R.; O'Brien, T.J.; Sander, J.W. Epilepsy in adults. *Lancet* **2019**, *393*, 689–701. [CrossRef]
20. Carona, A.; Bicker, J.; Silva, R.; Silva, A.; Santana, I.; Sales, F.; Falcão, A.; Fortuna, A. HPLC method for the determination of antiepileptic drugs in human saliva and its application in therapeutic drug monitoring. *J. Pharm. Biomed. Anal.* **2021**, *197*, 113961. [CrossRef]
21. Perucca, P.; Scheffer, I.E.; Kiley, M. The management of epilepsy in children and adults. *Med. J. Aust.* **2018**, *208*, 226–233. [CrossRef]
22. Vindenes, V.; Yttredal, B.; Oiestad, E.L.; Waal, H.; Bernard, J.P.; Mørland, J.G.; Christophersen, A.S. Oral fluid is a viable alternative for monitoring drug abuse: Detection of drugs in oral fluid by liquid chromatography-tandem mass spectrometry and comparison to the results from urine samples from patients treated with Methadone or Buprenorphine. *J. Anal. Toxicol.* **2011**, *35*, 32–39. [CrossRef]
23. Wallace, S.M.; Shah, V.P.; Riegelman, S. GLC analysis of acetazolamide in blood, plasma, and saliva following oral administration to normal subjects. *J. Pharm. Sci.* **1977**, *66*, 527–530. [CrossRef] [PubMed]
24. Hartley, R.; Lucock, M.; Becker, M.; Smith, I.J.; Forsythe, W.I. Solid-phase extraction of acetazolamide from biological fluids and subsequent analysis by high-performance liquid chromatography. *J. Chromatogr.* **1986**, *377*, 295–305. [CrossRef] [PubMed]
25. Nielsen, S. Benzodiazepines. *Curr. Top. Behav. Neurosci.* **2017**, *34*, 141–159. [PubMed]
26. Olkkola, K.T.; Ahonen, J. Midazolam and other benzodiazepines. *Handb. Exp. Pharmacol.* **2008**, *182*, 335–360.
27. Uddin, M.N.; Samanidou, V.F.; Papadoyannis, I.N. Validation of SPE-HPLC determination of 1,4-benzodiazepines and metabolites in blood plasma, urine, and saliva. *J. Sep. Sci.* **2008**, *31*, 3704–3717. [CrossRef]
28. Sverrisdóttir, E.; Lund, T.M.; Olesen, A.E.; Drewes, A.M.; Christrup, L.L.; Kreilgaard, M. A review of morphine and morphine-6-glucuronide's pharmacokinetic-pharmacodynamic relationships in experimental and clinical pain. *Eur. J. Pharm. Sci. Off. J. Eur. Fed. Pharm. Sci.* **2015**, *74*, 45–62. [CrossRef]
29. Bakke, E.; Høiseth, G.; Arnestad, M.; Gjerde, H. Detection of Drugs in Simultaneously Collected Samples of Oral Fluid and Blood. *J. Anal. Toxicol.* **2019**, *43*, 228–232. [CrossRef]
30. Gorodischer, R.; Burtin, P.; Verjee, Z.; Hwang, P.; Koren, G. Is saliva suitable for therapeutic monitoring of anticonvulsants in children: An evaluation in the routine clinical setting. *Ther. Drug Monit.* **1997**, *19*, 637–642. [CrossRef]
31. Bardy, A.H.; Seppälä, T.; Salokorpi, T.; Granström, M.L.; Santavuori, P. Monitoring of concentrations of clobazam and norclobazam in serum and saliva of children with epilepsy. *Brain Dev.* **1991**, *13*, 174–179. [CrossRef]
32. Hart, B.J.; Wilting, J.; de Gier, J.J. The stability of benzodiazepines in saliva. *Methods Find. Exp. Clin. Pharmacol.* **1988**, *10*, 21–26.
33. Moore, C.; Coulter, C.; Crompton, K.; Zumwalt, M. Determination of benzodiazepines in oral fluid using LC-MS-MS. *J. Anal. Toxicol.* **2007**, *31*, 596–600. [CrossRef]
34. Desharnais, B.; Lajoie, M.J.; Laquerre, J.; Mireault, P.; Skinner, C.D. A threshold LC-MS/MS method for 92 analytes in oral fluid collected with the Quantisal®device. *Forensic Sci. Int.* **2020**, *317*, 110506. [CrossRef]
35. Concheiro, M.; de Castro, A.; Quintela, O.; Cruz, A.; López-Rivadulla, M. Determination of illicit and medicinal drugs and their metabolites in oral fluid and preserved oral fluid by liquid chromatography-tandem mass spectrometry. *Anal. Bioanal. Chem.* **2008**, *391*, 2329–2338. [CrossRef]

36. Øiestad, E.L.; Johansen, U.; Christophersen, A.S. Drug screening of preserved oral fluid by liquid chromatography-tandem mass spectrometry. *Clin. Chem.* **2007**, *53*, 300–309. [CrossRef]
37. Gunnar, T.; Ariniemi, K.; Lillsunde, P. Validated toxicological determination of 30 drugs of abuse as optimized derivatives in oral fluid by long column fast gas chromatography/electron impact mass spectrometry. *J. Mass. Spectrom.* **2005**, *40*, 739–753. [CrossRef]
38. Hallstrom, C.; Lader, M.H. Diazepam and N-desmethyldiazepam concentrations in saliva, plasma and CSF. *Br. J. Clin. Pharmacol.* **1980**, *9*, 333–339. [CrossRef]
39. Gjerde, H.; Mordal, J.; Christophersen, A.S.; Bramness, J.G.; Mørland, J. Comparison of drug concentrations in blood and oral fluid collected with the Intercept sampling device. *J. Anal. Toxicol.* **2010**, *34*, 204–209. [CrossRef]
40. Christodoulides, N.; De La Garza, R.; Simmons, G.W.; McRae, M.P.; Wong, J.; Newton, T.F.; Smith, R.; Mahoney, J.J., III; Hohenstein, J.; Gomez, S.; et al. Application of programmable bio-nano-chip system for the quantitative detection of drugs of abuse in oral fluids. *Drug Alcohol. Depend.* **2015**, *153*, 306–313. [CrossRef] [PubMed]
41. Link, B.; Haschke, M.; Wenk, M.; Krähenbühl, S. Determination of midazolam and its hydroxy metabolites in human plasma and oral fluid by liquid chromatography/electrospray ionization ion trap tandem mass spectrometry. *Rapid Commun. Mass. Spectrom. RCM* **2007**, *21*, 1531–1540. [CrossRef]
42. Link, B.; Haschke, M.; Grignaschi, N.; Bodmer, M.; Aschmann, Y.Z.; Wenk, M.; Krähenbühl, S. Pharmacokinetics of intravenous and oral midazolam in plasma and saliva in humans: Usefulness of saliva as matrix for CYP3A phenotyping. *Br. J. Clin. Pharmacol.* **2008**, *66*, 473–484. [CrossRef]
43. Donzelli, M.; Derungs, A.; Serratore, M.G.; Noppen, C.; Nezic, L.; Krähenbühl, S.; Haschke, M. The basel cocktail for simultaneous phenotyping of human cytochrome P450 isoforms in plasma, saliva and dried blood spots. *Clin. Pharmacokinet.* **2014**, *53*, 271–282. [CrossRef] [PubMed]
44. Uehara, T.; Wang, Y.; Tong, W. Toxicogenomic and Pharmacogenomic Biomarkers for Drug Discovery and Personalized Medicine. In *General Methods in Biomarker Research and Their Applications*; Biomarkers in Disease: Methods, Discoveries and Applications; Preedy, V.R., Patel, V.B., Eds.; Springer Netherlands: Dordrecht, The Netherlands, 2015; pp. 75–109. Available online: http://link.springer.com/10.1007/978-94-007-7696-8_19 (accessed on 13 January 2023).
45. Smink, B.E.; Mathijssen, M.P.M.; Lusthof, K.J.; de Gier, J.J.; Egberts, A.C.G.; Uges, D.R.A. Comparison of urine and oral fluid as matrices for screening of thirty-three benzodiazepines and benzodiazepine-like substances using immunoassay and LC-MS(-MS). *J. Anal. Toxicol.* **2006**, *30*, 478–485. [CrossRef]
46. Lo Muzio, L.; Falaschini, S.; Rappelli, G.; Bambini, F.; Baldoni, A.; Procaccini, M.; Cingolani, M. Saliva as a diagnostic matrix for drug abuse. *Int. J. Immunopathol. Pharmacol.* **2005**, *18*, 567–573. [CrossRef] [PubMed]
47. Valen, A.; Leere Øiestad, Å.M.; Strand, D.H.; Skari, R.; Berg, T. Determination of 21 drugs in oral fluid using fully automated supported liquid extraction and UHPLC-MS/MS. *Drug Test. Anal.* **2017**, *9*, 808–823. [CrossRef] [PubMed]
48. Pil, K.; Verstraete, A. Current developments in drug testing in oral fluid. *Ther. Drug Monit.* **2008**, *30*, 196–202. [CrossRef]
49. Inscore, F.; Shende, C.; Sengupta, A.; Huang, H.; Farquharson, S. Detection of drugs of abuse in saliva by surface-enhanced Raman spectroscopy (SERS). *Appl. Spectrosc.* **2011**, *65*, 1004–1008. [CrossRef]
50. Rolan, P.; Sargentini-Maier, M.L.; Pigeolet, E.; Stockis, A. The pharmacokinetics, CNS pharmacodynamics and adverse event profile of brivaracetam after multiple increasing oral doses in healthy men. *Br. J. Clin. Pharmacol.* **2008**, *66*, 71–75. [CrossRef]
51. Patsalos, P.N.; Zugman, M.; Lake, C.; James, A.; Ratnaraj, N.; Sander, J.W. Serum protein binding of 25 antiepileptic drugs in a routine clinical setting: A comparison of free non-protein-bound concentrations. *Epilepsia* **2017**, *58*, 1234–1243. [CrossRef]
52. Patsalos, P.N. *Antiepileptic Drug Interactions*; Springer International Publishing: Cham, Switzerland, 2016. Available online: http://link.springer.com/10.1007/978-3-319-32909-3 (accessed on 12 July 2022).
53. Dordević, S.; Kilibarda, V.; Stojanović, T. Determination of carbamazepine in serum and saliva samples by high performance liquid chromatography with ultraviolet detection. *Vojnosanit. Pregl.* **2009**, *66*, 347–352.
54. Pujadas, M.; Pichini, S.; Civit, E.; Santamariña, E.; Perez, K.; de la Torre, R. A simple and reliable procedure for the determination of psychoactive drugs in oral fluid by gas chromatography-mass spectrometry. *J. Pharm. Biomed. Anal.* **2007**, *44*, 594–601. [CrossRef]
55. Djordjević, S.; Kilibarda, V.; Vucinić, S.; Stojanović, T.; Antonijević, B. Toxicokinetics and correlation of carbamazepine salivary and serum concentrations in acute poisonings. *Vojnosanit. Pregl.* **2012**, *69*, 389–393. [CrossRef]
56. Rosenthal, E.; Hoffer, E.; Ben-Aryeh, H.; Badarni, S.; Benderly, A.; Hemli, Y. Use of saliva in home monitoring of carbamazepine levels. *Epilepsia* **1995**, *36*, 72–74. [CrossRef]
57. Paxton, J.W.; Donald, R.A. Concentrations and kinetics of carbamazepine in whole saliva, parotid saliva, serum ultrafiltrate, and serum. *Clin. Pharmacol. Ther.* **1980**, *28*, 695–702. [CrossRef]
58. Vasudev, A.; Tripathi, K.D.; Puri, V. Correlation of serum and salivary carbamazepine concentration in epileptic patients: Implications for therapeutic drug monitoring. *Neurol. India* **2002**, *50*, 60–62.
59. Carvalho, J.; Rosado, T.; Barroso, M.; Gallardo, E. Determination of Antiepileptic Drugs Using Dried Saliva Spots. *J. Anal. Toxicol.* **2019**, *43*, 61–71. [CrossRef]
60. Chen, N.; Yuan, Y.; Lu, P.; Wang, L.; Zhang, X.; Chen, H.; Ma, P. Detection of carbamazepine in saliva based on surface-enhanced Raman spectroscopy. *Biomed. Opt. Express* **2021**, *12*, 7673–7688. [CrossRef]

61. Al Za'abi, M.; Deleu, D.; Batchelor, C. Salivary free concentrations of anti-epileptic drugs: An evaluation in a routine clinical setting. *Acta Neurol. Belg.* **2003**, *103*, 19–23.
62. Dziurkowska, E.; Wesolowski, M. Simultaneous Quantification of Antipsychotic and Antiepileptic Drugs and Their Metabolites in Human Saliva Using UHPLC-DAD. *Molecules* **2019**, *24*, 2953. [CrossRef]
63. Dwivedi, R.; Singh, M.; Kaleekal, T.; Gupta, Y.K.; Tripathi, M. Concentration of antiepileptic drugs in persons with epilepsy: A comparative study in serum and saliva. *Int. J. Neurosci.* **2016**, *126*, 972–978. [CrossRef]
64. Dziurkowska, E.; Wesolowski, M. Deproteinization as a Rapid Method of Saliva Purification for the Determination of Carbamazepine and Carbamazepine-10,11 Epoxide. *J. Clin. Med.* **2020**, *9*, 915. [CrossRef]
65. Capule, F.; Tragulpiankit, P.; Mahasirimongkol, S.; Jittikoon, J.; Wichukchinda, N.; Theresa Alentajan-Aleta, L.; James Barit, J.V.; Casanova-Gutierrez, J.; Cabral-Lim, L.; Baltazar Reyes, J.P.; et al. Association of carbamazepine-induced Stevens-Johnson syndrome/toxic epidermal necrolysis with the HLA-B75 serotype or HLA-B*15:21 allele in Filipino patients. *Pharm. J.* **2020**, *20*, 533–541. [CrossRef]
66. Berry, D.J.; Beran, R.G.; Plunkeft, M.J.; Clarke, L.A.; Hung, W.T. The absorption of gabapentin following high dose escalation. *Seizure* **2003**, *12*, 28–36. [CrossRef]
67. Brandt, C.; Bien, C.G.; Helmer, R.; May, T.W. Assessment of the correlations of lacosamide concentrations in saliva and serum in patients with epilepsy. *Epilepsia* **2018**, *59*, e34–e39. [CrossRef] [PubMed]
68. Greenaway, C.; Ratnaraj, N.; Sander, J.W.; Patsalos, P.N. Saliva and serum lacosamide concentrations in patients with epilepsy. *Epilepsia* **2011**, *52*, 258–263. [CrossRef] [PubMed]
69. Cawello, W.; Bökens, H.; Nickel, B.; Andreas, J.O.; Halabi, A. Tolerability, pharmacokinetics, and bioequivalence of the tablet and syrup formulations of lacosamide in plasma, saliva, and urine: Saliva as a surrogate of pharmacokinetics in the central compartment. *Epilepsia* **2013**, *54*, 81–88. [CrossRef]
70. Kuczynska, J.; Karas-Ruszczyk, K.; Zakrzewska, A.; Dermanowski, M.; Sienkiewicz-Jarosz, H.; Kurkowska-Jastrzebska, I.; Bienkowski, P.; Konopko, M.; Dominiak, M.; Mierzejewski, P. Comparison of plasma, saliva, and hair lamotrigine concentrations. *Clin. Biochem.* **2019**, *74*, 24–30. [CrossRef] [PubMed]
71. Tsiropoulos, I.; Kristensen, O.; Klitgaard, N.A. Saliva and serum concentration of lamotrigine in patients with epilepsy. *Ther. Drug Monit.* **2000**, *22*, 517–521. [CrossRef] [PubMed]
72. Malone, S.A.; Eadie, M.J.; Addison, R.S.; Wright, A.W.E.; Dickinson, R.G. Monitoring salivary lamotrigine concentrations. *J. Clin. Neurosci. Off. J. Neurosurg. Soc. Australas* **2006**, *13*, 902–907. [CrossRef]
73. Incecayir, T.; Agabeyoglu, I.; Gucuyener, K. Comparison of plasma and saliva concentrations of lamotrigine in healthy volunteers. *Arzneimittelforschung* **2007**, *57*, 517–521. [CrossRef]
74. Mallayasamy, S.R.; Arumugamn, K.; Jain, T.; Rajakannan, T.; Bhat, K.; Gurumadhavrao, P.; Devarakonda, R. A sensitive and selective HPLC method for estimation of lamotrigine in human plasma and saliva: Application to plasma-saliva correlation in epileptic patients. *Arzneimittelforschung* **2010**, *60*, 599–606. [CrossRef]
75. Ryan, M.; Grim, S.A.; Miles, M.V.; Tang, P.H.; Fakhoury, T.A.; Strawsburg, R.H.; DeGrauw, T.J.; Baumann, R.J. Correlation of lamotrigine concentrations between serum and saliva. *Pharmacotherapy* **2003**, *23*, 1550–1557. [CrossRef] [PubMed]
76. Grim, S.A.; Ryan, M.; Miles, M.V.; Tang, P.H.; Strawsburg, R.H.; deGrauw, T.J.; Fakhoury, T.A.; Baumann, R.J. Correlation of levetiracetam concentrations between serum and saliva. *Ther. Drug Monit.* **2003**, *25*, 61–66. [CrossRef]
77. Mecarelli, O.; Li Voti, P.; Pro, S.; Romolo, F.S.; Rotolo, M.; Pulitano, P.; Accornero, N.; Vanacore, N. Saliva and serum levetiracetam concentrations in patients with epilepsy. *Ther. Drug Monit.* **2007**, *29*, 313–318. [CrossRef] [PubMed]
78. Lins, R.L.; Otoul, C.; De Smedt, F.; Coupez, R.; Stockis, A. Comparison of plasma and saliva concentrations of levetiracetam following administration orally as a tablet and as a solution in healthy adult volunteers. *Int. J. Clin. Pharmacol. Ther.* **2007**, *45*, 47–54. [CrossRef] [PubMed]
79. Hamdan, I.I.; Alsous, M.; Masri, A.T. Chromatographic Characterization and Method Development for Determination of Levetiracetam in Saliva: Application to Correlation with Plasma Levels. *J. Anal. Methods Chem.* **2017**, *2017*, 7846742. [CrossRef]
80. Li, R.R.; Sheng, X.Y.; Ma, L.Y.; Yao, H.X.; Cai, L.X.; Chen, C.Y.; Zhu, S.N.; Zhou, Y.; Wu, Y.; Cui, Y.M. Saliva and Plasma Monohydroxycarbamazepine Concentrations in Pediatric Patients With Epilepsy. *Ther. Drug Monit.* **2016**, *38*, 365–370. [CrossRef]
81. Miles, M.V.; Tang, P.H.; Ryan, M.A.; Grim, S.A.; Fakhoury, T.A.; Strawsburg, R.H.; DeGrauw, T.J.; Baumann, R.J. Feasibility and limitations of oxcarbazepine monitoring using salivary monohydroxycarbamazepine (MHD). *Ther. Drug Monit.* **2004**, *26*, 300–304. [CrossRef]
82. Klitgaard, N.A.; Kristensen, O. Use of saliva for monitoring oxcarbazepine therapy in epileptic patients. *Eur. J. Clin. Pharmacol.* **1986**, *31*, 91–94. [CrossRef]
83. Cardot, J.M.; Degen, P.; Flesch, G.; Menge, P.; Dieterle, W. Comparison of plasma and saliva concentrations of the active monohydroxy metabolite of oxcarbazepine in patients at steady state. *Biopharm. Drug Dispos.* **1995**, *16*, 603–614. [CrossRef]
84. Kristensen, O.; Klitgaard, N.A.; Jönsson, B.; Sindrup, S. Pharmacokinetics of 10-OH-carbazepine, the main metabolite of the antiepileptic oxcarbazepine, from serum and saliva concentrations. *Acta Neurol. Scand.* **1983**, *68*, 145–150. [CrossRef]
85. Franco, V.; Gatti, G.; Mazzucchelli, I.; Marchiselli, R.; Fattore, C.; Rota, P.; Galimberti, C.A.; Capovilla, G.; Beccaria, F.; De Giorgis, V.; et al. Relationship between saliva and plasma rufinamide concentrations in patients with epilepsy. *Epilepsia* **2020**, *61*, e79–e84. [CrossRef]

86. Perucca, E.; Cloyd, J.; Critchley, D.; Fuseau, E. Rufinamide: Clinical pharmacokinetics and concentration-response relationships in patients with epilepsy. *Epilepsia* **2008**, *49*, 1123–1141. [CrossRef]
87. Mazzucchelli, I.; Rapetti, M.; Fattore, C.; Franco, V.; Gatti, G.; Perucca, E. Development and validation of an HPLC-UV detection assay for the determination of rufinamide in human plasma and saliva. *Anal. Bioanal. Chem.* **2011**, *401*, 1013–1021. [CrossRef]
88. Miles, M.V.; Tang, P.H.; Glauser, T.A.; Ryan, M.A.; Grim, S.A.; Strawsburg, R.H.; Ton, J.D.; Baumann, R.J. Topiramate concentration in saliva: An alternative to serum monitoring. *Pediatr. Neurol.* **2003**, *29*, 143–147. [CrossRef]
89. Dwivedi, R.; Gupta, Y.K.; Singh, M.; Joshi, R.; Tiwari, P.; Kaleekal, T.; Tripathi, M. Correlation of saliva and serum free valproic acid concentrations in persons with epilepsy. *Seizure* **2015**, *25*, 187–190. [CrossRef]
90. Tonic-Ribarska, J.; Haxhiu, A.; Sterjev, Z.; Kiteva, G.; Suturkova, L.; Trajkovic-Jolevska, S. Development and validation of a bioanalytical LC-UV method with solid-phase extraction for determination of valproic acid in saliva. *Acta Pharm. Zagreb. Croat.* **2012**, *62*, 211–220. [CrossRef]
91. Eadie, M.J. Plasma Level Monitoring of Anticonvulsants. *Clin. Pharmacokinet.* **1976**, *1*, 52–66. [CrossRef]
92. Aakerøy, R.; Stokes, C.L.; Tomić, M.; Hegstad, S.; Kristoffersen, A.H.; Ellekjær, H.; Schjøtt, J.; Spigset, O.; Helland, A. Serum or Plasma for Quantification of Direct Oral Anticoagulants? *Ther. Drug Monit.* **2022**, *44*, 578–584. [CrossRef]
93. Gross, A.S. Best practice in therapeutic drug monitoring. *Br. J. Clin. Pharmacol.* **2001**, *52* (Suppl. S1), 5S–10S.

Disclaimer/Publisher's Note: The statements, opinions and data contained in all publications are solely those of the individual author(s) and contributor(s) and not of MDPI and/or the editor(s). MDPI and/or the editor(s) disclaim responsibility for any injury to people or property resulting from any ideas, methods, instructions or products referred to in the content.

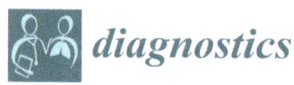 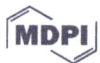

Article

The Role of Immunohistochemistry in the Differential Diagnosis between Intrahepatic Cholangiocarcinoma, Hepatocellular Carcinoma and Liver Metastasis, as Well as Its Prognostic Value

Lavinia Patricia Mocan [1,*], Ioana Rusu [2], Carmen Stanca Melincovici [1], Bianca Adina Boșca [1], Tudor Mocan [3,4], Rareș Crăciun [4,5], Zeno Spârchez [4,5], Maria Iacobescu [6] and Carmen Mihaela Mihu [1]

1. Department of Histology, "Iuliu Hațieganu" University of Medicine and Pharmacy, 400349 Cluj-Napoca, Romania
2. Department of Pathology, "Prof. Dr. Octavian Fodor" Regional Institute of Gastroenterology and Hepatology, 400162 Cluj-Napoca, Romania
3. UBBMed Department, Babeș-Bolyai University, 400347 Cluj-Napoca, Romania
4. Department of Gastroenterology, "Prof. Dr. Octavian Fodor" Regional Institute of Gastroenterology and Hepatology, 400162 Cluj-Napoca, Romania
5. 3rd Medical Department, "Iuliu Hațieganu" University of Medicine and Pharmacy, 400162 Cluj-Napoca, Romania
6. Department of Proteomics and Metabolomics, MedFUTURE Research Center for Advanced Medicine, "Iuliu Hațieganu" University of Medicine and Pharmacy, 400349 Cluj-Napoca, Romania
* Correspondence: trica.lavinia@umfcluj.ro

Abstract: Intrahepatic cholangiocarcinoma (iCCA) is the second most frequent primary hepatic malignant tumor, after hepatocellular carcinoma (HCC). Its incidence has risen worldwide, yet the only potentially curative treatment, surgical resection, is seldom applicable, and the median overall survival remains extremely low. So far, there are no personalized therapy regimens. This study investigated whether routine immunohistochemical stains have diagnostic and/or prognostic value in iCCA. Clinical, imaging, and pathology data were retrospectively gathered for patients diagnosed with iCCA, HCC, or liver metastases assessed using liver needle biopsies. Three study groups with an equal number of cases ($n = 65$) were formed. In the iCCA group, CK19, CA19-9, CK7, and CEA demonstrated the highest sensitivities (100%, 100%, 93.7%, and 82.6%, respectively). The most relevant stains used for diagnosing HCCs were Glypican 3, CD34 (sinusoidal pattern), and Hep Par 1, with corresponding sensitivities of 100%, 100%, and 98.2%. The immunohistochemical panels for diagnosing metastatic tumors were chosen after correlating the clinical data and morphologic H&E aspects. Moderate/intensely positive CK7 expression and absent/low amount of intratumoral immune cells were favorable prognostic factors and correlated with increased overall survival in both the univariate analysis and the multivariate regression adjusted for age, existence of cirrhosis, number of tumors, and tumor differentiation.

Keywords: intrahepatic cholangiocarcinoma; hepatocellular carcinoma; secondary tumor; needle biopsy; immunohistochemistry; CK7; intratumoral immune cells

Citation: Mocan, L.P.; Rusu, I.; Melincovici, C.S.; Boșca, B.A.; Mocan, T.; Crăciun, R.; Spârchez, Z.; Iacobescu, M.; Mihu, C.M. The Role of Immunohistochemistry in the Differential Diagnosis between Intrahepatic Cholangiocarcinoma, Hepatocellular Carcinoma and Liver Metastasis, as Well as Its Prognostic Value. *Diagnostics* **2023**, *13*, 1542. https://doi.org/10.3390/diagnostics13091542

Academic Editor: Gian Paolo Caviglia

Received: 3 March 2023
Revised: 20 April 2023
Accepted: 22 April 2023
Published: 25 April 2023

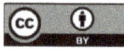

Copyright: © 2023 by the authors. Licensee MDPI, Basel, Switzerland. This article is an open access article distributed under the terms and conditions of the Creative Commons Attribution (CC BY) license (https://creativecommons.org/licenses/by/4.0/).

1. Introduction

Intrahepatic cholangiocarcinoma (iCCA), a tumor derived from the biliary epithelium, is the second most frequent primary liver malignancy after hepatocellular carcinoma (HCC) and accounts for 10–20% of primary hepatic malignancies [1]. Conventionally, iCCA is located in the hepatic parenchyma, proximal to the left and right hepatic ducts [2]. Although less frequent than perihilar and distal cholangiocarcinoma, both classified as extrahepatic cholangiocarcinoma (eCCA), the incidence of iCCA is rising worldwide at a much greater rate compared to the incidence of eCCA, with a striking difference of a 350% vs. 20% increase [3,4].

Most risk factors for iCCA are associated with chronic liver inflammation: primary sclerosing cholangitis, hepatolithiasis, bile duct cysts and malformations, and liver flukes. The latter account for the development of most cholangiocarcinoma cases in endemic areas [5] but can also sporadically occur in Caucasian patients. Some authors include hepatitis B virus (HBV) and hepatitis C virus (HCV), chronic viral hepatitis, cirrhosis, non-alcoholic fatty liver disease, obesity, and diabetes among the risk factors [6–8]. Typically, both iCCA and HCC occur in the setting of chronic liver disease. In such cases, serum liver function tests, serology for viral hepatitis, alpha-fetoprotein (AFP), carcinoembryonic antigen (CEA), carbohydrate antigen 19-9 (CA19-9), and imaging studies with tumor characterization are part of the initial diagnostic workup.

In particular, imaging tests have a pivotal role in the diagnostic process. Differently from any other cancer entity, the diagnosis of HCC can be made based only on imaging if the hallmarks of HCC are present: arterial phase hyperenhancement (APHE), with washout in the portal venous or delayed phases on CT and MRI, using extracellular contrast agents or gadobenate dimeglumine; APHE with washout in the portal venous phase on MRI using gadoxetic acid; and APHE with late-onset (>60 s) washout of mild intensity on CEUS [9]. In the context of compensated advanced chronic liver disease (cACLD) and in the absence of non-invasive criteria, a liver tumor has the same probability of being either HCC or iCCA, and a liver biopsy (LB) is mandatory for a definite diagnosis [10]. Among the different HCC histological subtypes, steatohepatitic HCC, scirrhous HCC, and the macrotrabecular massive HCC do not display typical HCC features on imaging [11]. In the clinical context of a patient with cACLD, one should rarely consider a secondary liver tumor, since this situation is infrequent in clinical practice. According to one metanalysis, only 1.7% of liver masses from 1453 cirrhotic livers were metastases [12]. One should, however, bear in mind the possibility of the association between non-Hodgkin B-cell lymphoma and hepatitis C virus infection [13]. On the other hand, when cACLD is not present, a liver nodule has the same chance of being an HCC, an iCCA, or a secondary tumor. Clinical data and imaging tools can be helpful in this setting, but the final diagnosis relies on LB. For example, a prior history of malignant disease in a patient with liver nodules might hint at secondary tumors, or sectional imaging might incidentally reveal the presence of the primary tumor, and depending on the location, endoscopy might confirm the final diagnosis.

As seen above, LB is necessary in some clinical scenarios. However, assessing whether a LB is necessary in a case-by-case manner is essential, given that it is an invasive procedure that exposes the patient to risks such as bleeding and seeding [14]. LB only offers a small tumor fragment, while pressuring the pathologist to extract maximal information. Differential diagnosis between iCCA, HCC, and liver metastases is sometimes not straightforward. Moreover, discriminating between the three types of tumor using only the basic hematoxylin and eosin (H&E) stain can be difficult. One can perform a limited number of immunohistochemical stains on such a small sample. Therefore, it is vital to know the complete clinical history and only afterward choose the correct immunohistochemical markers. Moreover, the immunohistochemical spectrum has tremendous potential for clinical practice, since multiple markers can have diagnostic, theranostic, or prognostic power. Nevertheless, prognostic biomarkers in liver cancer are a necessity. Current iCCA prognostic predictors include large tumor size (tumor > 5 cm, as stated in the current 8th edition of the AJCC staging system), multiple tumors, vascular invasion, perineural infiltration, and positive regional lymph nodes (N1) [15,16]. However, the evidence supporting these predictors is not unanimous, as not all authors reached a consensus in extensive multicentric studies. One striking example is related to tumor size, which was associated with survival only in univariate analysis in a large multi-institutional study that included 449 iCCA resection specimens. This correlation was not maintained in the multivariate regression model [17]. Some immunohistochemical markers already used in daily practice to diagnose HCC or iCCA might also have prognostic potential.

Therefore, our primary aim was to investigate which markers can aid the discrimination between the three entities, based on the experience of a tertiary hepatobiliary healthcare facility. Our second aim was to investigate whether certain immunohistochemical stains have a prognostic role correlating with patient survival and whether other readily-available pathological parameters could represent prognostic markers for iCCA or HCC.

2. Materials and Methods

2.1. Case Selection

Three Caucasian cohorts, including a matching number of cases ($n = 65$) with pathologic diagnosis of iCCA (group 1), HCC (group 2), and metastatic hepatic tumors (group 3), established with a needle biopsy performed during 2014–2021 were retrospectively selected from the hospital's database. Groups 1 and 2 only included patients with advanced, unresectable tumors. We decided to only include patients with advanced HCC or iCCA because (a) we rarely perform LB in patients with resectable HCC or iCCA at our center; (b) the majority of iCCA are diagnosed at an advanced stage, and we decided to compare them with advanced HCC (and not with early HCC) and, therefore, to avoid potential bias; and (c) the patients with liver metastases were already at an advanced stage, and therefore we wanted to avoid further bias. Clinical data and imaging studies were further analyzed for each patient, to ensure correct assignment to the study groups. Alive/dead status and the date of death were obtained in December 2022, and overall survival (OS) (from initial diagnosis until death) was determined. For the patients in group 3, an additional survival period (from the secondary hepatic tumor diagnosis to the time of death) was calculated. Data from patients alive at the end of follow-up were censored in the statistical analysis. In total, 15 patients were excluded: six patients with metachronous iCCA and HCC, two patients with combined hepatocellular–cholangiocarcinoma, and seven cases where the diagnosis was established without the use of immunohistochemical stains.

2.2. Data Gathering and Interpretation of Pathology Slides

Clinical, laboratory, and imaging characteristics were recorded for each case. They included general demographic parameters, relevant clinical characteristics, associated diseases, nonspecific serum tumoral markers, number of tumors (solitary or multifocal), and tumor size. The pathological parameters available in small biopsies were as follows: final diagnosis (iCCA, HCC, or histologic type of metastasis along with primary site), tumor differentiation (well, moderate, or weak), and intratumoral immune infiltrate (absent, weak, moderate, or abundant). The immunohistochemical stains used for diagnostic purposes were performed on 3 μm tissue sections, using completely automated systems (Leica Bond-Max Immunostainer; Leica Biosystems, Nussloch, Germany), according to the manufacturer's instructions. Two pathologists reevaluated all slides blind to the clinical data, to ensure uniformity of stain intensity interpretation. Stains were scored using a four-tier system: negative, weakly positive, medium positive, and intensely positive. Pathologists requested all immunohistochemical stains made during the initial case evaluation, for diagnostic purposes.

2.3. Statistical Analysis

Categorical data were presented as counts and percentages. Comparisons of categorical data were performed using a Chi-square or Fisher's exact test in case of low expected frequencies. Continuous normally distributed data were reported as means and standard deviations, and skewed data as medians and quartiles. Comparisons of continuous skewed data were performed with a Wilcoxon rank sum test. Spearman's correlation coefficient and its associated statistical test assessed the correlation between continuous skewed data. The OS was defined as the time from diagnosis until death or the study end date (December 2022). Survival data were graphically presented using the Kaplan–Meier method. Univariate proportional Cox regression verified the relationship between various immunohistochemical markers and survival. To confirm that these relations were not spurious, we further added known predictors of survival as adjustment variables in the multivariate Cox regression models. The proportional hazard assumption was checked with a formal statistical test for all these models, while the linear functional form for continuous variables was checked using model residual plot inspection. For multivariate models, multicollinearity was assessed with variance inflation factors. The two-tailed p-value was computed for all statistical tests, and the results were considered statistically significant for values below 0.05. All analyses were computed using the R environment for statistical computing and graphics (R Foundation for Statistical Computing, Vienna, Austria), version 3.6.3, R Core Team. R: A Language and Environment for Statistical Computing (Internet), Vienna, Austria; 2019.

2.4. Ethics Committee

Approvals from the Ethics Committees of both "Iuliu Hațieganu" University of Medicine and Pharmacy (34/13 December 2021) and "Octavian Fodor" Regional Institute of Gastroenterology and Hepatology (165/9 December 2021) were obtained. All biopsies analyzed in this study were performed for diagnostic purposes; consequently, patient consent was waived.

3. Results

3.1. General Findings

A total of 195 patients were included in the study. The baseline patient characteristics are depicted in Table 1.

Table 1. Baseline characteristics of the study population.

Patient Characteristics	Intrahepatic Cholangiocarcinoma	Hepatocellular Carcinoma	Liver Secondary Tumors	p Value
Number of patients	65	65	65	ns
Clinical parameters				
Age				
Mean ± SD	64.42 ± 9.23	65.57 ± 6.49	63.06 ± 9.78	ns
Range	41–84	51–80	39–85	
Sex, n (%)				
Male	34 (52.3)	50 (76.92)	31 (47.69)	ns
Female	31 (47.69)	15 (23.08)	34 (52.3)	
Environment, n (%)				
Urban	35 (53.85)	45 (69.23)	50 (76.92)	0.0013
Rural	30 (46.15)	20 (30.77)	15 (23.08)	
Associated diseases, n (%)				
Obesity	6 (9.23)	8 (12.3)	9 (13.84)	ns
Diabetes mellitus	13 (20)	15 (23.07)	13 (20)	ns
Liver steatosis	16 (24.61)	15 (23.07)	13 (20)	ns
Chronic Hepatitis				
HBV	7 (10.77)	11 (16.92)	1 (1.53)	0.01
HCV	10 (15.38)	31 (47.69)	2 (3.07)	<0.001
Alcohol abuse	3 (4.61)	15 (23.07)	3 (4.61)	<0.001
Liver cirrhosis	12 (18.46)	53 (81.53)	4 (61.53)	<0.001
Ethanolic	3 (4.61)	14 (21.53)	1 (1.53)	<0.001
HBV	3 (4.61)	8 (12.3)	-	nc
HCV	5 (7.69)	29 (44.61)	1 (1.53)	<0.001
Autoimmune	1 (1.53)	-	-	ns
Metabolic	-	1 (1.53)	-	nc

Table 1. Cont.

Patient Characteristics		Intrahepatic Cholangiocarcinoma	Hepatocellular Carcinoma	Liver Secondary Tumors	p Value
	Idiopathic	1 (1.53)	3 (4.61)	1 (1.53)	nc
Overall survival (months)					
	Mean ± SD	9.25 ± 9.65	31.22 ± 24.9	31.85 ± 44.47	<0.001
	Range	0.1–38.66	0.16–84	0.5–192	
Serum tumoral markers					
	AFP	72.59 ± 139.51	95.74 ± 151.93	24.84 ± 90.93	nc
	CEA	8.84 ± 13.32	3.65 ± 4.02	40.64 ± 58.23	nc
	CA 19-9	202.14 ± 162.71	98.36 ± 95.12	146.84 ± 170.3	nc
Morphologic parameters					
Tumor size (cm)					
	Mean ± SD	8.05 ± 3.58	5.45 ± 4.11	4.86 ± 3.81	<0.001
	Range	0.6–16	1.3–19	0.5–18	
Number of tumors, n (%)					
	Solitary	26 (40)	28 (43.07)	5 (7.7)	<0.001
	Multiple	39 (60)	37 (56.92)	60 (92.3)	
Tumor differentiation, n (%)					
	Good	12 (18.46)	6 (9.24)	16 (24.61)	<0.001
	Moderate	23 (35.38)	45 (69.24)	17 (26.16)	
	Poor	15 (23.07)	3 (4.62)	8 (12.31)	
	N/A	14 (21.53)	11 (16.9)	24 (36.92)	
Tumor infiltrating lymphocytes count, n (%)					
	Low	38 (58.46)	26 (40)	23 (35.38)	<0.001
	Moderate	17 (26.15)	5 (7.69)	13 (20)	
	Abundant	0	1 (1.54)	1 (1.54)	
	Absent	3 (4.62)	0	0	
	N/A	7 (10.77)	33 (50.77)	28 (43.08)	
Number of immunohistochemical stains used (Mean ± SD)		8 ± 3	4 ± 1.67	6 ± 3.62	nc

nc = not calculated due to low sample size, ns = not significant.

Most patients with metastatic liver disease (group 3) had multifocal lesions (92.3%). This was also the case in primary tumors, since more than half (60% iCCAs and 56.92% HCCs) had multiple tumors. Liver metastases originated from the following primary tumors (in descending order): colorectal carcinomas (25 cases, 38.45%), neuroendocrine carcinomas (10 cases, 15.38% with pancreatic, pulmonary or unassigned primary location), pancreatic ductal adenocarcinomas (9 cases, 13.85%), invasive breast carcinomas (7 cases, 10.78%), and gastric adenocarcinomas (3 cases, 4.61%).

3.2. Immunohistochemical Markers Expressed in HCC, iCCA, and Liver Metastases

The most relevant antibodies for iCCA were CK19, CA19-9, CK7, and CEA; the corresponding sensitivity of each marker was 100%, 100%, 93.7%, and 82.6%, respectively. The most relevant antibodies for HCC were Glypican 3, CD34 (with sinusoidal pattern), and Hep Par 1; the corresponding sensitivity of each marker was 100%, 100%, and 98.2%, respectively. One case with iCCA tested positive for Hep Par 1 (low intensity), and one iCCA tested positive for Gypican 3 (low intensity). Three cases with iCCA expressed CD34 but none showed a sinusoidal pattern. Four cases from the iCCA group were CK20-positive, but three of the four only expressed a weak intensity, while the other expressed a moderate intensity. From the HCC cohort, only one case was positive for CK7 (weak intensity), and three cases were CK19-positive, all with weak intensity.

The most used markers in liver metastases were CDX2, CK7, CK20, and CK AE1/AE3. No case from the liver metastases group tested positive for Hep Par 1 or Glypican 3. Four cases from iCCA were CK20-positive (three of four cases showed weak intensity and one moderate intensity). In the iCCA group, 11 cases tested positive for CDX2, while ten had weak intensity and only one had moderate intensity. The most important and highly expressed immunohistochemical markers in each cancer entity (HCC, iCCA, and liver metastases) are depicted in Table 2.

Table 2. The most common immunohistochemistry markers expressed in the different types of liver cancer.

Marker	iCCA	HCC	Liver Metastases	p Value
CK7, n (%) *	59 (93.7)	1 (14.3)	25 (80.6)	<0.001
CK19, n (%)	43 (100)	3 (37.5)	6 (54.5)	<0.001
CEA, n (%)	19 (82.6)	4 (44.4)	5 (50)	<0.001
CA19-9, n (%)	9 (100)	0	6 (100)	<0.001
Hep Par 1, n (%)	1 (3.3)	55 (98.2)	0	<0.001
Glypican 3, n (%)	1 (16.7)	44 (100)	0	<0.001
CD34, n (%)	3 (37.5)	54 (100)	0	<0.001
CDX2, n (%)	12 (28.6)	0	36 (94.7)	<0.001
CK20, n (%)	4 (9.8%)	0	18 (94.7)	<0.001

In blue—the most frequently expressed markers in intrahepatic cholangiocarcinoma; in red—the most frequently expressed markers in hepatocellular carcinoma; in green—the most frequently expressed markers in liver metastases from colorectal carcinoma; HCC = hepatocellular carcinoma, iCCA = intrahepatic cholangiocarcinoma; n = number, % = per cent; p = level of significance, CK = cytokeratin; CA = carcinogenic antigen; CEA = carcinoembryonic antigen; CD = cluster of differentiation; * a marker expressed in both iCCA and liver metastases from colorectal carcinoma.

3.3. Prognostic Markers of iCCA

The subsequent focus was to identify histological or immunohistochemical-based prognostic biomarkers. We first compared the OS between the two most frequent primary liver cancers. As shown in Figure 1, patients diagnosed with iCCA had a strikingly lower OS than HCC patients (months, interquartile range): 38.1 (27.81–52.19), 18.31 (10.58–31.69), 7.12 (2.54–19.97), and 3.56 (0.63–20.03) for the iCCA group; compared to 79.91 (70.72–90.3), 73.25 (63.11–85.03), 57.85 (46.67–71.72), and 43.2 (31.77–58.76) for the HCC group at 12, 24, 36, and 48 months, respectively, $p < 0.001$ (log-rank test).

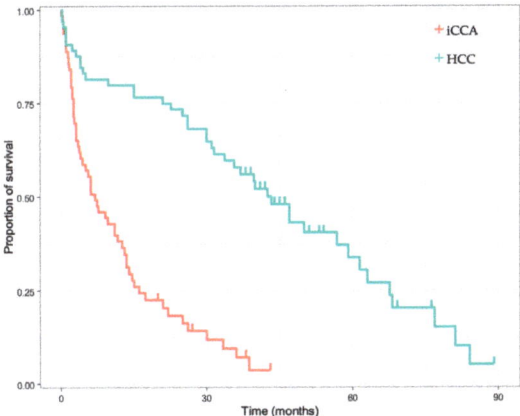

Figure 1. Kaplan–Meier survival analysis regarding the pathology-confirmed diagnosis of intrahepatic cholangiocarcinoma (iCCA) versus hepatocellular carcinoma (HCC); $p < 0.001$ (log-rank test).

Next, we performed a univariate analysis, to search for prognostic biomarkers. Among the multiple biomarkers included in the analyses (tumor size, age, tumor number, tumor differentiation, tumor size, presence of cirrhosis, CDX2, CK19, CK7, pCEA, mCEA, CA19-9), only CK7 (Figure 2) and the presence of immune cell infiltrates (Figure 3) were correlated with OS ($p = 0.016$, $p = 0.0028$). Furthermore, both moderate/intense CK7 positivity and absence/low amount of immune cell infiltrate remained as positive prognostic biomarkers in the multivariate analysis (Table 3).

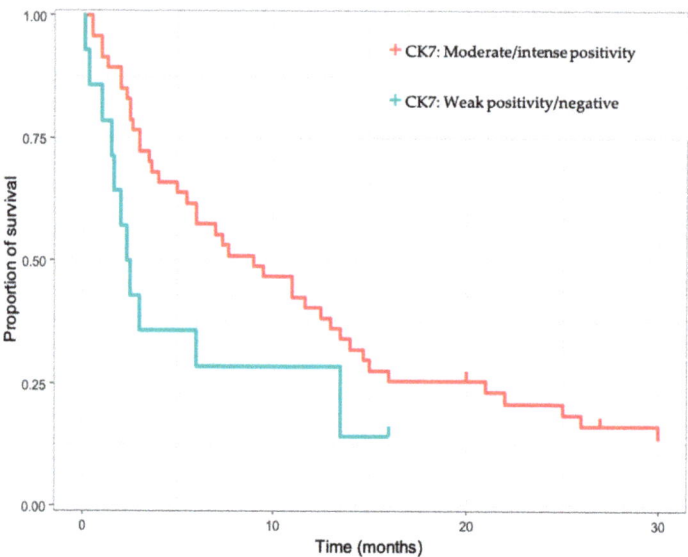

Figure 2. Kaplan–Meier survival analysis for intrahepatic cholangiocarcinoma (iCCA) cases, regarding CK7 immunoexpression.

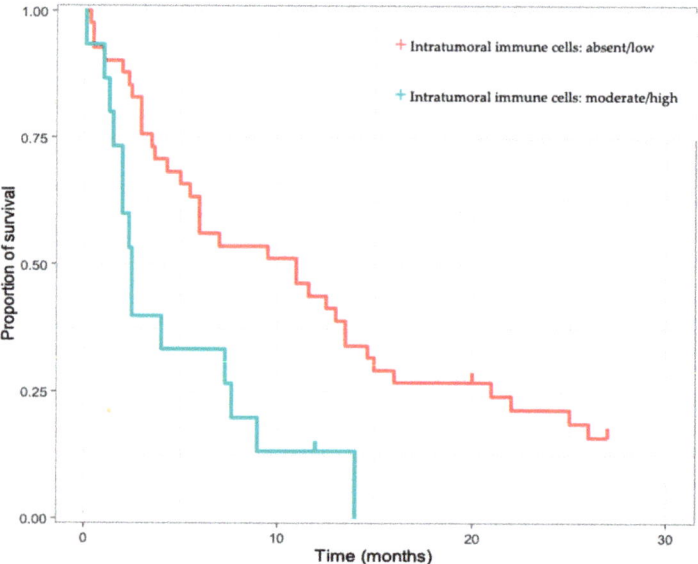

Figure 3. Kaplan–Meier survival analysis for intrahepatic cholangiocarcinoma (iCCA) cases based on the amount of intratumoral immune cells.

Table 3. Univariate and multivariate analysis of overall survival in intrahepatic cholangiocarcinoma (iCCA) patients.

OS	Univariate Analysis			Multivariate Analysis		
	HR	95% CI	p	HR	95% CI	p
Age	0.97	0.94–1	0.076			
Tumor number (multiple vs. single)	1.42	0.82–2.46	0.208			
Liver cirrhosis (yes vs. no)	0.93	0.46–1.85	0.828			
Immune cell infiltrate (yes vs. no) *	2.68	1.38–5.2	0.004	3.64	1.67–7.9	0.001
Tumor differentiation **	1.11	0.56–2.18	0.771			
CDX2 (positive vs. negative)	1.84	0.88–3.85	0.108			
CK7 negative (yes vs. no) ***	1.82	0.92–3.6	0.087	2.42	1.1–5.33	0.028
CK19 negative (yes vs. no) #	0.48	0.22–1.03	0.06			

* we compared intense and moderate with low or negative; ** we compared well-differentiated with moderate and poor differentiation; *** patients CK7-negative or with a weak staining were compared with moderate or intense staining; # patients CK19-negative or with a weak staining were compared with moderate or intense staining; p = level of significance; CI = confidence interval; HR = hazard ratio.

3.4. Prognostic Markers of HCC

The subsequent focus was to identify histological- or immunohistochemical-based prognostic markers. Therefore, we performed an univariate analysis. None of the multiple biomarkers included in the analyses (age, tumor number, intratumoral lymphocytes, liver cirrhosis, Hep Par 1, CD34, Glypican 3) reached statistical significance (p = 0.68, p = 0.22, p = 0.54, p = 0.60, p = 0.68, p = 0.79, and p = 0.53, respectively).

4. Discussion

4.1. Diagnostic Perspectives

4.1.1. iCCA vs. HCC

Hepatocyte paraffin 1 (Hep Par 1) demonstrates the hepatocellular origin of tumor cells, dyes normal and neoplastic hepatocytes, and should be considered positive in cytoplasmic, diffuse, granular staining. Both the sensitivity and specificity of Hep Par 1 exceed 90% [18,19]. Similarly to in our study, where one iCCA case showed weak Hep Par 1 positivity, other authors reported Hep Par 1 positivity in small subsets of cholangiocarcinomas [18,19]. These data suggest that diagnosis of cholangiocarcinoma should not be ruled out solely based on Hep Par 1 positivity but it is highly unlikely in cases with high-intensity staining. Conversely, poorly differentiated HCCs can lose Hep Par 1 expression [20]. Moreover, small HCC needle biopsies can result in false-negative interpretations due to discontinuous staining. Hep Par 1 can show positivity in scarce hepatoid variants of gastrointestinal and pancreatic adenocarcinomas [21]. Our series had no Hep Par 1-positive cases among the metastatic tumors.

Glypican 3 is highly expressed in embryonal tissue and should be considered positive in cases with strong and diffuse cytoplasmic staining, with or without membranous staining. The sensitivity ranges between 53% and 100% in resection specimens with low values for well-differentiated HCCs, but percentages reach 100% in poorly differentiated tumors [22]. This particularity confers Glypican 3 a substantial discriminative value in poorly differentiated HCCs, since Hep Par 1 frequently loses expression in these scenarios. Sensitivity is lower in needle biopsies [23] and the specificity is also low, since Glypican 3 marks other hepatic or extrahepatic tumors, such as hepatoblastomas, ovarian clear cell carcinomas, testicular yolk sac tumors, choriocarcinomas, and specific subsets of melanomas and lung squamous cell carcinomas [24]. Glypican 3 discriminates well between HCC and cholangiocarcinoma (intrahepatic and extrahepatic), since its expression is downregulated in the latter [25]. In our study, all HCC cases (irrespective of their histologic differentiation) were Glypican 3-positive, while only one iCCA case showed weak Glypican 3 positivity.

CD34 marks sinusoidal capillarization in HCC, with uniform intensity and distribution, while normal sinusoidal endothelial cells are CD34-negative. In our study, all HCC cases demonstrated CD34 positivity with a sinusoidal pattern. Three iCCA cases were positive for CD34. Nevertheless, none showed a sinusoidal pattern.

Cytokeratin 7 (CK7) and Cytokeratin 20 (CK20) display various patterns in the epithelia throughout the human body. Hence pathologists frequently describe them in conjunction. CK7 is expressed in normal bile duct epithelia but not in hepatocytes. CK20 shows a variable expression, generally positive in extrahepatic bile duct tumors, including gall bladder carcinoma, but negative in both HCC and iCCA [26]. Our findings were in accordance with this. CK7 was utilized in 96.92% of iCCA cases, among which 59 cases (93.65%) were positive, while four cases (6.77%) were CK7-negative. A single HCC case was CK7-positive but showed weak intensity. CK20 was utilized in 41 iCCA cases (63.07%). Among these, only four cases (9.75%) were CK20-positive, showing a weak intensity in three cases and moderate intensity in one case.

Cytokeratin 19 (CK19) stains bile ducts in cirrhotic nodules and is generally CK19-negative in HCC. In a study by Durnez et al., 16% of HCC cases were CK19-positive [27]. In our study, three cases from the HCC group stained positive for CK19, all showing weak intensity.

Polyclonal carcinoembryonic antigen (pCEA) displays a canalicular staining pattern in HCC, with a sensitivity ranging between 50 and 96%, with higher percentages in well- and moderately differentiated tumors. However, it shows a diffuse cytoplasmic and luminal pattern in iCCA and part of metastatic tumors [26,28]. Monoclonal carcinoembryonic antigen (mCEA) is usually positive in iCCA and negative in HCC [29]. We analyzed pCEA in 23 iCCA cases, among which 19 (82.61%) were positive.

Although not an immunohistochemical stain, Alcian blue can aid in distinguishing poorly differentiated HCC from iCCA, by highlighting mucus secretion within the cytoplasm of tumoral cells and thus confirming a glandular phenotype in the latter, but not in HCC [30].

4.1.2. iCCA vs. Metastatic Tumors

In the metastatic tumor group, immunoassays were requested in concordance with existing clinical data, pursuing tissue-specific markers.

CDX2 is a transcription factor expressed in the small intestine and colon. It stains normal intestinal epithelium, hyperplastic colonic polyps [31], and colorectal adenocarcinoma. Consequently, it is the first choice and sometimes the only immunostaining required to confirm the clinical diagnosis, but it is a highly non-specific marker for colorectal adenocarcinoma. CDX2 marks 86–100% [32] well- and moderately-differentiated colorectal adenocarcinomas but is also immune-positive in intestinal metaplasia, wherever it occurs. Therefore, it can serve as a marker for intestinal differentiation. However, there is evidence that CDX2 is positive in subgroups of ovarian mucinous adenocarcinomas; 30% of cervical mucinous adenocarcinomas [33]; small intestine carcinoma; 36–70% of gastric adenocarcinomas, including signet ring cell adenocarcinomas, urothelial carcinoma, and pancreatic [34], ileal, and appendicular neuroendocrine tumors. CDX2 also stains over one-third (37.3%) of eCCAs and gall bladder carcinomas [35]. Thus, CDX2 is considered less specific than the CK7-negative/CK20-positive panel for colorectal carcinoma [36]. In our study, CDX2 was performed in 42 iCCA cases (64.61%), among which 11 cases (26.19%) were CDX2-positive. However, 10 out of 11 cases showed weak positivity, and one showed moderate positivity. In group 3, CDX2 staining was performed in all metastases with colorectal primaries. All cases (n = 25) showed CDX2 positivity. Among these, 24 cases demonstrated moderate- and high-intensity staining, while only one showed weak CDX2 staining. Among the pancreatic ductal adenocarcinoma cases, 71.42% demonstrated weak CDX2 positivity (80%) or moderate CDX2 positivity (20%).

A major shortcoming is the lack of reliable biomarkers for distinguishing iCCA from gastric and pancreatic adenocarcinomas and between iCCA, eCCA, and gall bladder carcinomas. Indeed some markers are undergoing evaluation [37,38] but have yet to reach clinical practice. Until then, the clinical context and the proper use of paraclinical tools are crucial. For instance, when discriminating between iCCA and gastric cancer, the epistemologically sound approach should always include an upper gastrointestinal endoscopy to settle diagnostic doubts. Following the same rationale, discriminating between iCCA and pancreatic adenocarcinoma should, at least in theory, be facilitated by imaging tools to pinpoint the primary tumor.

Finally, if the immune profile is extremely ambiguous or inconclusive, we recommend returning to the H&E morphology.

4.2. Prognostic Perspectives

Our results confirmed that advanced iCCA has a worse prognosis when compared to advanced HCC, which is concordant with existing literature data. This statement further reinforces the importance of accurate early diagnosis. Several studies have focused on identifying biomarkers for iCCA patients using various omics methods [39]. However, little attention, if any, has been given to developing immunohistochemical-based biomarkers for the prognoses that are already available in clinical practice and with which the pathologist has had time to familiarize. A meta-analysis that evaluated 77 different proteins within 73 research studies listed five immunohistochemical markers associated with patient outcome: EGFR, MUC1, MUC4, p27, and fascein [40]. Among these, only MUC1 (also known as EMA) has entered routine practice and promises to ensure reproducibility in large case series.

A recent study conducted by He et al. demonstrated a significant association between the post-surgery survival of iCCA patients and two immunohistochemical markers: while SATB1 indicated poor survival (median survival of 122 days vs. 347 days in SATB1-negative cases, $p = 0.04$), Villin-positive cases were associated with better OS, with direct correlation with Villin intensity ($p = 0.002$). This study recommended CK7 assessment in iCCA cases, since it was negatively correlated with lymphatic metastasis in their case series [41]. An interesting study conducted by Yeh et al. in Taipei validated C-reactive protein (CRP) as a highly performant diagnostic marker for iCCA, with a 93.3% sensitivity and an 88.2% specificity. CRP also correlated with better OS ($p = 0.002$) and longer postoperative recurrence-free time ($p = 0.032$) [42].

Our study showed that CK7-positive iCCA patients had a better OS. Until now, only one study has evaluated the prognostic potential of CK7 and CK19 in surgically resected iCCA patients. Based on the mARN levels of both CK7 and CK19, the authors showed that the CK7-positive/CK19-positive index was an independent adverse prognostic factor for survival in iCCA [43]. In addition, our study has shown that the presence of intratumoral immune cells bears a negative prognostic significance. While the results from this dataset appear to contrast with a previously published report from our study group, in which PD-L1-positive intratumoral cells had a positive predictive impact, the difference is more nuanced and resides in PD-L1 staining, the types of immune cell studied, and population selection (early vs. advanced disease) [44]. For a further expansion on this topic, one systematic review discussed the discrepancy between intratumoral immune cells and the prognosis of iCCA patients (some studies describe intratumoral immune cells as positive prognostic markers, while others as negative prognostic markers) [45]. The type of lymphocytes infiltrating iCCA is also important: Dong Liu et al. compared CD8-positive with Foxp3-positive lymphocytes, the latter having a positive prognostic value [45]. We did not evaluate the type of intratumoral lymphocytes in our study. However, our findings are significant, since tumor-infiltrating lymphocytes might correlate with the response to durvalumab, a checkpoint inhibitor recently approved for the systemic treatment of iCCA, based on a presumption extrapolated from HCC [46].

Our study has several limitations. First, it was a retrospective study, with all the limitations derived from this. The study only included advanced epithelial primary liver tumors and did not analyze other malignant liver tumors, such as hemangioendothelioma, lymphoma, or angiosarcoma. However, the three entities included represent the vast majority of those encountered in daily clinical practice. Second, we analyzed only the immunohistochemical markers routinely used for diagnostic purposes; therefore, other prognostic markers frequently analyzed in experimental settings could not be assessed. Third, a thorough analysis of the tumoral microenvironment was not an essential step in the study design. Hence, the reporting on tumor-infiltrating immune cells should be interpreted cautiously, since this represents only a quantitative estimate, with no in-depth reporting on the type of cells and expression.

Nonetheless, despite all the limitations, some important conclusions can be made. First, for a definite diagnosis, knowing the clinical context of each patient is mandatory. None of the immunohistochemical markers evaluated in our study showed a perfect delineation between the three cancer entities, and therefore one should only perform a LB when necessary. In some situations, LB is unnecessary (e.g., liver nodule with typical HCC features on imaging), while in others LB is not feasible (e.g., small tumors or tumors located in segment VI or VIII) [47]. Moreover, LB is an invasive procedure, which poses non-negligible risks, despite an overall safe profile [48]. Last, LB offers a limited tissue fragment, so one should maximize the amount of data extracted from it. Unfortunately, a biopsy cannot be repeated ad libitum, and the number of immunohistochemical stains per fragment is finite. Therefore, using a panel of carefully selected immunohistochemical markers can facilitate a less expensive and laborious final diagnosis.

5. Conclusions

Immunohistochemical stains should be assessed, first and foremost, in conjunction with morphology and clinical data. Nothing is black and white in microscopy, and immunohistochemistry is no exception. In liver tumors, as in other sites, immuno-histochemical panels remain superior to single colorations. Furthermore, apart from diagnosis, immunohistochemical studies can also provide prognostic information. Lastly, we strongly recommend mentioning both the presence and the amount of intratumoral immune infiltrate in routine pathologic reports.

Author Contributions: Conceptualization, L.P.M. and C.M.M.; methodology, L.P.M., I.R. and B.A.B.; software, T.M.; validation, I.R. and B.A.B.; formal analysis, L.P.M., T.M. and M.I.; investigation, L.P.M. and M.I.; resources, L.P.M., T.M. and Z.S.; data curation, L.P.M., I.R. and C.S.M.; writing—original draft preparation, L.P.M., M.I., R.C., T.M. and C.S.M.; writing—review and editing, C.M.M., T.M., R.C. and B.A.B.; visualization, L.P.M.; supervision, C.M.M. and Z.S. All authors have read and agreed to the published version of the manuscript.

Funding: This research received no external funding.

Institutional Review Board Statement: The study was conducted in accordance with the Declaration of Helsinki, and approved by the Ethics Committee of both "Iuliu Hatieganu" University of Medicine and Pharmacy (protocol code 34, date of approval 13 December 2021) and "Octavian Fodor" Regional Institute of Gastroenterology and Hepatology (protocol code 165, date of approval 9 December 2021).

Informed Consent Statement: Patient consent was waived because the material used in this study was obtained for diagnostic purposes.

Data Availability Statement: The data presented in this study are available on request from the corresponding author.

Conflicts of Interest: The authors declare no conflict of interest.

References

1. Shaib, Y.; El-Serag, H. The Epidemiology of Cholangiocarcinoma. *Semin. Liver Dis.* **2004**, *24*, 115–125. [CrossRef] [PubMed]
2. WHO Classification of Tumours Editorial Board. *Digestive System Tumours, WHO Classification of Tumours*, 5th ed.; World Health Organization: Lyon, France; IARC Publications: Lyon, France, 2019; ISBN 978-92-832-4499-8.
3. Saha, S.K.; Zhu, A.X.; Fuchs, C.S.; Brooks, G.A. Forty-Year Trends in Cholangiocarcinoma Incidence in the U.S.: Intrahepatic Disease on the Rise. *Oncologist* **2016**, *21*, 594–599. [CrossRef] [PubMed]
4. Mukkamalla, S.K.R.; Naseri, H.M.; Kim, B.M.; Katz, S.C.; Armenio, V.A. Trends in Incidence and Factors Affecting Survival of Patients with Cholangiocarcinoma in the United States. *J. Natl. Compr. Cancer Netw.* **2018**, *16*, 370–376. [CrossRef] [PubMed]
5. Tyson, G.L.; El-Serag, H.B. Risk Factors for Cholangiocarcinoma. *Hepatology* **2011**, *54*, 173–184. [CrossRef] [PubMed]

6. Shaib, Y.H.; El-Serag, H.B.; Nooka, A.K.; Thomas, M.; Brown, T.D.; Patt, Y.Z.; Hassan, M.M. Risk Factors for Intrahepatic and Extrahepatic Cholangiocarcinoma: A Hospital-Based Case?Control Study. *Am. J. Gastroenterol.* **2007**, *102*, 1016–1021. [CrossRef]
7. Wongjarupong, N.; Assavapongpaiboon, B.; Susantitaphong, P.; Cheungpasitporn, W.; Treeprasertsuk, S.; Rerknimitr, R.; Chaiteerakij, R. Non-Alcoholic Fatty Liver Disease as a Risk Factor for Cholangiocarcinoma: A Systematic Review and Meta-Analysis. *BMC Gastroenterol.* **2017**, *17*, 149. [CrossRef]
8. Welzel, T.M.; Graubard, B.I.; El-Serag, H.B.; Shaib, Y.H.; Hsing, A.W.; Davila, J.A.; McGlynn, K.A. Risk Factors for Intrahepatic and Extrahepatic Cholangiocarcinoma in the United States: A Population-Based Case-Control Study. *Clin. Gastroenterol. Hepatol.* **2007**, *5*, 1221–1228. [CrossRef]
9. Galle, P.R.; Forner, A.; Llovet, J.M.; Mazzaferro, V.; Piscaglia, F.; Raoul, J.-L.; Schirmacher, P.; Vilgrain, V. EASL Clinical Practice Guidelines: Management of Hepatocellular Carcinoma. *J. Hepatol.* **2018**, *69*, 182–236. [CrossRef]
10. Marrero, J.A.; Kulik, L.M.; Sirlin, C.B.; Zhu, A.X.; Finn, R.S.; Abecassis, M.M.; Roberts, L.R.; Heimbach, J.K. Diagnosis, Staging, and Management of Hepatocellular Carcinoma: 2018 Practice Guidance by the American Association for the Study of Liver Diseases. *Hepatology* **2018**, *68*, 723–750. [CrossRef]
11. State-of-the-Art Review on the Correlations between Pathological and Magnetic Resonance Features of Cirrhotic Nodules. *Histol. Histopathol.* **2022**, *37*, 1151–1165. [CrossRef]
12. Mahdi, Z.; Ettel, M.G.; Gonzalez, R.S.; Hart, J.; Alpert, L.; Fang, J.; Liu, N.; Hammer, S.T.; Panarelli, N.; Cheng, J.; et al. Metastases Can Occur in Cirrhotic Livers with Patent Portal Veins. *Diagn. Pathol.* **2021**, *16*, 18. [CrossRef] [PubMed]
13. Ronot, M.; Burgio, M.D.; Purcell, Y.; Pommier, R.; Brancatelli, G.; Vilgrain, V. Focal Lesions in Cirrhosis: Not Always HCC. *Eur. J. Radiol.* **2017**, *93*, 157–168. [CrossRef] [PubMed]
14. Sparchez, Z.; Mocan, T.; Hagiu, C.; Kacso, G.; Zaharie, T.; Rusu, I.; Al Hajjar, N.; Leucuta, D.C.; Sparchez, M. Real-Time Contrast-Enhanced–Guided Biopsy Compared with Conventional Ultrasound–Guided Biopsy in the Diagnosis of Hepatic Tumors on a Background of Advanced Chronic Liver Disease: A Prospective, Randomized, Clinical Trial. *Ultrasound Med. Biol.* **2019**, *45*, 2915–2924. [CrossRef]
15. Endo, I.; Gonen, M.; Yopp, A.C.; Dalal, K.M.; Zhou, Q.; Klimstra, D.; D'Angelica, M.; DeMatteo, R.P.; Fong, Y.; Schwartz, L.; et al. Intrahepatic Cholangiocarcinoma: Rising Frequency, Improved Survival, and Determinants of Outcome After Resection. *Ann. Surg.* **2008**, *248*, 84–96. [CrossRef]
16. Fisher, S.B.; Patel, S.H.; Kooby, D.A.; Weber, S.; Bloomston, M.; Cho, C.; Hatzaras, I.; Schmidt, C.; Winslow, E.; Staley, C.A.; et al. Lymphovascular and Perineural Invasion as Selection Criteria for Adjuvant Therapy in Intrahepatic Cholangiocarcinoma: A Multi-Institution Analysis. *HPB* **2012**, *14*, 514–522. [CrossRef] [PubMed]
17. de Jong, M.C.; Nathan, H.; Sotiropoulos, G.C.; Paul, A.; Alexandrescu, S.; Marques, H.; Pulitano, C.; Barroso, E.; Clary, B.M.; Aldrighetti, L.; et al. Intrahepatic Cholangiocarcinoma: An International Multi-Institutional Analysis of Prognostic Factors and Lymph Node Assessment. *JCO* **2011**, *29*, 3140–3145. [CrossRef]
18. Chu, P.G.; Ishizawa, S.; Wu, E.; Weiss, L.M. Hepatocyte Antigen as a Marker of Hepatocellular Carcinoma: An Immunohistochemical Comparison to Carcinoembryonic Antigen, CD10, and Alpha-Fetoprotein. *Am. J. Surg. Pathol.* **2002**, *26*, 978–988. [CrossRef] [PubMed]
19. Fan, Z.; van de Rijn, M.; Montgomery, K.; Rouse, R.V. Hep Par 1 Antibody Stain for the Differential Diagnosis of Hepatocellular Carcinoma: 676 Tumors Tested Using Tissue Microarrays and Conventional Tissue Sections. *Mod. Pathol.* **2003**, *16*, 137–144. [CrossRef]
20. Butler, S.L.; Dong, H.; Cardona, D.; Jia, M.; Zheng, R.; Zhu, H.; Crawford, J.M.; Liu, C. The Antigen for Hep Par 1 Antibody Is the Urea Cycle Enzyme Carbamoyl Phosphate Synthetase 1. *Lab. Investig.* **2008**, *88*, 78–88. [CrossRef]
21. Maitra, A.; Murakata, L.A.; Albores-Saavedra, J. Immunoreactivity for Hepatocyte Paraffin 1 Antibody in Hepatoid Adenocarcinomas of the Gastrointestinal Tract. *Am. J. Clin. Pathol.* **2001**, *115*, 689–694. [CrossRef]
22. Shafizadeh, N.; Ferrell, L.D.; Kakar, S. Utility and Limitations of Glypican-3 Expression for the Diagnosis of Hepatocellular Carcinoma at Both Ends of the Differentiation Spectrum. *Mod. Pathol.* **2008**, *21*, 1011–1101. [CrossRef] [PubMed]
23. Anatelli, F.; Chuang, S.-T.; Yang, X.J.; Wang, H.L. Value of Glypican 3 Immunostaining in the Diagnosis of Hepatocellular Carcinoma on Needle Biopsy. *Am. J. Clin. Pathol.* **2008**, *130*, 219–223. [CrossRef] [PubMed]
24. Ho, M.; Kim, H. Glypican-3: A New Target for Cancer Immunotherapy. *Eur. J. Cancer* **2011**, *47*, 333–338. [CrossRef] [PubMed]
25. Kandil, D.H.; Cooper, K. Glypican-3: A Novel Diagnostic Marker for Hepatocellular Carcinoma and More. *Adv. Anat. Pathol.* **2009**, *16*, 125–129. [CrossRef]
26. Chan, E.S.; Yeh, M.M. The Use of Immunohistochemistry in Liver Tumors. *Clin. Liver Dis.* **2010**, *14*, 687–703. [CrossRef]
27. Durnez, A.; Verslype, C.; Nevens, F.; Fevery, J.; Aerts, R.; Pirenne, J.; Lesaffre, E.; Libbrecht, L.; Desmet, V.; Roskams, T. The Clinicopathological and Prognostic Relevance of Cytokeratin 7 and 19 Expression in Hepatocellular Carcinoma. A Possible Progenitor Cell Origin. *Histopathology* **2006**, *49*, 138–151. [CrossRef]
28. Morrison, C.; Marsh, W.; Frankel, W.L. A Comparison of CD10 to PCEA, MOC-31, and Hepatocyte for the Distinction of Malignant Tumors in the Liver. *Mod. Pathol.* **2002**, *15*, 1279–1287. [CrossRef]
29. Kakar, S.; Gown, A.M.; Goodman, Z.D.; Ferrell, L.D. Best Practices in Diagnostic Immunohistochemistry: Hepatocellular Carcinoma Versus Metastatic Neoplasms. *Arch. Pathol. Lab. Med.* **2007**, *131*, 1648–1654. [CrossRef]
30. Guedj, N. Pathology of Cholangiocarcinomas. *Curr. Oncol.* **2022**, *30*, 370–380. [CrossRef]

31. Wu, J.M.; Montgomery, E.A.; Iacobuzio-Donahue, C.A. Frequent β-Catenin Nuclear Labeling in Sessile Serrated Polyps of the Colorectum with Neoplastic Potential. *Am. J. Clin. Pathol.* **2008**, *129*, 416–423. [CrossRef]
32. Saad, R.S. CDX2 as a Marker for Intestinal Differentiation: Its Utility and Limitations. *WJGS* **2011**, *3*, 159. [CrossRef] [PubMed]
33. Sullivan, L.M.; Smolkin, M.E.; Frierson, H.F.; Galgano, M.T. Comprehensive Evaluation of CDX2 in Invasive Cervical Adenocarcinomas: Immunopositivity in the Absence of Overt Colorectal Morphology. *Am. J. Surg. Pathol.* **2008**, *32*, 1608–1612. [CrossRef]
34. Schmitt, A.M.; Riniker, F.; Anlauf, M.; Schmid, S.; Soltermann, A.; Moch, H.; Heitz, P.U.; Klöppel, G.; Komminoth, P.; Perren, A. Islet 1 (Isl1) Expression Is a Reliable Marker for Pancreatic Endocrine Tumors and Their Metastases. *Am. J. Surg. Pathol.* **2008**, *32*, 420–425. [CrossRef] [PubMed]
35. Hong, S.-M.; Cho, H.; Moskaluk, C.A.; Frierson, H.F.; Yu, E.; Ro, J.Y. CDX2 and MUC2 Protein Expression in Extrahepatic Bile Duct Carcinoma. *Am. J. Clin. Pathol.* **2005**, *124*, 361–370. [CrossRef] [PubMed]
36. Bayrak, R.; Haltas, H.; Yenidunya, S. The Value of CDX2 and Cytokeratins 7 and 20 Expression in Differentiating Colorectal Adenocarcinomas from Extraintestinal Gastrointestinal Adenocarcinomas: Cytokeratin 7−/20+ Phenotype Is More Specific than CDX2 Antibody. *Diagn. Pathol.* **2012**, *7*, 9. [CrossRef]
37. Ferrone, C.R.; Ting, D.T.; Shahid, M.; Konstantinidis, I.T.; Sabbatino, F.; Goyal, L.; Rice-Stitt, T.; Mubeen, A.; Arora, K.; Bardeesey, N.; et al. The Ability to Diagnose Intrahepatic Cholangiocarcinoma Definitively Using Novel Branched DNA-Enhanced Albumin RNA In Situ Hybridization Technology. *Ann. Surg. Oncol.* **2016**, *23*, 290–296. [CrossRef]
38. Lok, T.; Chen, L.; Lin, F.; Wang, H.L. Immunohistochemical Distinction between Intrahepatic Cholangiocarcinoma and Pancreatic Ductal Adenocarcinoma. *Hum. Pathol.* **2014**, *45*, 394–400. [CrossRef]
39. Mocan, L.-P.; Ilieș, M.; Melincovici, C.S.; Spârchez, M.; Crăciun, R.; Nenu, I.; Horhat, A.; Tefas, C.; Spârchez, Z.; Iuga, C.A.; et al. Novel Approaches in Search for Biomarkers of Cholangiocarcinoma. *WJG* **2022**, *28*, 1508–1525. [CrossRef]
40. Ruys, A.T.; Groot Koerkamp, B.; Wiggers, J.K.; Klümpen, H.-J.; ten Kate, F.J.; van Gulik, T.M. Prognostic Biomarkers in Patients with Resected Cholangiocarcinoma: A Systematic Review and Meta-Analysis. *Ann. Surg. Oncol.* **2014**, *21*, 487–500. [CrossRef]
41. He, J.; Zhang, C.; Shi, Q.; Bao, F.; Pan, X.; Kuai, Y.; Wu, J.; Li, L.; Chen, P.; Huang, Y.; et al. Association between Immunohistochemistry Markers and Tumor Features and Their Diagnostic and Prognostic Values in Intrahepatic Cholangiocarcinoma. *Comput. Math. Methods Med.* **2022**, *2022*, 8367395. [CrossRef]
42. Yeh, Y.-C.; Lei, H.-J.; Chen, M.-H.; Ho, H.-L.; Chiu, L.-Y.; Li, C.-P.; Wang, Y.-C. C-Reactive Protein (CRP) Is a Promising Diagnostic Immunohistochemical Marker for Intrahepatic Cholangiocarcinoma and Is Associated with Better Prognosis. *Am. J. Surg. Pathol.* **2017**, *41*, 1630–1641. [CrossRef] [PubMed]
43. Liu, L.-Z.; Yang, L.-X.; Zheng, B.-H.; Dong, P.-P.; Liu, X.-Y.; Wang, Z.-C.; Zhou, J.; Fan, J.; Wang, X.-Y.; Gao, Q. CK7/CK19 Index: A Potential Prognostic Factor for Postoperative Intrahepatic Cholangiocarcinoma Patients. *J. Surg. Oncol.* **2018**, *117*, 1531–1539. [CrossRef] [PubMed]
44. Mocan, L.P.; Craciun, R.; Grapa, C.; Melincovici, C.S.; Rusu, I.; Al Hajjar, N.; Sparchez, Z.; Leucuta, D.; Ilies, M.; Sparchez, M.; et al. PD-L1 Expression on Immune Cells, but Not on Tumor Cells, Is a Favorable Prognostic Factor for Patients with Intrahepatic Cholangiocarcinoma. *Cancer Immunol. Immunother.* **2022**, *72*, 1003–1014. [CrossRef]
45. Liu, D.; Heij, L.R.; Czigany, Z.; Dahl, E.; Lang, S.A.; Ulmer, T.F.; Luedde, T.; Neumann, U.P.; Bednarsch, J. The Role of Tumor-Infiltrating Lymphocytes in Cholangiocarcinoma. *J. Exp. Clin. Cancer Res.* **2022**, *41*, 127. [CrossRef] [PubMed]
46. Merters, J.; Lamarca, A. Integrating Cytotoxic, Targeted and Immune Therapies for Cholangiocarcinoma. *J. Hepatol.* **2022**, *78*, 652–657. [CrossRef]
47. Renzulli, M.; Pecorelli, A.; Brandi, N.; Brocchi, S.; Tovoli, F.; Granito, A.; Carrafiello, G.; Ierardi, A.M.; Golfieri, R. The Feasibility of Liver Biopsy for Undefined Nodules in Patients under Surveillance for Hepatocellular Carcinoma: Is Biopsy Really a Useful Tool? *J. Clin. Med.* **2022**, *11*, 4399. [CrossRef]
48. Giorgio, A.; Tarantino, L.; de Stefano, G.; Francica, G.; Esposito, F.; Perrotta, A.; Aloisio, V.; Farella, N.; Mariniello, N.; Coppola, C.; et al. Complications After Interventional Sonography of Focal Liver Lesions: A 22-Year Single-Center Experience. *J. Ultrasound Med.* **2003**, *22*, 193–205. [CrossRef]

Disclaimer/Publisher's Note: The statements, opinions and data contained in all publications are solely those of the individual author(s) and contributor(s) and not of MDPI and/or the editor(s). MDPI and/or the editor(s) disclaim responsibility for any injury to people or property resulting from any ideas, methods, instructions or products referred to in the content.

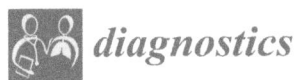

Article

Chitotriosidase and Neopterin as Two Novel Potential Biomarkers for Advanced Stage and Survival Prediction in Gastric Cancer—A Pilot Study

Vlad-Ionuț Nechita [1,2], Nadim Al Hajjar [2,3,*], Cristina Drugan [4,*], Cristina-Sorina Cătană [4], Emil Moiș [2,3], Mihaela-Ancuța Nechita [5] and Florin Graur [2,3]

1. Department of Medical Informatics and Biostatistics, "Iuliu Hațieganu" University of Medicine and Pharmacy, Louis Pasteur Str., No. 6, 400349 Cluj-Napoca, Romania; nechita.vlad@umfcluj.ro
2. "Octavian Fodor" Regional Institute of Gastroenterology and Hepatology, 010336 Cluj-Napoca, Romania
3. Department of Surgery, "Iuliu Hațieganu" University of Medicine and Pharmacy, Croitorilor Str., No. 19–21, 400162 Cluj-Napoca, Romania
4. Department of Medical Biochemistry, "Iuliu Hațieganu" University of Medicine and Pharmacy Cluj-Napoca, Louis Pasteur Str., No. 6, 400349 Cluj-Napoca, Romania
5. "Ion Chiricuță" Oncology Institute, Republicii Str., No. 34–36, 400015 Cluj-Napoca, Romania
* Correspondence: na_hajjar@yahoo.com (N.A.H.); cdrugan@umfcluj.ro (C.D.)

Abstract: Gastric cancer is the fifth type of neoplasia most frequently diagnosed and the fourth cause of death among other cancers. Prevalence is around two times higher for males than females. Chitotriosidase and neopterin are two molecular biomarkers with potential diagnostic and prognostic use in malignant pathology. We conducted a longitudinal prospective cohort study on thirty-nine patients with gastric adenocarcinoma, with a male-to-female ratio of 1.78 and an average age of 64.3 ± 9.97 years. No statistically significant differences in biomarker levels at presentation were observed between curative-intent surgery (28 patients) and advanced cases, suited only for palliative procedures (11 patients). Biomarker values were not significantly different for the advanced T stage and the presence of metastasis ($p > 0.05$—Mann Whitney test). The patients that died in the first 30 days after surgery did not present significantly different values at baseline, in comparison with those that had longer survival times, though a significant cut-off value was observed for chitotriosidase activity at 310 nmol/mL/h [AUC (area under the curve) = 0.78; 95% CI (0.61–0.92)]. The cut-off values corresponding to death after the first year, tumor invasion, and metastasis were not statistically significant. In the COX multivariate model, neopterin did not validate itself as a prognostic biomarker, however, chitotriosidase activity before surgery was significantly associated with overall survival (HR = 1.0038, $p = 0.03$). We conclude that chitotriosidase may have the potential to improve the prognostic model for gastric adenocarcinoma.

Keywords: gastric cancer; neopterin; chitotriosidase; stadialisation; resectability; survival

Citation: Nechita, V.-I.; Hajjar, N.A.; Drugan, C.; Cătană, C.-S.; Moiș, E.; Nechita, M.-A.; Graur, F. Chitotriosidase and Neopterin as Two Novel Potential Biomarkers for Advanced Stage and Survival Prediction in Gastric Cancer—A Pilot Study. Diagnostics 2023, 13, 1362. https://doi.org/10.3390/diagnostics13071362

Academic Editor: Costin Teodor Streba

Received: 21 March 2023
Revised: 31 March 2023
Accepted: 4 April 2023
Published: 6 April 2023

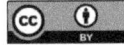

Copyright: © 2023 by the authors. Licensee MDPI, Basel, Switzerland. This article is an open access article distributed under the terms and conditions of the Creative Commons Attribution (CC BY) license (https://creativecommons.org/licenses/by/4.0/).

1. Introduction

Gastric cancer is the fifth most frequently diagnosed type of neoplasia (5.6%) after mammary (11.7%), lung (11.4%), colorectal (10%), and prostate (7.3%) cancer, being the fourth cause of death due to neoplasia (after lung, colorectal, and liver cancer) [1]. Gastric cancer affects the male population about two times more frequently than females [1,2]. Higher incidence and prevalence of gastric cancer were observed in Eastern Asia and Eastern Europe, while in Northern America, Africa, and Northern Europe, the rates are lower [3].

Survival in gastric cancer is poor for advanced stages. Katai et al., working on a cohort of over 100,000 patients, reported a five years survival rate of 71.1%, 95% CI (70.9–71.3%) for patients with surgical resection. From 118,367 patients with gastrectomy, 587 died in the first 30 days after the intervention, leading to short-term postoperative mortality of 0.5%.

For stages I and II, the five-year overall survival was above 68.9%; for stages IIIA and IIIB it was above 32.3%, while for stage IV it dropped to only 17%. The presence of metastasis reduces the five-year survival rate to 11.5% for liver metastasis and 9.5% for peritoneal metastasis [4]. According to Isobe et al., the 30 days postoperative mortality was 0.6% for patients who had undergone gastrectomy [5].

Chitotriosidase and neopterin are molecular biomarkers for cellular immune response activation. Activated macrophages are responsible for the secretion of both molecules [6,7]. Neopterin, a pteridine derivative that results after GTP (guanosine triphosphate) catabolism, is a product of monocyte and macrophage activation, after stimulation with gamma interferon, a proinflammatory cytokine [7–9].

Murr et al. suggested that malignant cells present a modified cell surface that can trigger specific cellular immune system activation and neopterin production. Otherwise, they considered this biomarker to be inadequate for screening or diagnostic purposes in malignant pathology, as the frequency of higher serum levels of neopterin is related to tumor type (with over 90% frequency of increased neopterin for hematologic neoplasms, such as Hodgkin and non-Hodgkin lymphoma, and less than 20% for breast cancer, respectively). On the other hand, the utility of neopterin can be relevant for the prognostic estimation at the moment of diagnosis, as the tumor stage can influence neopterin elevation [10].

According to Unal et al., neopterin levels for subjects with gastric cancer (15.26 ± 11.46 nmol/L) were significantly higher than for healthy age and gender-matched subjects in the control group (9.87 ± 2.90 nmol/L), without malignancy, infections, or inflammatory pathology [11].

Hacisevki et al. also suggested that neopterin levels (mean ± standard error) before intervention can be a possible biomarker for gastrointestinal tumors, including gastric cancer (4.84 ± 0.74 ng/mL), colorectal cancer (4.20 ± 0.68 ng/mL), and oesophageal, pancreatic, or liver cancer (4.67 ± 0.45 ng/mL), with a significant elevation ($p < 0.001$) in comparison with a healthy control group (1.57 ± 0.13). The differences between different types of gastrointestinal tumors were not significant [12].

Chitotriosidase is an enzyme belonging to the chitinase family, involved in the protection against pathogens with a chitin cell wall [13]. Chitotriosidase is considered an important biomarker for inherited lysosomal storage disorders such as Gaucher disease [14]. Its synthesis takes place in both physiological and pathological conditions, predominantly in activated macrophages, neutrophils, Kupffer cells, or bronchial epithelial cells [15]. According to van Eijk et al., chitotriosidase production can be triggered by the granulocyte-macrophage colony-stimulating factor (GM-CSF) [16].

Thein et al. evaluated chitotriosidase and neopterin levels in patients with primary breast cancer and prostatic cancer in different evolutive stages [17]. The diagnostic capacity of the two biomarkers was evaluated with the ROC (receiver operating characteristics) curve. Patients with breast cancer presented a significantly higher chitotriosidase activity in comparison with control females without cancer ($p < 0.0001$). Patients with prostate cancer also presented a significantly higher chitotriosidase activity in comparison with control, cancer-free males ($p < 0.05$). For neopterin values in breast cancer, the differences with gender-matched controls were not statistically significant, though median neopterin was significantly higher ($p < 0.0001$) in prostate cancer subjects in comparison to the healthy males' group. No significant differences were observed between male and female controls for both biomarkers. For the diagnosis of breast cancer, the AUC (area under the curve) was 0.97, indicating significance ($p < 0.0001$) for chitotriosidase at the cut-off value of 13.80 nmol/mL/h, though not for neopterin (AUC = 0.68, $p = 0.88$). For prostate cancer diagnosis, chitotriosidase presented a significant AUC of 0.64 ($p < 0.05$) at the cut-off value of 13.80 nmol/mL/h, and also neopterin had a significant ($p < 0.0001$) AUC of 0.76, at the cut-off value of 7.6 nmol/L.

Kukur et al. also described a significantly ($p < 0.05$) higher chitotriosidase activity in patients with primary prostate cancer (91.33 ± 8.32 nmol/mL/h), compared to those with biopsy-certified benign prostatic hyperplasia (69.72 ± 8.69 nmol/mL/h). In addition, a higher chitotriosidase activity was observed in the group with a higher Gleason score (118.18 ± 10.28 nmol/mL/h) [18].

This study aimed to evaluate the association of chitotriosidase and neopterin (two novel molecular biomarkers) with tumor pathological characteristics (TNM stadialisation) and prognosis at the presentation of gastric cancer in a surgical department. Our hypothesis was that elevated levels of neopterin and chitotriosidase might be related to more advanced tumors and poor survival rates.

2. Materials and Methods

2.1. Participants, Setting, and Study Design

The cohort was evaluated in an observational, longitudinal, prospective study. Participants were selected from the patients presenting with surgery indication for gastric cancer at the "Prof. Dr. Octavian Fodor" Regional Institute of Gastroenterology and Hepatology, Cluj-Napoca, Romania, between 8 August 2019 to 28 January 2021, who gave their informed consent for participation. Only thirty-nine patients with gastric adenocarcinoma confirmed by pathology report were included, whereas other types of tumors were excluded.

The sample was divided into multiple subgroups according to the following criteria: resectability (patients with gastrectomy and patients with palliative procedure), survival in the first 30 days and in the first year, the TNM (tumor-node-metastasis) stage, the T (tumor) stage, class, and the presence of metastasis (M1). Neopterin levels and chitotriosidase activity were compared between groups. All patients had at least one open laparotomy and the presence of metastasis was confirmed during surgery and in the pathology report for unresectable cases.

2.2. Variables, Data Source, and Collection

Demographic data (age, sex, and urban setting), routine blood test results to evaluate nutritional status, blood group and anemia (albumin, total proteins, and hemoglobin levels), information about the surgical procedure, intraoperative findings, tumor extension or metastasis, as well as pathology reports regarding tumor type and stage, were collected. Data about preoperative neoadjuvant treatment were also considered.

Overall survival represented the interval between the date of surgical intervention and the date of death. To evaluate survival, patients or their contact relatives received 4 phone calls during the follow-up period. For surviving patients, the last information about survival was obtained up to 20 January 2023.

To determine neopterin levels and chitotriosidase activity, fresh blood samples were collected in EDTA vacutainers (4 mL) for each patient at hospital admission, before surgery, after agreeing to participate in the study and signing the informed consent. The samples were centrifuged within 15 min after collection (3000 rpm, 4 °C, 10 min). The separated plasma was stored at −20 °C. Neopterin quantitation was performed using the Neopterin ELISA kit (Wuhan Fine Biotech, China), according to the manufacturer's instructions. To measure plasma chitotriosidase activity (expressed as nanomoles of hydrolyzed substrate per milliliter per hour—nmol/mL/h) we used an artificial fluorescent substrate (4-methylumbelliferyl-chitotrioside), according to the method described by Hollak et al. [19].

2.3. Statistical Methods

The statistical analysis was performed with R Commander (R version 4.0.5). To evaluate the distribution of quantitative data, we used skewness, kurtosis, and the Shapiro–Wilk test. Quantitative data were presented as mean and standard deviation or as median and interquartile range. To compare quantitative data for independent groups, we used the Mann–Whitney test. The log-rank test was used to compare median survival time, according to the procedure and the median values of the biomarkers.

The effect of molecular biomarkers on overall survival (OS) was evaluated with Cox proportional hazard regressions; we presented the hazard ratio with the 95% confidence interval, respectively, the p-value. To build the univariate models, we used the absolute values of the determined biomarkers and the values dichotomized with medians. Multivariate models were built that adjusted the previous values for the TNM stage and neoadjuvant chemotherapy. Differences were considered statistically significant at a two-tailed p-value of less than 0.05.

To find the best cut-off values and the ability of the studied biomarkers in the prediction of advanced tumor stage (T4), the presence of metastasis (M1), and short time survival (at thirty days and at one year after the intervention), we used the ROC (receiver operating characteristics) curves and the maximum Youden index. The AUC (areas under the curve) computed with bootstrap with 95% confidence intervals were also presented.

We hypothesized that neopterin levels (nmol/L) and chitotriosidase activity (nmol/mL/h) values at presentation were increased in advanced cases (i.e., subjects with higher TNM stages and those with unresectable tumors). We also assumed that these values could be related to patients' short and long-term outcomes (overall survival).

2.4. Ethical Statement

Conducted according to the revised Helsinki Declaration of 2000, this research received approval from the "Iuliu Hațieganu" Ethics Committee (no. 121/24.04.2019) and from the Ethics Committee of the "Prof. Dr. Octavian Fodor" Regional Institute of Gastroenterology and Hepatology (no. 8900/10.07.2019). Before the investigation, all the participants agreed and signed the informed consent form.

3. Results

Forty-two patients signed the informed consent and were evaluated; three patients were excluded after the pathology result, two of them with GIST (gastrointestinal stromal tumor) tumors and one with a neuroendocrine tumor. The male-to-female ratio was 1.78 (25/14), and 18 subjects originated from an urban area (46.15%). The average age for the sample was 64.3 + 9.97 years. According to blood group, we had 22 (56.41%) A (II) group patients, 8 (20.51%) O (I) group patients, 7 (17.94%) B (III) patients, and 2 subjects (5.12%) with the AB (IV) blood group. Six patients had a negative Rh factor.

Within the chosen sample, 28 patients (71.79%) had benefitted from gastrectomy (11 total and 17 subtotal gastrectomies), and 11 patients (28.2%) had had palliative procedures. One patient (3.57%) had a positive resection margin. Eight patients (20.51%) received neoadjuvant chemotherapy before surgery. Regarding the TNM stage, at presentation, three patients (7.69%) were in stage I, eight patients (20.51%) in stage II, seventeen patients (43.58%) in stage III, and eleven patients (28.2%) in stage IV. At presentation, eleven patients (28.2%) had metastasis. The mortality in the first 30 days after surgery was 7.6% (3/39 patients); two patients, representing 18.18%, had a palliative approach, and one patient, representing 3.5% of the resected group, had a gastrectomy. The survival rate in the first year after surgery was 56.41% (representing 9% of the subjects with palliative surgery and 75% of the cases with resection).

The differences in neopterin levels and chitotriosidase activity, according to the optimal procedure, were not statistically significant. However, the differences regarding nutritional status were important (Table 1). For neopterin values ($p = 0.07$, Mann–Whitney test) or chitotriosidase activity ($p = 0.82$, Mann–Whitney test) no statistically significant differences were observed between patients who benefitted from neoadjuvant chemotherapy and those without preoperative treatment at presentation.

Comparing the values of the biomarkers between the individual T-groups (T1 vs. T2 vs. T3 vs. T4), the differences were not significant for both chitotriosidase ($p = 0.3977$—Kruskal–Wallis test) and neopterin ($p = 0.15$—Kruskal–Wallis test). The differences in the values of the studied biomarkers between the individual N stages (N1 vs. N2 vs. N3) were not significant for either chitotriosidase ($p = 0.6374$—Kruskal–Wallis test) and neopterin ($p = 0.51$—Kruskal–Wallis test). The differences in chitotriosidase activity and neopterin levels, according to the subgroups of different T stages, the presence of metastasis, and the length of survival (30 days and one-year survival), are presented in Table 2.

Table 1. Laboratory findings according to the optimal procedure (n = 39).

	All Subjects (n = 39)	Curative Resection (n = 28)	Palliative Surgery (n = 11)	p-Value
Chitotriosidase (nmol/mL/h)	270.00 (130.00–395.00)	290.00 (137.50–400.00)	230.00 (107.50–297.50)	0.23
Neopterin (nmol/L)	10.06 (5.31–18.15)	10.49 (5.61–20.95)	7.12 (5.31–10.50)	0.21
Total proteins (g/dL)	6.50 (5.70–7.25)	7.05 (6.00–7.50)	5.70 (5.45–6.55)	0.01
Albumin (g/dL)	3.90 (3.60–4.10)	4.00 (3.80–4.23)	3.70 (3.35–3.90)	0.04
Haemoglobin (g/dL)	10.9 (9.3–12.85)	11.35 (10.20–13.38)	10.00 (9.05–11.70)	0.16

Values presented as the median and interquartile range (Q1–Q3); p value (Mann–Whitney test) represents the comparison between the group with curative resection and the group with palliative surgery.

Table 2. The association of chitotriosidase activity (nmol/mL/h) and neopterin levels (nmol/L) at presentation with tumor characteristics and short-term survival.

Group of Patients (n = 39)	Neopterin (nmol/L) Yes*	Neopterin (nmol/L) No**	p-Value	Chitotriosidase (nmol/mL/h) Yes*	Chitotriosidase (nmol/mL/h) No**	p-Value
T34 vs. T12 (n = 23)	8.47 (5.31–18.27)	11.09 (8.43–13.72)	1	280 (125–395)	250 (220–295)	1
T4 vs. T123 (n = 29)	7.12 (5.21–11.73)	16.42 (7.25–25.62)	0.1	255 (127.5–333.75)	300 (145–400)	0.45
M1 vs. M0 (n = 11)	7.11 (5.31–10.5)	10.49 (5.61–20.95)	0.21	230 (107.5–297.5)	290 (137.5–400)	0.23
Death during the first 30 days (n = 3)	7.12 (6.47–8.59)	10.22 (5.21–19.55)	0.54	490 (405–525)	250 (127.5–367.5)	0.12
Death during the first year (n = 17)	7.12 (5.33–16.22)	10.22 (5.32–19.67)	0.65	270 (170–360)	270 (130–397.5)	0.91

Yes*—values for subjects with more advanced T or M stage, or death within the first 30 days or the first year, respectively. No**—values for subjects with lower T stage, without metastasis and improved survival. Results are presented as median and interquartile range.

In univariate analysis, neopterin levels and chitotriosidase activity were not significantly associated with poor survival. For the multivariate model, only the chitotriosidase activity was significantly associated with poor outcomes (Table 3).

Table 3. Univariate and multivariate Cox proportional hazard regressions on chitotriosidase activity (nmol/mL/h) and neopterin levels (nmol/L) at presentation, adjusted for TNM stage and neoadjuvant chemotherapy.

	HR Unadjusted	(95% CI)	p	HR Adjusted *	(95% CI)	p
Neopterin (nmol/L)	1.002	(0.9659–1.04)	0.9	1.0012	(0.952–1.0523)	0.96
Chitotriosidase (nmol/mL/h)	1.001	(0.9988–1.003)	0.37	1.0038	(1.00023–1.007)	0.03
Neopterin ≥ median	0.62	(0.267–1.48)	0.29	0.52	(0.18–1.46)	0.22
Chitotriosidase ≥ median	1.038	(0.43–2.507)	0.99	3.101	(0.758–12.69)	0.11

HR—hazard ratio; 95% CI—95% confidence interval; * Adjusted for TNM stage (I + II, III, and IV) and neoadjuvant chemotherapy.

The ROC (receiver operating characteristic) analysis for patients that died in the first 30 days after intervention showed a cut-off value of 10.22 nmol/L for neopterin levels [AUC = 0.61; 95% CI (0.43–0.78)] and 310 nmol/mL/h for chitotriosidase activity [AUC = 0.78; 95% CI (0.61–0.92)] at presentation (Figure 1). For patients who died within the first year after the intervention, the cut-off values were 7.15 nmol/L for neopterin [AUC = 0.54; 95% CI (0.35–0.72)] and 105 nmol/mL/h for chitotriosidase activity [AUC = 0.51; 95% CI (0.32–0.70)]. For the presence of metastasis (M1), the cut-off value for neopterin was 7.15 [AUC = 0.63; 95% CI (0.43–0.81)] and 275 nmol/mL/h for chitotriosidase activity [AUC = 0.62; 95% CI (0.42–0.81)]. For the T4 stage, the cut-off value for neopterin was 16.32 [AUC = 0.66; 95% CI (0.46–0.83)] and 342.5 nmol/mL/h for chitotriosidase activity [AUC = 0.57; 95% CI (0.37–0.77)].

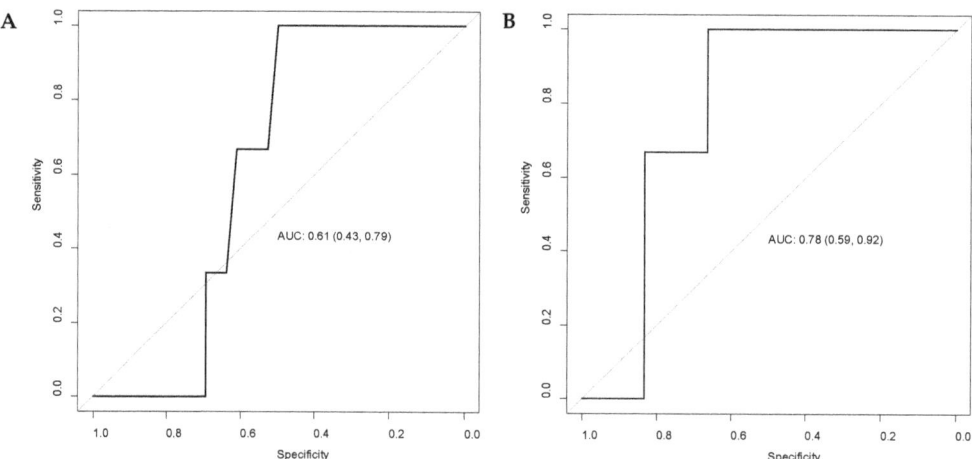

Figure 1. ROC (receiver operating characteristic) curves for neopterin levels (**A**) and chitotriosidase activity (**B**), at presentation, considering patients' death in the first 30 days after the intervention. AUC = area under the curve, with 95% confidence intervals.

A significant difference in survival was observed between the patients with curative resection (median survival time 309 days), compared to those with palliative procedures (median survival time 159 days, $p = 0.006$–logrank test). No significant difference in survival ($p = 0.28$–logrank test) was observed between patients with neopterin levels below (median survival time 215 days) and above (median survival time 299 days) the sample's median value (10.06 nmol/L). For the patients with chitotriosidase activity above the sample's median value (270 nmol/mL/h), the median survival time was 159 days, whereas, for those with chitotriosidase activity below the median value, the median survival time was 282 days, without statistical significance at the logrank test ($p = 0.93$).

4. Discussion

This study evaluated two novel inflammatory biomarkers, still insufficiently investigated in gastric cancer, the fifth most common type of cancer worldwide and the fourth cause of death among cancers [1], with a poor prognosis in advanced stages [4,5]. As an Eastern European country, Romania has a high incidence of gastric cancer, according to the Global Cancer Observatory [3]. In our patient sample, the number of male patients was almost double the number of females, in accordance with the higher prevalence of gastric cancer in males described in the literature [1,2]. The predominant blood group in our sample was A (II) for more than half of the subjects (56.41%), while the AB (IV) blood group was less represented (5.12%), corresponding to the findings of Yu et al., who indicated a higher risk of gastric cancer for people with the A blood group and a lower risk for the AB blood group [20].

In our patient sample, the mortality in the first 30 days after gastrectomy was 3.5%, higher than the postoperative mortality described in other studies [4,5]. This can be explained by the high percentage of patients with advanced-stage cancers (43.58% stage III and 28.2% stage IV, due to locally advanced tumors or the presence of metastasis confirmed by pathology reports). Isobe et al. reported first-year and five-year survival rates at 88.6% and 70.9%, respectively, for patients with surgical resection, respectively, and 23% and 5.6%, for unresected cases [5]. Due to the short period of follow up, we were able to evaluate only the first-year survival rate, which proved to be lower, at only 75% for surgical resection patients. For patients with metastasis and palliative surgical intervention, the first-year survival rate was 9%, close to the values found by Katai et al. [4]. As expected, a significant difference ($p = 0.006$—logrank test) was observed between the median survival time for patients with curative resection (309 days) and median survival for those with palliative surgery (159 days).

At presentation, there were no significant differences in the values of the studied biomarkers between the patients that benefitted from curative-intent resection and those with a palliative approach (Table 1). A significant difference was observed in the nutritional status, as patients with advanced gastric cancers that were suited only for a palliative approach presented lower albumin and total protein levels. On the other hand, Hacisevki et al. found a significant ($p = 0.002$) negative correlation between neopterin and albumin levels in patients with gastrointestinal cancer. The authors suggested that neopterin and inflammation could contribute to the alteration of serum albumin and total proteins [12]. For Unal et al. [11], neopterin levels were higher in the group with unresectable gastric cancer, advanced stage, or metastasis, though without reaching statistical significance ($p > 0.05$). On the contrary, in our sample, neopterin median values were apparently increased in patients that qualified for curative resection and not in those with palliative surgery, though without a statistical significance between these variations (Table 1). The potential effect of neoadjuvant treatment over the biomarker values was equally not significant in our study.

Gastric cancer TNM (tumor-node-metastasis) stadialisation for the included subjects was performed according to the 8th edition AJCC (the American Joint Committee on Cancer) staging system [21,22], where the presence of metastasis leads to patient inclusion in stage IV. Tumor invasion in nearby organs (T4b), and the presence of 16 or more positive lymph nodes (N3b), but without metastasis, is indicative of stage IIIC. We have to mention that all palliative cases in our cohort were a direct cause of metastatic disease. Patients with tumor invasion benefitted from curative-intent resection, and only one of them presented R1 positive resection margins, as shown in the results section. The N-stage data were available only for patients with resection and a complete pathology report. This did not influence the TNM stadialisation, as for unresectable subjects, it was attributed according to the presence of metastasis. Considering the low number of subjects, the T classes were also grouped as low (stages T1, T2, and T3) and high (stage T4), with serosa or other organ invasion. We also grouped the TNM stage for COX regressions on the same principle.

Chitotriosidase and neopterin have been previously evaluated together as biomarkers of macrophage activation in infectious diseases such as brucellosis [23], ankylosing spondylitis [24], microvascular complications of type I diabetes [6], and even lung [25], breast [17], and prostate [17] cancer. Chitotriosidase and CHI3L1 (Chitinase-3-like-1 protein) are part of the same family of chitinases [26]. CHI3L1 is more frequently evaluated in the scientific literature. Some tumor-promoting mechanisms were highlighted. CHI3L1 (known also as YKL-40) was associated with angiogenesis and bad prognosis in tumors such as breast, lung, and cervical cancers [27–29]. Also, according to the literature, IL-8 (Interleukin-8) and VEGFA (vascular endothelial growth factor) angiogenic properties may be influenced by CHI3L1 to promote cancer progression [30–32].

According to Thein et al., significantly higher ($p < 0.005$) neopterin levels were observed in breast cancer patients with metastasis (10.02 nmol/L), in comparison with localized tumors (6.34 nmol/L). The same pattern was observed for prostate cancer, with significantly ($p < 0.0005$) higher median neopterin levels (21.7 nmol/L) for metastatic tumors, in comparison to localized prostate cancer (8.26 nmol/L). The chitotriosidase activity was higher in the group with metastasis, in comparison with localized disease, for both breast and prostate cancer, though without statistical significance [17]. In our cohort, the biomarkers' values were higher in the groups without metastasis and lower tumor stage (Table 2), but without a significant difference between the groups. This could be attributed to a better immune response in less advanced stages, as well as to the attenuation of inflammatory activation in higher-stage or metastatic cancer. A few studies [11,12,17,18] suggested elevated chitotriosidase activity or neopterin levels in patients with neoplasia and indicated the utility of these molecular biomarkers in the diagnostic process.

On the other hand, Murr et al. argued that neopterin levels at presentation could be relevant for prognosis due to its association with tumor stage, though they also mentioned that this approach would be difficult to use for screening and diagnostic purposes [10]. Due to altered cell surface compared to normal cells, the malignant cells can lead to an activation of the cellular immune system and neopterin release. It is possible that the cellular immune reaction towards the tumor, which may be stronger in individuals with more aggressive tumors, explains why those with higher neopterin production have a higher tumor stage and a poorer prognosis [10]. According to this study, the frequency of elevated serum levels of this biomarker is related to tumor type; it has been observed in 42% of cases with gastric cancer, which is lower than the frequency of increased levels in hematological malignancies, but above that of reported elevations in prostate, breast cancer, or malignant melanoma [10]. The cut-off values were computed in our study for the pathological proof of advanced stages, such as the presence of metastasis and local tumor invasion (T4), however, the values were not statistically significant.

No statistically significant differences in biomarker values were observed between short-term (30 days) and first-year survival (Table 2). In gastric cancer, Unal et al. described a better survival (42.05 months) when serum neopterin levels were below the cut-off value of 11.15 nmol/L, compared to the subjects with serum neopterin values above the cut off (28.53 months, $p < 0.05$) [11]. In our study, the cut-off values for survival at 30 days and at one year after the intervention were computed with the ROC curves and maximum Youden index. Chitotriosidase activity over 310 nmol/mL/h was significant for short-term survival (Figure 1). For one-year survival, the cut-off values of neopterin indicated a poor AUC and no statistical significance. In a multivariate Cox regression, neopterin levels proved to be an independent factor for the prediction of overall survival in gastric cancer, with an HR of 1.052; 95% CI (1.014–1.092), $p = 0.007$ [11]. In the univariate model, the individual effect of the studied biomarkers on overall survival did not reach statistical significance (Table 3).

Due to the low number of subjects, in order to prevent overfitting, the important tumor pathological characteristics were considered together as the TNM stage. Moreover, stages I and II were grouped together, as they were poorly represented. In this model, we appreciated that the maximum number of covariates is two, and we also considered the impact of neoadjuvant therapy. Contrary to the findings of Unal et al. [11], according to our results, neopterin did not prove to have a prognostic value, though chitotriosidase activity presented a significant influence (HR = 1.0038, $p = 0.03$).

This research, however, is subject to several limitations: (one) other comorbidities, treatments, or inflammatory disorders were not taken into account before patient selection; (two) the study was based on a single-center's experience; (three) the low number of subjects.

Being largely accessible with reduced measuring costs, chitotriosidase, and neopterin may have the potential to improve, not only the diagnostic methods but also the prognostic models in multiple malignant pathologies [11,12,17,18]. According to our knowledge, neopterin and chitotriosidase have not been evaluated yet in Romanian patients with gastric cancer. Our study attempted to evaluate the association of the circulating levels of these molecular biomarkers with tumor characteristics and to establish their prognostic value for patient survival.

5. Conclusions

In the present study, neopterin did not display significantly higher values in patients with advanced-stage gastric cancer or poor prognosis; on the contrary, lower values (without statistical significance) were associated with higher T-stage, the presence of metastasis, and poor survival. The chitotriosidase activity was also lower in the group with palliative interventions, without reaching statistical significance, but displayed higher values in the groups with poor survival and was significantly associated with poor outcome, according to the multivariate model regression. We speculate that chitotriosidase may be a useful biomarker to evaluate the prognosis of gastric adenocarcinoma, though larger studies comprising a higher number of subjects are necessary for confirmation.

Author Contributions: Conceptualization, N.A.H., C.D., C.-S.C., V.-I.N. and F.G.; methodology, V.-I.N., C.D., C.-S.C., F.G. and N.A.H.; project administration, N.A.H., F.G. and V.-I.N.; validation, N.A.H., C.D., C.-S.C., F.G. and E.M.; formal analysis, V.-I.N., M.-A.N. and E.M.; investigation, V.-I.N., M.-A.N. and E.M.; software, V.-I.N. and M.-A.N.; writing—original draft preparation, V.-I.N. and M.-A.N.; writing—review and editing, F.G., C.D., C.-S.C., N.A.H. and E.M.; visualization, V.-I.N. and M.-A.N.; supervision, N.A.H. and F.G.; funding acquisition, V.-I.N. All authors have read and agreed to the published version of the manuscript.

Funding: This research was funded by "Iuliu Hațieganu" University of Medicine and Pharmacy Cluj-Napoca, Romania, Doctoral Research Program, through the project PCD 1529/50/18.01.2019.

Institutional Review Board Statement: The approval of "Octavian Fodor" Regional Institute of Gastroenterology and Hepatology Ethics Committee (no. 8900/10.07.2019) and Iuliu Hațieganu Ethics Committee (no. 121/24.04.2019) were obtained for this study.

Informed Consent Statement: Informed consent was obtained from all subjects involved in the study.

Data Availability Statement: The data presented in this study are available on request from the corresponding author. The data are not publicly available due to restrictions both of privacy and ethics.

Conflicts of Interest: The authors declare no conflict of interest.

References

1. Sung, H.; Ferlay, J.; Siegel, R.L.; Laversanne, M.; Soerjomataram, I.; Jemal, A.; Bray, F. Global Cancer Statistics 2020: GLOBOCAN Estimates of Incidence and Mortality Worldwide for 36 Cancers in 185 Countries. *CA A Cancer J. Clin.* **2021**, *71*, 209–249. [CrossRef] [PubMed]
2. Rawla, P.; Barsouk, A. Epidemiology of gastric cancer: Global trends, risk factors and prevention. *Gastroenterol. Rev.* **2019**, *14*, 26–38. [CrossRef] [PubMed]
3. Ferlay, J.; Ervik, M.; Lam, F.; Soerjomataram, I.; Mery, L.; Bray, F. (Eds.) Global Cancer Observatory: Cancer Today. Available online: http://gco.iarc.fr/today/home (accessed on 20 January 2023).
4. Katai, H.; Registration Committee of the Japanese Gastric Cancer Association; Ishikawa, T.; Akazawa, K.; Isobe, Y.; Miyashiro, I.; Oda, I.; Tsujitani, S.; Ono, H.; Tanabe, S.; et al. Five-year survival analysis of surgically resected gastric cancer cases in Japan: A retrospective analysis of more than 100,000 patients from the nationwide registry of the Japanese Gastric Cancer Association (2001–2007). *Gastric Cancer* **2018**, *21*, 144–154. [CrossRef] [PubMed]
5. Isobe, Y.; Nashimoto, A.; Akazawa, K.; Oda, I.; Hayashi, K.; Miyashiro, I.; Katai, H.; Tsujitani, S.; Kodera, Y.; Seto, Y.; et al. Gastric cancer treatment in Japan: 2008 annual report of the JGCA nationwide registry. *Gastric Cancer* **2011**, *14*, 301–316. [CrossRef] [PubMed]
6. Cutaș, A.; Drugan, C.; Roman, G.; Rusu, A.; Cătană, C.; Achimaș-Cadariu, A.; Drugan, T. Evaluation of Chitotriosidase and Neopterin as Biomarkers of Microvascular Complications in Patients with Type 1 Diabetes Mellitus. *Diagnostics* **2021**, *11*, 263. [CrossRef]
7. Fuchs, D.; Weiss, G.; Wachter, H. Neopterin, biochemistry andclinical use as a marker for cellular immune reactions. *Int. Arch. Allergy Immunol.* **1993**, *101*, 1–6. [CrossRef]
8. Oxenkrug, G.; Tucker, K.L.; Requintina, P.; Summergrad, P. Neopterin, a Marker of Interferon-Gamma-Inducible Inflammation, Correlates with Pyridoxal-5′-Phosphate, Waist Circumference, HDL-Cholesterol, Insulin Resistance and Mortality Risk in Adult Boston Community Dwellers of Puerto Rican Origin. *Am. J. Neuroprot. Neuroregen.* **2011**, *3*, 48–52. [CrossRef]
9. Pingle, S.K.; Tumane, R.G.; Jawade, A.A. Neopterin: Biomarker of Cell-Mediated Immunity and Potent Usage as Biomarker in Silicosis and Other Occupational Diseases. *Indian J. Occup. Environ. Med.* **2008**, *12*, 107–111. [CrossRef]
10. Murr, C.; Widner, B.; Wirleitner, B.; Fuchs, D. Neopterin as a marker for immune system activation. *Curr. Drug Metab.* **2002**, *3*, 175–187. [CrossRef]
11. Unal, B.; Kocer, B.; Altun, B.; Surmeli, S.; Aksaray, S.; Balci, M.; Ozlu, B.; Cengiz, O. Serum Neopterin as a Prognostic Indicator in Patients with Gastric Carcinoma. *J. Investig. Surg.* **2009**, *22*, 419–425. [CrossRef]
12. Hacisevki, A.; Baba, B.; Aslan, S.; Ozkan, Y. Neopterin: A Possible Biomarker In Gastrointestinal Cancer. *J. Fac. Pharm. Ank. Univ.* **2018**, *42*, 32–41.
13. Kumar, A.; Zhang, K.Y.J. Human Chitinases: Structure, Function, and Inhibitor Discovery. *Adv. Exp. Med. Biol.* **2019**, *1142*, 221–251. [CrossRef]
14. Kzhyshkowska, J.; Gratchev, A.; Goerdt, S. Human Chitinases and Chitinase-like Proteins as Indicators for Inflammation and Cancer. *Biomark. Insights* **2007**, *2*, 128–146. [CrossRef]
15. Mazur, M.; Zielińska, A.; Grzybowski, M.M.; Olczak, J.; Fichna, J. Chitinases and Chitinase-Like Proteins as Therapeutic Targets in Inflammatory Diseases, with a Special Focus on Inflammatory Bowel Diseases. *Int. J. Mol. Sci.* **2021**, *22*, 36966. [CrossRef]

16. Van Eijk, M.; van Roomen, C.P.A.A.; Renkema, G.H.; Bussink, A.P.; Andrews, L.; Blommaart, E.F.C.; Sugar, A.; Verhoeven, A.J.; Boot, R.G.; Aerts, J.M.F.G. Characterization of Human Phagocyte-Derived Chitotriosidase, a Component of Innate Immunity. *Int. Immunol.* **2005**, *17*, 1505–1512. [CrossRef]
17. Thein, M.S.; Kohli, A.; Ram, R.; Ingaramo, M.C.; Jain, A.; Fedarko, N.S. Chitotriosidase, a marker of innate immunity, is elevated in patients with primary breast cancer. *Cancer Biomark.* **2017**, *19*, 383–391. [CrossRef]
18. Kucur, M.; Isman, F.K.; Balcı, C.; Onal, B.; Hacıbekiroglu, M.; Ozkan, F.; Ozkan, A. Serum YKL-40 Levels and Chitotriosidase Activity as Potential Biomarkers in Primary Prostate Cancer and Benign Prostatic Hyperplasia. *Urol. Oncol. Semin. Orig. Investig.* **2008**, *26*, 47–52. [CrossRef]
19. Hollak, C.E.; Van Weely, S.; Van Oers, M.H.; Aerts, J.M. Marked elevation of plasma chitotriosidase activity. A novel hallmark of Gaucher disease. *J. Clin. Investig.* **1994**, *93*, 1288–1292. [CrossRef]
20. Yu, H.; Xu, N.; Li, Z.-K.; Xia, H.; Ren, H.-T.; Li, N.; Wei, J.-B.; Bao, H.-Z. Association of ABO Blood Groups and Risk of Gastric Cancer. *Scand. J. Surg.* **2020**, *109*, 309–313. [CrossRef]
21. Amin, M.B.; Edge, S.B.; Greene, F.L.; Byrd, D.R.; Brookland, R.K.; Washington, M.K.; Gershenwald, J.E.; Compton, C.C.; Hess, K.R.; Sullivan, D.C.; et al. (Eds.) *AJCC Cancer Staging Manual*, 8th ed.; 2017, Corr. 3rd Printing 2018 Edition; Springer: Chicago, IL, USA, 2016; ISBN 978-3-319-40617-6.
22. Stomach (Gastric) Cancer Stages | How Far Has Stomach Cancer Spread? Available online: https://www.cancer.org/cancer/stomach-cancer/detection-diagnosis-staging/staging.html (accessed on 2 February 2023).
23. Coskun, O.; Oter, S.; Yaman, H.; Kilic, S.; Kurt, I.; Eyigun, C.P. Evaluating the Validity of Serum Neopterin and Chitotriosidase Levels in Follow-Up Brucellosis Patients. *Intern. Med.* **2010**, *49*, 1111–1118. [CrossRef]
24. Yavuz, F.; Kesikburun, B.; Öztürk, Ö.; Güzelküçük, Ü. Serum Chitotriosidase and Neopterin Levels in Patients with Ankylosing Spondylitis. *Ther. Adv. Musculoskelet.* **2019**, *11*, 1759720X1983232. [CrossRef] [PubMed]
25. Crintea, A.; Drugan, C.; Constantin, A.-M.; Lupan, I.; Fekete, Z.; Silaghi, C.N.; Crăciun, A.M. Assessment of Specific Tumoral Markers, Inflammatory Status, and Vitamin D Metabolism before and after the First Chemotherapy Cycle in Patients with Lung Cancer. *Biology* **2022**, *11*, 1033. [CrossRef] [PubMed]
26. Di Rosa, M.; Malaguarnera, G.; De Gregorio, C.; Drago, F.; Malaguarnera, L. Evaluation of CHI3L-1 and CHIT-1 Expression in Differentiated and Polarized Macrophages. *Inflammation* **2013**, *36*, 482–492. [CrossRef] [PubMed]
27. Shao, R.; Cao, Q.J.; Arenas, R.B.; Bigelow, C.; Bentley, B.; Yan, W. Breast Cancer Expression of YKL-40 Correlates with Tumour Grade, Poor Differentiation, and Other Cancer Markers. *Br. J. Cancer* **2011**, *105*, 1203–1209. [CrossRef]
28. Wang, X.-W.; Cai, C.-L.; Xu, J.-M.; Jin, H.; Xu, Z.-Y. Increased Expression of Chitinase 3-like 1 Is a Prognosis Marker for Non-Small Cell Lung Cancer Correlated with Tumor Angiogenesis. *Tumour Biol.* **2015**, *36*, 901–907. [CrossRef]
29. Ngernyuang, N.; Francescone, R.; Jearanaikoon, P.; Daduang, J.; Supoken, A.; Yan, W.; Shao, R.; Limpaiboon, T. Chitinase 3 like 1 Is Associated with Tumor Angiogenesis in Cervical Cancer. *Int. J. Biochem. Cell Biol.* **2014**, *51*, 45–52. [CrossRef]
30. Francescone, R.A.; Scully, S.; Faibish, M.; Taylor, S.L.; Oh, D.; Moral, L.; Yan, W.; Bentley, B.; Shao, R. Role of YKL-40 in the Angiogenesis, Radioresistance, and Progression of Glioblastoma. *J. Biol. Chem.* **2011**, *286*, 15332–15343. [CrossRef]
31. Kawada, M.; Seno, H.; Kanda, K.; Nakanishi, Y.; Akitake, R.; Komekado, H.; Kawada, K.; Sakai, Y.; Mizoguchi, E.; Chiba, T. Chitinase 3-like 1 Promotes Macrophage Recruitment and Angiogenesis in Colorectal Cancer. *Oncogene* **2012**, *31*, 3111–3123. [CrossRef]
32. Tang, H.; Sun, Y.; Shi, Z.; Huang, H.; Fang, Z.; Chen, J.; Xiu, Q.; Li, B. YKL-40 Induces IL-8 Expression from Bronchial Epithelium via MAPK (JNK and ERK) and NF-KB Pathways, Causing Bronchial Smooth Muscle Proliferation and Migration. *J. Immunol.* **2013**, *190*, 438–446. [CrossRef]

Disclaimer/Publisher's Note: The statements, opinions and data contained in all publications are solely those of the individual author(s) and contributor(s) and not of MDPI and/or the editor(s). MDPI and/or the editor(s) disclaim responsibility for any injury to people or property resulting from any ideas, methods, instructions or products referred to in the content.

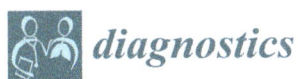

Article

Relationship between Systemic Inflammatory Markers, GLUT1 Expression, and Maximum 18F-Fluorodeoxyglucose Uptake in Non-Small Cell Lung Carcinoma and Their Prognostic Significance

Sonya Youngju Park [1], Deog-Gon Cho [2], Byoung-Yong Shim [3] and Uiju Cho [4,*]

1. Department of Nuclear Medicine, Seoul St. Mary's Hospital, College of Medicine, The Catholic University of Korea, Seoul 06591, Republic of Korea
2. Department of Thoracic Surgery, St. Vincent's Hospital, College of Medicine, The Catholic University of Korea, Seoul 06591, Republic of Korea
3. Division of Medical Oncology, Department of Internal Medicine, St. Vincent's Hospital, College of Medicine, The Catholic University of Korea, Seoul 06591, Republic of Korea
4. Department of Pathology, St. Vincent's Hospital, College of Medicine, The Catholic University of Korea, Seoul 06591, Republic of Korea
* Correspondence: hailtoya@catholic.ac.kr; Tel.: +83-31-249-7647; Fax: +82-31-244-6786

Abstract: Background: Factors involved in inflammation and cancer interact in various ways with each other, and biomarkers of systemic inflammation may have a prognostic value in cancer. Glucose transporter 1 (GLUT1) plays a pivotal role in glucose transport and metabolism and it is aberrantly expressed in various cancer types. We evaluated the differential expression of GLUT1, along with 18F-fluorodeoxyglucose positron emission tomography (FDG-PET) in non-small-cell lung cancer (NSCLC), and then analyzed their prognostic significance. Methods: A total of 163 patients with resectable NSCLC were included in this study. Tumor sections were immunohistochemically stained for GLUT1 and GLUT3. Maximum standardized uptake value (SUV_{max}) was measured by preoperative FDG-PET, and neutrophil–lymphocyte ratio (NLR), platelet–lymphocyte ratio (PLR), and lymphocyte–monocyte ratio (LMR) were derived from pretreatment blood count. Results: GLUT1 and GLUT3 was positively expressed in 74.8% and 6.1% of the NSCLC tissues, respectively. GLUT1 expression was significantly correlated with squamous cell carcinoma histology, poor differentiation, high pathologic stage, old age, male, smoking, and high SUV_{max} (>7) (all $p < 0.05$). The squamous cell carcinoma and smoker group also showed significantly higher SUV_{max} (both $p < 0.001$). Systemic inflammation markers, including NLR, PLR, and LMR, were positively correlated with high SUV_{max} (all $p < 0.05$). High GLUT1 expression, high SUV_{max}, high NLR, and low LMR, were significantly associated with poor overall survival in patients with NSCLC. However, in the multivariate survival analysis, LMR was an independent prognostic factor overall (HR 1.86, 95% CI 1.05–3.3) and for the stage I/II cohort (HR 2.3, 95% CI 1.24–4.3) (all $p < 0.05$). Conclusions: Systemic inflammatory markers—NLR, PLR, and LMR are strongly correlated with the SUV_{max} and are indicators of aggressive tumor behavior. Specifically, LMR is a promising prognostic biomarker in NSCLC patients.

Keywords: inflammation; monocyte; GLUT1; PET-CT scan; non-small cell lung cancer; prognosis; survival

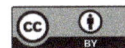

1. Introduction

Despite recent therapeutic advances, the prognosis of non-small-cell lung cancer (NSCLC) is still poor, and it is a leading cause of cancer death worldwide [1]. The diverse nature of this cancer contributes to its high mortality rate [2]. Therefore, understanding the biology of NSCLC and its patient stratification is important for designing optimal treatments.

The hallmarks of cancer are distinctive capabilities that make tumor growth and metastasis possible [3]. They include sustaining proliferative signaling, evading growth suppressors, activating invasion and metastasis, enabling replicative immortality, inducing angiogenesis, and resisting cell death. In addition to these classic hallmarks, two new hallmarks are emerging: reprogramming energy metabolism and avoiding immune destruction [3]. Cancer cells' ability to reprogram their glucose metabolism was first discovered by Otto Warburg and is called the Warburg Effect [4]. The Warburg Effect is characterized by increased glycolysis in cancer cells, even in the presence of oxygen. This metabolic switch in cancer cells is accomplished in part by upregulating glucose transporters, especially glucose transporter-1 (GLUT1), and increases glucose influx into the cytoplasm [4].

GLUT1 is a member of a glucose transporter family (GLUT), which transports glucose across the cell membrane. Seven glucose transporters in this family have been discovered [5]. GLUT1 is overexpressed in various cancers, including lung, colorectal, and breast cancers [6–9]. Increased uptake and utilization of glucose have also been observed by noninvasively visualizing glucose uptake using a radiolabeled analog of glucose (18F-fluorodeoxyglucose, FDG) and positron emission tomography (PET). FDG-PET parameters are tumor glucose metabolic markers. Typically, the maximum standardized uptake value (SUV_{max}) has been associated with the progression, metastasis, and prognosis of various cancer types, including lung cancer [10–15].

Another emerging hallmark of cancer is its evasion of immune responses [3]. Cancer cells are suspected of having mechanisms that help them evade immunological monitoring or limit the extent of immunological killing [3,16,17]. Recent studies have reported new findings regarding this ability of cancer cells, as well as the interaction between tumor cells and immune cells in the tumor microenvironment and the relationship between tumor cells and systemic inflammatory responses [18,19]. One of the human body's immune responses to cancer is changing the populations of circulating leukocytes and platelets. Similar to bacterial or virus infections, patients with cancer often develop thrombocytosis or neutrophilia, and these immune responses are reflected by systemic inflammatory markers such as the neutrophil–lymphocyte ratio (NLR), the platelet–lymphocyte ratio (PLR), and the lymphocyte–monocyte ratio (LMR) [20,21]. Interestingly, high NLR and PLR are increasingly reported to be associated with poor prognosis in different cancers [22–27]. Although LMR has been reported as a prognostic marker for several cancers, including lung cancer, there is currently a lack of sufficient evidence [28,29]. While it is not a novel concept, the association of systemic inflammation with cancer has increasingly become the subject of current research [30].

The clinical meaning of tumor metabolic activity and systemic inflammation in lung cancer has been extensively investigated in previous studies. However, the relationship of these key features has not been clearly elucidated, and only few studies have evaluated these hallmarks in NSCLC rather than in small-cell carcinoma [15]. Therefore, herein, we evaluated 18-F-FDG PET-CT, GLUT1 expression, NLR, PLR, and LMR, among other indicators of tumor metabolic activity and systemic inflammation, for their association with NSCLC and compared their prognostic values. Since these factors can be easily examined in a clinical context, our findings are valuable for the therapeutic management of NSCLC.

2. Methods

2.1. Patients

A total of 163 patients diagnosed with NSCLC in St. Vincent's Hospital between 2006 and 2016 were included in the study. All patients underwent surgical resection or excisional biopsy. The patients' clinical information and pathological data were obtained from hospital medical records. The patients were classified by cancer stage at the time of the surgery, and patients diagnosed before the announcement of staging guidelines of the 7th American Joint Committee on Cancer were restaged according to the 7th edition of the TNM classification of malignant tumors [31]. Pure ground-glass lesions were excluded from the study. Patients did not receive neoadjuvant chemotherapy or radiotherapy.

Using patients' medical reports, we recorded their differential white blood cell (WBC) counts, taken within one month of surgery or excisional biopsy as part of a preoperative workup. Inflammatory markers were defined as follows: NLR (absolute neutrophil count/absolute lymphocyte count), PLR (absolute platelet count/absolute lymphocyte count), and LMR (absolute lymphocyte count/absolute monocyte count).

The study was conducted according to the World Medical Association Declaration of Helsinki and the study protocol was approved by the Institutional Review Board (IRB) of St. Vincent's Hospital at The Catholic University of Korea (IRB No. VC20SISI0017). Written informed consent was obtained from all patients.

2.2. FDG/PET-CT Protocol and Image Analysis

After the patients fasted for a minimum of six hours, 3.7–5.5 MBq/kg of 18F-FDG was injected intravenously. None of the patients had a blood glucose level exceeding 130 mg/dL pre-injection. No contrast agent was given. Studies were acquired using a combined PET/CT in-line system (Biograph TruePoint, Siemens Medical Solutions, Knoxville, TN, USA), for 2–3 min per bed position.

FDG PET/CT images were reviewed by an expert nuclear medicine physician (S.Y.P.). FDG avidity was defined as showing discrete uptake exceeding the background soft tissue visual. The maximum standardized uptake value (SUV_{max}) of the primary lung lesion was calculated from the injected dose and body weight. When there were multifocal lesions, the region of interest was drawn for the largest lesion. The SUV_{max} was calculated as follows:

$$SUV = C/(Di/W)$$

C is the decay-corrected tracer tissue concentration (kBq/mL), Di is the injected dose (MBq), and W is the body weight (kg).

2.3. Immunohistochemistry

For the construction of tissue microarrays (TMAs), the most representative areas were identified on a slide stained with hematoxylin and eosin and marked by a pathologist (U.C.). One core measuring 5.0 mm in diameter was obtained and arrayed onto a paraffin block. Each sample was tested using primary antibodies for GLUT1 (Abcam, Cambridge, UK; diluted 1:200) and GLUT3 (Abcam; diluted 1:200). Briefly, 4-μm sections were deparaffinized in xylene and then rehydrated through a graded ethanol series. Slides were loaded into a BenchMark XT automated slide stainer (Ventana Medical Systems, Inc., Oro Valley, AZ, USA) and then incubated for 16 min at 37 °C with each primary antibody. Immunoreactivity was detected using an ultraView Universal DAB detection kit (Ventana Medical Systems, Inc.) and 3,3′-diaminobenzidine, followed by counterstaining with hematoxylin and a bluing agent.

An expert pathologist (U.C.) performed immunohistochemical assessments. For the evaluation of immunoreactivity in tumor cells, a dichotomized scoring system was used as follows: GLUT1 and GLUT3 positivity was determined if ≥10% of tumor cells demonstrated either membranous and/or cytoplasmic staining.

2.4. Statistical Analysis

We applied chi-squared tests to compare categorical variables. Overall survival (OS) was defined from the date of the initial diagnosis to the date of death. Progression-free survival was defined from the date of the initial diagnosis to the data of progression. Survival estimates were analyzed based on the Kaplan–Meier method and compared using the log-rank test and univariate Cox proportional hazard regression analysis. Factors that were significant according to univariate analysis or factors that were considered clinically important were subjected to Cox proportional hazards regression multivariate analysis.

The ideal cutoff value for the FDG-PET SUV_{max} was determined via receiver operating characteristic (ROC) curve analysis. A score closest to the point of maximum sensitivity and specificity was selected, leading to the largest group of tumors that correctly predicted the survival event. Median values were used as cutoffs for NLR, PLR, and LMR. A nomogram for possible prognostic factors used the R packages survival and rms. The performance of the nomogram for predicting survival was evaluated with Harrell's concordance index (C-index). The bootstrapping method was used for internal validation of the nomogram. A two-sided p value < 0.05 was considered significant. R software (version 4.2.2) was used for the statistical analyses.

3. Results

3.1. Study Population: Demographic and Clinical Features

This study cohort included 105 adenocarcinoma (105/163, 64.4%), 49 squamous cell carcinoma (49/163, 30.1%), and nine other histological types of cancer (e.g., large cell carcinoma and pleomorphic carcinoma: 9/163; 5.5%) cases. The mean age was 64.8 years (ranging from 36 to 82), and males outnumbered females (male/female ratio: 2.13). Records showed that 43.6% of patients involved in the study had never smoked, and patients were distributed among each discrete cancer staging category as follows: IA: 21.5%, IB: 16.6%, IIA: 16.6%, IIB: 8.6%, IIIA: 18.4%, IIIB: 2.5%, and IV: 16.0%. About two-thirds (103/163, 63.2%) of patients received adjuvant therapy, including chemotherapy, radiation therapy, combined chemoradiation therapy, or tyrosine kinase inhibitor therapy, while others (60/163, 36.8%) received only surgery.

3.2. GLUT1 and GLUT3 Expression and FDG-PET SUV_{max} Characterization

GLUT1 and GLUT3 were positively expressed in 74.8% and 6.1% of patients, respectively. GLUT1 expression was significantly correlated with male patients, smokers, and squamous cell carcinomas with poor histologic differentiation (all $p < 0.05$) (Figure 1). The average FDG-PET SUV_{max} was 7.1 ± 3.8, and it was significantly higher in the GLUT1-positive compared to the GLUT1-negative group ($p < 0.001$) (Table 1). FDG-PET SUV_{max} values ranged from 0.6 to 19.6 (median 5.9), and the mean was 6.4 (standard deviation 3.83). On the other hand, GLUT3 expression did not correlate with any clinicopathologic features (all $p > 0.05$). A high SUV_{max} value (>7) also significantly correlated with male patients, smokers, squamous cell carcinomas with poor differentiation, as well as patients in advanced T stage or AJCC stage (all $p < 0.05$) (Table 1).

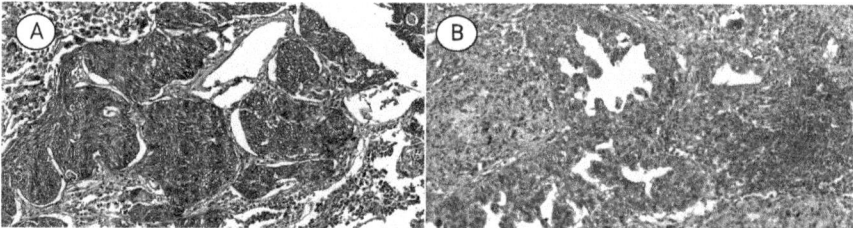

Figure 1. Micrograph of non-small cell lung cancer-expressing (**A**) GLUT1 and (**B**) GLUT3 (×400).

3.3. NLR and PLR Characterization and Their Association with Clinicopathologic Characteristics

Among all patients with NSCLC, the mean white blood cell count was $7.7 \pm 2.6 \times 10^6$/mL, and the mean NLR, PLR, and LMR were 2.8 ± 3.0, 4.0 ± 1.8, and 133.8 ± 84.8, respectively. Patients with elevated NLR had a more advanced AJCC stage, and mean FDG-PET SUV_{max} and PLR were higher in the high NLR group (all $p < 0.05$). The mean LMR was significantly lower in the high NLR group ($p < 0.001$). Elevated PLR was associated with high FDG-PET SUV_{max} and high LMR (all $p < 0.05$). Elevated LMR was correlated with females and a less advanced AJCC stage (all $p < 0.05$). The mean FDG-PET SUV_{max}, NLR, and PLR were significantly lower in the high LMR group (all $p < 0.05$) (Table 2).

Table 1. Relationship between metabolic markers and clinicopathologic features in patients with non-small cell lung carcinoma.

	GLUT1			GLUT3			FDG-PET SUV$_{max}$		
	Negative (n = 41)	Positive (n = 122)	p	Negative (n = 153)	Positive (n = 10)	p	Low (<7) (n = 99)	High (≥7) (n = 64)	p
Age (years)	63.2 ± 9.4	65.3 ± 10.1	0.236	64.6 ± 9.8	67.7 ± 11.9	0.337	63.7 ± 9.7	66.5 ± 10.1	0.082
Sex									
Male (n = 111, 68.1%)	17 (41.5%)	94 (77.0%)	<0.001	103 (67.3%)	8 (80%)	0.629	58 (58.6%)	53 (82.8%)	0.002
Female (n = 52, 31.9%)	24 (58.5%)	28 (23.0%)		50 (32.7%)	2 (20%)		41 (41.4%)	11 (17.2%)	
Smoking Status									
Never smoker (n = 71, 43.6%)	27 (65.9%)	44 (36.1%)	0.002	67 (43.8%)	4 (40%)	0.999	53 (53.5%)	18 (28.1%)	0.002
Ever smoker (n = 92, 56.4%)	14 (34.1%)	78 (63.9%)		86 (56.2%)	6 (60%)		46 (46.5%)	46 (71.9%)	
Histology									
Non-SqCC (n = 115 70.6%)	40 (97.6%)	75 (61.5%)	<0.001	106 (69.3%)	8 (80%)	0.719	80 (80.8%)	34 (53.1%)	<0.001
SqCC (n = 48, 29.4%)	1 (2.44%)	47 (38.5%)		47 (30.7%)	2 (20%)		19 (19.2%)	30 (46.9%)	
Tumor differentiation									
WD and MD (n = 133, 81.6%)	39 (95.1%)	94 (77.0%)	0.019	127 (83.0%)	6 (60%)	0.162	87 (87.9%)	46 (71.9%)	0.018
PD (n = 30, 18.4%)	2 (4.88%)	28 (23.0%)		26 (17.0%)	4 (40%)		12 (12.1%)	18 (28.1%)	
Lymphovascular invasion									
Absent (n = 125, 76.7%)	34 (82.9%)	91 (74.6%)	0.380	117 (76.5%)	8 (80.0%)	0.999	77 (77.8%)	48 (75.0%)	0.826
Present (n = 38, 23.3%)	7 (17.1%)	31 (25.4%)		36 (23.5%)	2 (20.0%)		22 (22.2%)	16 (25.0%)	
T stage *									
1 (n = 50, 30.7%)	18 (46.2%)	32 (32.3%)	0.129	50 (38.2%)	0	0.164	40 (46.5%)	10 (19.2%)	0.007
2 (n = 66, 40.5%)	19 (48.7%)	47 (47.5%)		60 (45.8%)	6 (85.7%)		37 (43.0%)	29 (55.8%)	
3 (n = 18, 6.7%)	2 (5.1%)	16 (16.2%)		17 (13.0%)	1 (14.3%)		7 (8.1%)	11 (21.2%)	
4 (n = 4, 2.5%)	0	4 (4.0%)		4 (3.1%)	0		2 (2.3%)	2 (3.8%)	
N stage †									
0 (n = 77, 47.2%)	26 (66.7%)	51 (52.0%)	0.139	72 (55.4%)	5 (71.4%)	0.558	52 (61.2%)	25 (48.1%)	0.37
1 (n = 30, 18.4%)	6 (15.4%)	24 (24.5%)		28 (21.5%)	2 (28.6%)		16 (18.8%)	14 (26.9%)	
2 (n = 29, 17.8%)	6 (15.4%)	23 (23.5%)		29 (22.3%)	0		16 (18.8%)	13 (25.0%)	
3 (n = 1, 0.6%)	1 (2.6%)	0		1 (0.8%)	0		1 (1.2%)	0	
AJCC Stage									
I (n = 62, 38.0%)	22 (53.7%)	40 (32.8%)	0.084	58 (37.9%)	4 (40.0%)	0.302	47 (47.5%)	15 (23.4%)	0.022
II (n = 41, 25.2%)	9 (22.0%)	32 (26.2%)		38 (24.8%)	3 (30.0%)		21 (21.2%)	20 (31.2%)	
III (n = 34, 20.9%)	7 (17.1%)	27 (22.1%)		34 (22.2%)	0		18 (18.2%)	16 (25.0%)	
IV (n = 30, 18.4%)	3 (7.3%)	23 (18.9%)		23 (15.0%)	3 (30.0%)		13 (13.1%)	13 (20.3%)	
SUV$_{max}$	4.2 ± 2.9	7.1 ± 3.8	<0.001	6.3 ± 3.8	8.1 ± 3.5	0.157	-	-	-
NLR	2.9 ± 3.4	2.8 ± 2.9	0.915	2.9 ± 3.1	2.6 ± 1.3	0.579	2.5 ± 2.6	3.4 ± 3.4	0.091
PLR	120.8 ± 57.8	138.1 ± 91.9	0.16	131.8 ± 85.8	164.3 ± 64.5	0.241	119.2 ± 60.4	156.4 ± 109.4	0.015
LMR	4.4 ± 1.7	3.9 ± 1.8	0.148	4.1 ± 1.8	3.2 ± 1.1	0.12	4.2 ± 1.6	3.7 ± 2.1	0.085

SqCC, squamous cell carcinoma; WD, well differentiated; MD, moderately differentiated; PD, poorly differentiated; AJCC, American Joint Committee on Cancer; SUV$_{max}$, maximum standardized uptake value; NLR, Neutrophil–lymphocyte ratio; PLR, Platelet–lymphocyte ratio; LMR, Lymphocyte–monocyte ratio. * Twenty-five patients have missing pathologic T stage data. † Twenty-six patients have missing pathologic N stage data.

Table 2. Relationship between systemic inflammatory markers and clinicopathologic features in patients with non-small cell lung carcinoma.

	NLR Low (n = 82)	NLR High (n = 81)	p	PLR Low (n = 81)	PLR High (n = 82)	p	LMR Low (n = 81)	LMR High (n = 82)	p
Age (years)	65.5 ± 9.3	64.0 ± 10.5	0.353	65.3 ± 9.1	64.3 ± 10.7	0.511	65.2 ± 10.5	64.3 ± 9.4	0.552
Sex			0.262			0.999			0.005
Male (n = 111, 68.1%)	30 (36.6%)	59 (72.8%)		55 (67.9%)	56 (68.3%)		64 (79.0%)	47 (57.3%)	
Female (n = 52, 31.9%)	52 (63.4%)	22 (27.2%)		26 (32.1%)	26 (31.7%)		17 (21.0%)	35 (42.7%)	
Smoking Status			0.232			0.483			0.379
Never smoker (n = 71, 43.6%)	40 (48.8%)	31 (38.3%)		43 (53.1%)	33 (40.2%)		32 (39.5%)	39 (47.6%)	
Ever smoker (n = 92, 56.4%)	42 (51.2%)	50 (61.7%)		38 (46.9%)	49 (59.8%)		49 (60.5%)	43 (52.4%)	
Histology			0.156			0.156			0.463
Non-SqCC (n = 115 70.6%)	62 (75.6%)	52 (64.2%)		52 (64.2%)	62 (75.6%)		54 (66.7%)	60 (73.2%)	
SqCC (n = 48, 29.4%)	20 (24.4%)	29 (35.8%)		29 (35.8%)	20 (24.4%)		27 (33.3%)	22 (26.8%)	
Tumor differentiation			0.52			0.33			0.146
WD and MD (n = 133, 81.6%)	69 (84.1%)	64 (79.0%)		69 (85.2%)	64 (78.0%)		62 (76.5%)	71 (86.6%)	
PD (n = 30, 18.4%)	13 (15.9%)	17 (21.0%)		12 (14.8%)	18 (22.0%)		19 (23.5%)	11 (13.4%)	
Lymphovascular invasion			0.332			0.377			0.887
Absent (n = 125, 76.7%)	66 (80.5%)	59 (72.8%)		65 (80.2%)	60 (73.2%)		63 (77.8%)	62 (75.6%)	
Present (n = 38, 23.3%)	16 (19.5%)	22 (27.2%)		16 (19.8%)	22 (26.8%)		18 (22.2%)	20 (24.4%)	
T stage *			0.138			0.156			0.693
1 (n = 50, 30.7%)	30 (40.0%)	20 (31.7%)		28 (38.4%)	22 (33.8%)		22 (34.9%)	28 (37.3%)	
2 (n = 66, 40.5%)	38 (50.7%)	28 (44.4%)		34 (46.6%)	32 (49.2%)		30 (47.6%)	36 (48.0%)	
3 (n = 18, 6.7%)	6 (8.0%)	12 (19.0%)		11 (15.1%)	7 (10.8%)		8 (12.7%)	10 (13.3%)	
4 (n = 4, 2.5%)	1 (1.3%)	3 (4.8%)		0 (0.0%)	4 (6.2%)		3 (4.8%)	1 (1.3%)	
N stage †			0.145			0.784			0.626
0 (n = 77, 47.2%)	47 (62.7%)	30 (48.4%)		40 (55.6%)	37 (56.9%)		34 (54.0%)	43 (58.1%)	
1 (n = 30, 18.4%)	16 (21.3%)	14 (22.6%)		15 (20.8%)	15 (23.1%)		13 (20.6%)	17 (23.0%)	
2 (n = 29, 17.8%)	11 (14.7%)	18 (29.0%)		16 (22.2%)	13 (20.0%)		15 (23.8%)	14 (18.9%)	
3 (n = 1, 0.6%)	1 (1.3%)	0 (0.0%)		1 (1.4%)	0 (0.0%)		1 (1.6%)	0 (0.0%)	
AJCC Stage			0.012			0.207			0.032
I (n = 62, 38.0%)	40 (48.8%)	22 (27.2%)		34 (42.0%)	28 (34.1%)		26 (32.1%)	36 (43.9%)	
II (n = 41, 25.2%)	21 (25.6%)	20 (24.7%)		21 (25.9%)	20 (24.4%)		17 (21.0%)	24 (29.3%)	
III (n = 34, 20.9%)	13 (15.9%)	21 (25.9%)		18 (22.2%)	16 (19.5%)		19 (23.5%)	15 (18.3%)	
IV (n = 30, 18.4%)	8 (9.8%)	18 (22.2%)		8 (9.9%)	18 (22.0%)		19 (23.5%)	7 (8.5%)	
SUV$_{max}$	5.5 ± 3.5	7.3 ± 3.9	0.003	5.5 ± 3.6	7.3 ± 3.8	0.004	7.0 ± 3.8	5.8 ± 3.8	0.032
NLR	-	-	-	1.6 ± 0.7	4.0 ± 3.8	<0.001	3.8 ± 3.6	1.8 ± 1.7	<0.001
PLR	96.5 ± 32.2	171.5 ± 103.2	<0.001	-	-	-	166.2 ± 104.8	101.7 ± 38.0	<0.001
LMR	4.8 ± 1.8	3.2 ± 1.4	<0.001	4.9 ± 1.9	3.2 ± 1.2	<0.001	-	-	-

SqCC—squamous cell carcinoma; WD—well differentiated; MD—moderately differentiated; PD—poorly differentiated; AJCC—American Joint Committee on Cancer; SUV$_{max}$—maximum standardized uptake value; NLR—neutrophil–lymphocyte ratio; PLR—platelet–lymphocyte ratio; LMR—lymphocyte–monocyte ratio. * Twenty-five patients have missing pathologic T stage data. † Twenty-six patients have missing pathologic N stage data.

3.4. Correlation of Metabolic Markers and Systemic Inflammatory Markers in Patients with Stage I and II NSCLC

Additionally, we performed a subgroup analysis in 103 patients with AJCC Stage I and II low-stage groups. As among all patients with NSCLC, GLUT1 expression was correlated with high FDG-PET SUV_{max} (6.8 ± 3.6 vs. 3.3 ± 2.5, $p < 0.001$), but GLUT3 expression showed no correlation with any other markers. NLR and PLR were also positively corelated with the FDG-PET SUV_{max} (all $p < 0.05$). However, LMR had no correlation with FDG-PET SUV_{max} in this subgroup ($p = 0.498$).

3.5. Survival Analysis

The follow-up period ranged from 1 to 139.9 months (median 5.8 months). Ninety patients (55.2%) died during the follow-up, and the median OS was 55.0 months. The survival rates at 2 and 5 years after diagnosis were 71.2% (standard error 3.6%) and 51.7% (standard error 4.0%), respectively. After surgery, 26.4% of the patients received adjuvant chemotherapy, radiotherapy, or chemoradiotherapy.

In the univariate analysis, poor tumor differentiation, high GLUT1 expression, high SUV_{max}, high NLR, low LMR, and advanced T, N, and AJCC stage were associated with worse OS (all $p < 0.05$) (Figure 2). However, age, sex, smoking history, squamous cell carcinoma histology, lymphovascular invasion, GLUT3 expression, and high PLR demonstrated no prognostic significance (all $p > 0.05$). In a multivariate analysis, old age, AJCC stage, and LMR were independent prognostic factors that were associated with OS (all $p < 0.05$) (Figure 3).

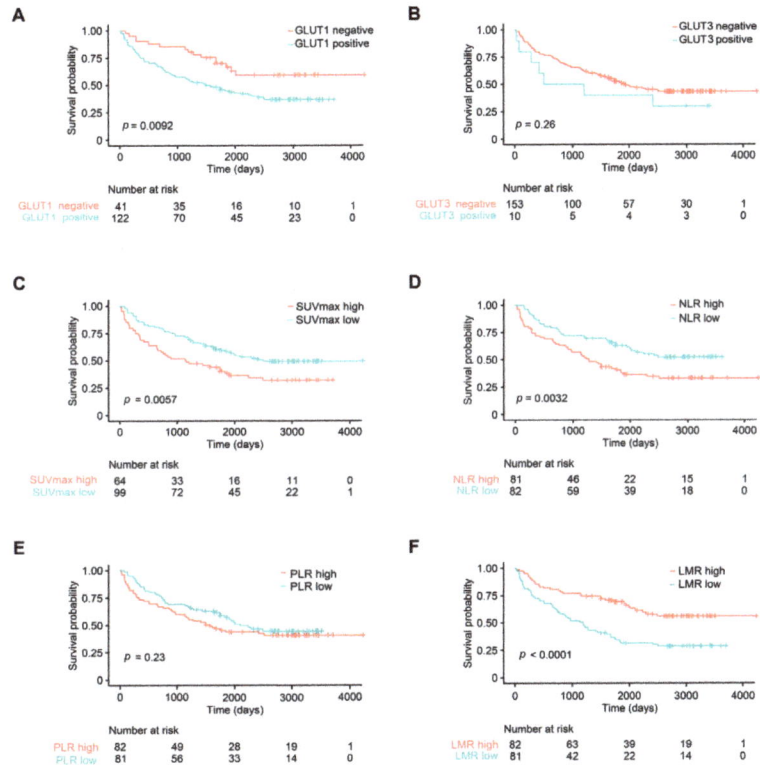

Figure 2. Kaplan–Meier survival curves of different parameters in patients with non-small cell carcinoma. (**A**) GLUT1 expression, (**B**) GLUT3 expression, (**C**) FDG-PET SUV_{max}, (**D**) neutrophil–lymphocyte ratio (NLR), (**E**) platelet–lymphocyte ratio (PLR), and (**F**) lymphocyte–monocyte ratio (LMR). FDG-PET SUV_{max}, fluoro-D-glucose-positron emission tomography maximum uptake value.

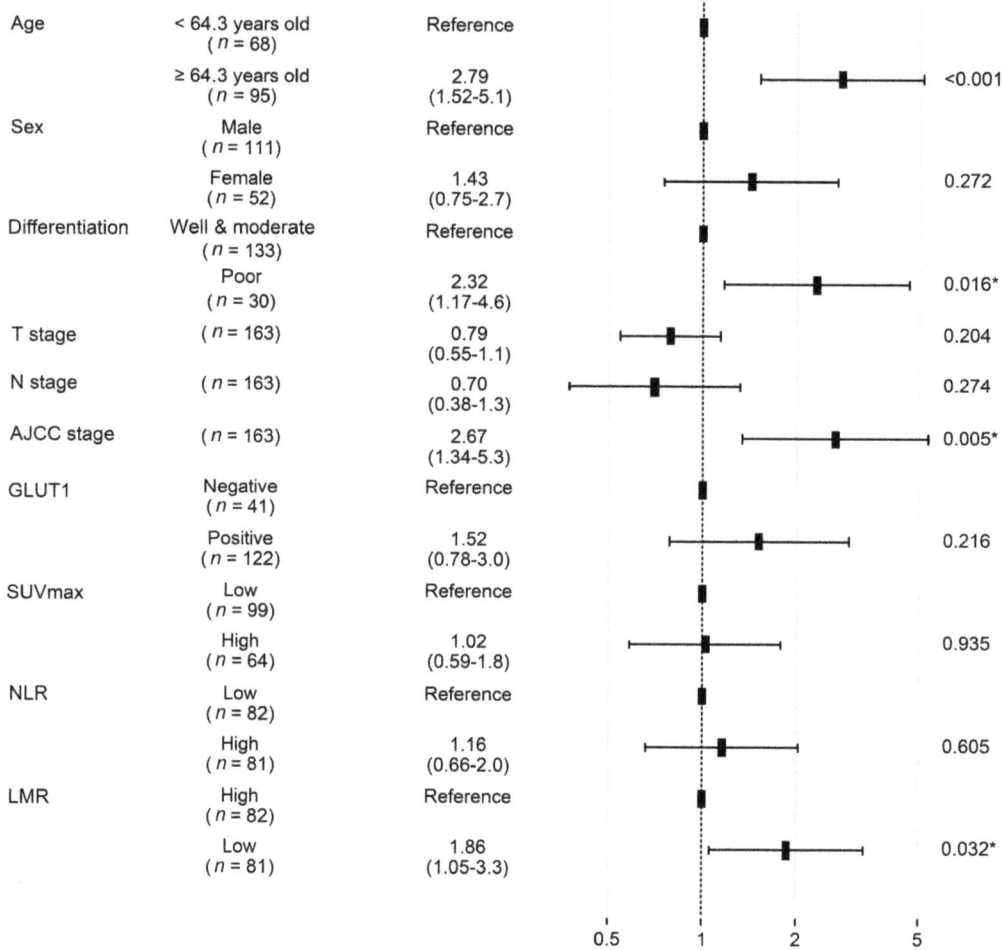

Figure 3. Forest plot showing hazard ratios obtained by multivariate Cox regression for overall survival in patients with non-small cell carcinoma. SUV_{max}, fluoro-D-glucose-positron emission tomography maximum uptake value; NLR—neutrophil–lymphocyte ratio; LMR—lymphocyte–monocyte ratio. * Indicates factors with significant p values.

Survival analysis was then performed in patients with AJCC stage I, II, and III NSCLC and in patients with AJCC stage IV NSCLCL, i.e., with metastasis. In the patient with AJCC stage I, II, and III NSCLC, old age, poor histologic differentiation, AJCC stage, and LMR were independent prognostic factors with regard to OS (all $p < 0.05$) (Table 3). Progression-free survival was analyzed in the patient with AJCC stage IV NSCLC, and none of the clinicopathologic, metabolic, or systemic inflammatory markers were associated with progression (all $p > 0.05$).

Table 3. Univariate and multivariate Cox regression analysis for overall survival in 137 Stage I, II and III non-small cell lung cancer patients.

	Univariate Analysis			Multivariate Analysis		
	HR	95% CI	p	HR	95% CI	p
Age (reference: <64.3 years old)	3.51	1.16–3.51	0.009	3.11	1.67–5.8	<0.001
Sex (reference: male)	1.45	0.83–2.53	0.2	1.79	0.91–3.52	0.09
Smoking Status (reference: never smoker)	1.25	0.76–2.04	0.4	-	-	-
Histology (reference: non-SqCC)	1.4	0.85–2.30	0.2	-	-	-
Differentiation (reference: WD and MD)	2.34	1.25–4.38	0.006	2.89	1.43–5.83	<0.001
Lymphovascular invasion (reference: absent)	1.51	0.88–2.58	0.10	-	-	-
T stage (reference: 1)			0.003			
2	1.03	0.59–1.81		0.7	0.38–1.29	0.25
3	3.02	1.54–5.91		1.37	0.52–3.63	0.53
4	1.17	0.28–4.99		0.48	0.08–2.73	0.41
N stage * (reference:0)			0.01			
1	1.65	0.90–3.05		1.07	0.37–3.08	0.9
2	2.26	1.25–4.09		2.54	0.30–21.43	0.39
3	3.15	0.43–23.28		1.93	0.12–31.83	0.64
AJCC stage (reference: I)			<0.001			
Stage II	2.48	1.37–4.50		3.41	1.18–9.91	0.02
Stage III	2.86	1.54–5.30		1.52	0.16–14.39	0.72
GLUT1 (reference: negative)	1.96	1.04–3.66	0.036	1.76	0.88–3.53	0.11
GLUT3 (reference: negative)	1.25	0.45–3.44	0.67	-	-	-
FDG-PET SUV$_{max}$ (reference: low)	0.71	0.44–1.16	0.2	-	-	-
NLR (reference: low)	1.59	0.97–2.59	0.06	-	-	-
PLR (reference: low)	1.01	0.62–1.65	0.961	-	-	-
LMR (reference: high)	2.04	1.24–3.34	0.04	2.23	1.28–3.86	<0.001

HR—hazard ratio; CI—confidence interval; SqCC—squamous cell carcinoma; WD—well differentiated; MD—moderately differentiated; AJCC—American Joint Committee on Cancer; SUV$_{max}$—maximum standardized uptake value; NLR—Neutrophil–lymphocyte ratio; PLR—Platelet–lymphocyte ratio; LMR—Lymphocyte-monocyte ratio. * One patient has missing pathologic N stage data.

In the subgroup of patients with stage I and II NSCLC, 42.7% of the patients died during the follow-up period, and the median OS was 65.3 months (range 1 to 139.9 months). The 2-year survival rate was 81.6% (standard error 3.8%) and the 5-year survival rate was 65.8% (standard error 4.7%). In this group, histological differentiation, lymphovascular invasion, old age, T stage, and LMR were associated with OS (all $p < 0.05$) (Figure 4). The 2-year survival rate of patients with low LMR was 74.4%, which was significantly lower when compared to that of the high-LMR group, which was 86.7% ($p = 0.002$). GLUT1 expression, GLUT3 expression, squamous cell carcinoma histology, sex, high SVU$_{max}$, N stage, NLR, and PLR were not significant prognostic factors in stage I and II group (all $p > 0.05$). According to multivariate Cox proportional hazards analysis, old age, poor differentiation, lymphovascular invasion, and low LMR remained independent prognostic factors associated with poor OS in patients with stage I/II NSCLC (all $p < 0.05$). Low LMR was a particularly poor prognostic factor, with a hazard ratio of 2.3 (95% CI 1.2–4.3, $p = 0.008$) (Figure 5).

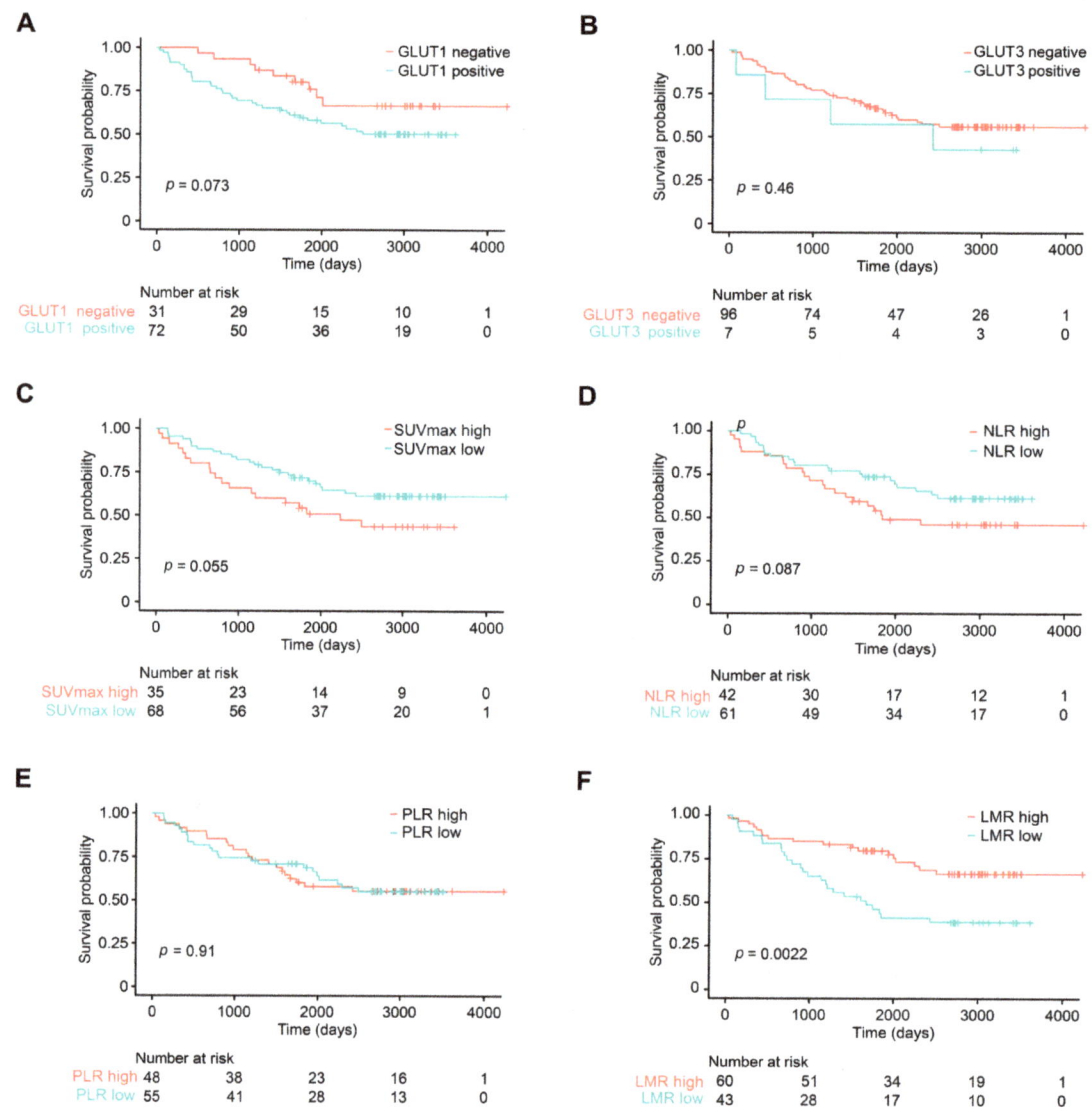

Figure 4. Kaplan–Meier survival curves of different parameters in patients with stage I/II non-small cell carcinoma. (**A**) GLUT1 expression, (**B**) GLUT3 expression, (**C**) FDG-PET SUV$_{max}$, (**D**) neutrophil–lymphocyte ratio (NLR), (**E**) platelet–lymphocyte ratio (PLR), and (**F**) lymphocyte–monocyte ratio (LMR). FDG-PET SUV$_{max}$, fluoro-D-glucose-positron emission tomography maximum uptake value.

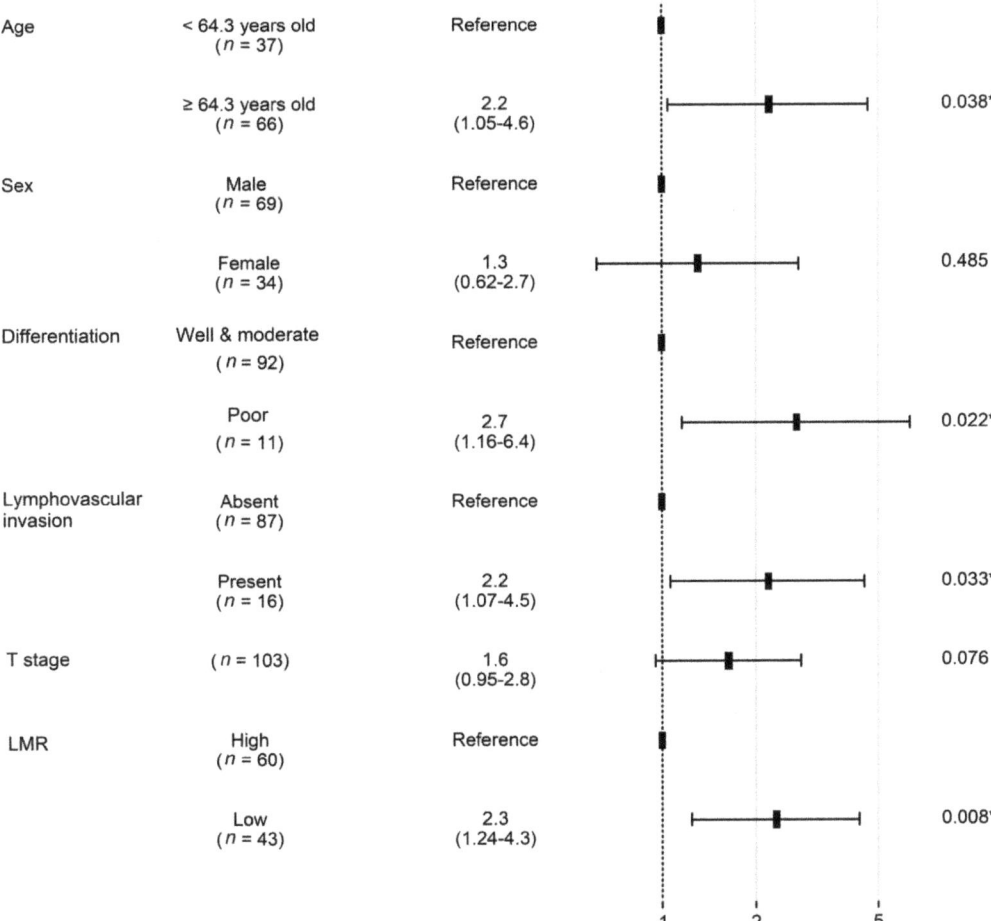

Figure 5. Forest plot showing hazard ratios obtained by multivariate Cox regression for overall survival in patients with stage I/II non-small cell carcinoma. LMR—lymphocyte–monocyte ratio. * Indicates factors with significant *p* values.

3.6. Nomogram for Prediction of OS

A prognostic nomogram of patients with NSCLC was established using a Cox regression model according to significant independent prognostic factors of OS (age, AJCC stage, and LMR). Each factor in the nomogram was assigned a weighted number of points. The sum of points for each patient was in accordance with a specific predicted 3- and 5-year OS. A nomogram predicting OS was also established in the group of patients with stage I and II NSCLC (Figure 6). Independent prognostic factors in this group—such as age, histologic differentiation, lymphovascular invasion, and LMR—were incorporated in the nomogram. The C-index of the multivariate prognostic model slightly improved from 0.75 (standard error 0.02) to 0.65 (standard error 0.04) when LMR was added to the model, which was developed based on age, histological differentiation, and lymphovascular invasion.

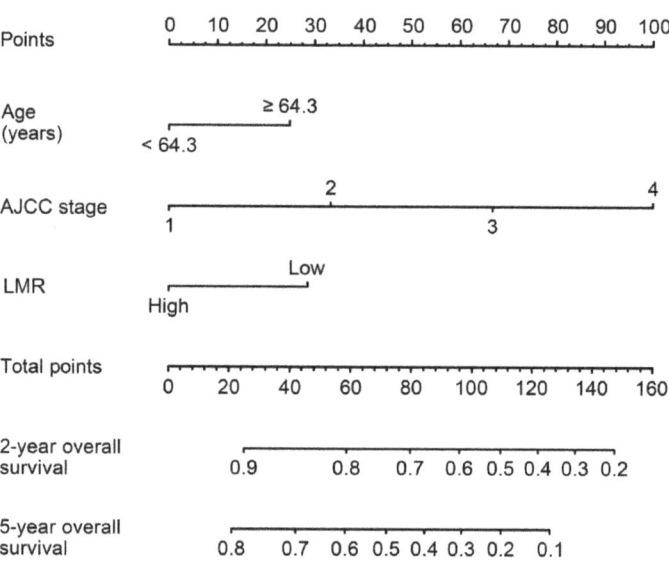

Figure 6. Nomogram for overall survival of patients with stage I/II non-small cell carcinoma. LMR—lymphocyte–monocyte ratio.

4. Discussion

In this paper, we investigated the clinical significance of 18-F-FDG PET-CT SUV_{max}, NLR, PLR, LMR, and expression of GLUT1 and GLUT3, which can easily be measured in clinical settings, among various tumor metabolic activity and systemic inflammation markers, in patients with NSCLC. Our findings showed that GLUT1 expression, NLR, and LMR are prognostic factors predicting the OS of patients with NSCLC.

Changes in metabolic activity can be measured in vivo via metabolomics, magnetic resonance spectroscopy, PET, and stable isotope tracing [32]. In particular, 18-F-FDG PET-CT is not only used to diagnose malignant tumors of different cancers, but also reflects treatment response [33], while parameters such as SUV_{max}, metabolic tumor volume, and total lesion glycolysis are associated with the prognosis of patients with cancer [10–14,34]. Previous findings suggest that the uptake of 18F-FDG has an independent prognostic value in patients newly diagnosed with NSCLC [35]. However, in our study, PET SUV_{max} was not a significant prognostic factor. FDG-PET parameters are related to and affected by different tumor markers or biomarkers such as CFLYRA21-1, NSE, SCC-ag, ki67, and p53 [36], and MTV is known to better reflect the prognosis of patients with cancer when compared to SUV_{max} [14]. In general, 18F-FDG-PET is a promising biomarker in cancer prognosis; however, its statistical significance as a prognostic factor has not been demonstrated. Thus, further studies must be conducted to confirm the power of 18F-FDG-PET as a prognostic factor [37].

We investigated the expression and clinical significance of two representative GLUT family proteins, GLUT1 and GLUT2. Only the expression of GLUT1, not GLUT3, was associated with a shorter OS. Interestingly, GLUT1 expression and SUV_{max} significantly differed according to the tumor histology and smoking history of patients with NSCLC. Herein, both GLUT1 expression and SUV_{max} were higher in patients who had squamous histology and who were smokers. These results are in line with those of previous studies [38]. In a previous study that analyzed differential gene expression in lung squamous cell carcinoma and adenocarcinoma using The Cancer Genome Atlas datasets, GLUT1 had the highest mRNA expression level among GLUT family proteins in squamous cell carcinoma. Similarly, GLUT1 overexpression was phenotypically and specifically linked to the squamous cell carcinoma subtype rather than the adenocarcinoma patient group [38]. Additionally, in a cell line study, squamous cell carcinoma was a more glycolysis-reliant histological phenotype than adenocarcinoma, and lung squamous cell carcinoma had higher 18F-FDG uptake than adenocarcinoma [38]. In a study by Koh et al., immunohistochemical evaluation of GLUT1 expression also demonstrated close association with a squamous phenotype, micropapillary/solid histology, lymphovascular invasion, and advanced pTNM stage in NSCLC [7]. Based on these previous findings and our data, we conclude that GLUT1 contributes to tumor aggressiveness, especially in squamous cells. GLUT1 immunohistochemical staining does not reflect the in vivo metabolic activity, but it can easily be conducted as an ancillary test during surgery or biopsies. We conclude that GLUT1 is an important indicator that can reflect the metabolic activity of NSCLC.

Analysis of the relationship between systemic inflammatory markers and other clinicopathological factors revealed interesting findings. Increases in neutrophil, platelet, and monocyte counts in relation to lymphocyte counts were generally correlated with an advanced stage, tumor aggressiveness, and markers of tumor metabolic activity, e.g., SUV_{max} and GLUT1 expression. NLR, PLR, and LMR were indicators of aggressive tumor behavior.

In our study, NLR, PLR, and LMR correlated with SUV_{max}, in agreement with previous studies. In one study of head and neck cancer, NLR was positively correlated with FDG-PET metabolic markers, including SUV_{max} [39]. In NSCLC, LMR and NLR showed a weak significant correlation with SUV_{max} [15]. In another study, SUV_{max} and LMR were independent prognostic factors in patients with stage IIIB-IV NSCLC. A novel score combining these two factors was developed and was useful for prognostication [39]. Some researchers have suggested that the underlying mechanism of such correlations is the nonspecific inflammatory response, which may reflect increased metabolism in the primary tumor [40]. Another hypothesis is related to tumor oxygenation and suggests that larger, poorly oxygenated tumors show increased FDG uptake and metabolism, which may then induce a systemic inflammatory response [15]. Our findings support such a relationship in which the pretreatment systemic inflammatory markers correlate positively with cancer's FDG metabolism markers.

The association and interaction between systemic inflammatory markers and another metabolic marker, GLUT1 expression, remains to be unexplored. The direct relationship of NLR, PLR, LMR, and GLUT1 expression in NSCLC tissues has not been studied. In our data, these systemic inflammatory marker levels were not associated with GLUT1 expression status. However, one study showed the link between GLUT1 copy number and immune biomarkers of various immune cells, such as CD20, CD8A, and CD68 [41]. In this study, GLUT1 overexpression had a negative relationship with tumor-infiltrating T-cells but a positive relationship with tumor-infiltrating neutrophils and dendritic cells [41]. The researchers of this study hypothesized that GLUT1 influences the immune microenvironment with yet unrevealed mechanisms [41].

Based on our findings, LMR was an independent prognostic factor not only in the total patient group, but also in early stage (stage I and II) patient groups. Conventionally, treatment for patients with stage I or II NSCLC is surgical resection, but it is possible that resected early stage patients with adverse prognostic factors, such as lymphovascular invasion, would benefit more from adjuvant treatment than those without [42]. In such patients, risk stratification is fundamental for adequate adjuvant therapy. In addition to conventional pathologic high-risk factors, such as lymphovascular invasion and differentiation, using systemic inflammatory factors that do not require additional tests can greatly help in designing a treatment plan. When comparing nomograms with and without LMR, the inclusion of LMR showed an increase in the C-index value from 0.65 to 0.75, representing a more accurate prediction. In individual patients with NSCLC, low LMR adds 28.7 points to the total score—that is, a decrease of approximately 5.7%—for the 2-year survival rate.

The interaction between tumors and inflammation has been studied in various cancers, including NSCLC [43]. Inflammatory cells are now thought to promote cancer onset and progression through disruption of the anti-tumor immune system and regulation of the tumor microenvironment and epigenetic alterations [44]. Monocytes are inflammatory cells that produce reactive oxygen species, reactive nitrogen species, and other cytokines, promoting DNA mutation and eventually leading to tumor progression [45]. Monocytes can potentially differentiate into tumor-associated macrophages (TAM). TAM may promote cancer progression, metastasis, and immune evasion via angiogenesis, secreting epithelial and vascular endothelial growth factors, extracellular matrix remodeling, and upregulating PD-1 expression [46]. With this underlying mechanism, a relative increase in the monocyte to lymphocyte count—that is, lower LMR—may be associated with cancer prognosis. LMR has been demonstrated as a promising prognostic marker in various solid cancers, including NSCLC [29].

Our study was limited because EGFR mutation test results were unavailable for most patients in the cohort. Most administered adjuvant therapies were non-tyrosine kinase inhibitors (TKI) and were conventional, but a few patients who experienced cancer recurrence underwent EGFR testing and received TKI therapy. Such heterogeneity in treatment methods may have affected the survival data and is thus a limitation of this study. However, a review of medical records showed that only a small number of patients (five in total) underwent TKI therapy, suggesting that the potential effects on the results of this study would have been minimal.

5. Conclusions

In this study, we showed that markers of tumor metabolic activity—GLUT1 and SUV_{max}—were positively correlated with neutrophil, platelet, and monocyte count increases in relation to lymphocyte count. GLUT1, NLR, and LMR are predictors of OS in NSCLC patients, helping to identify high-risk patients in need of close surveillance and adjuvant therapy. Further studies are warranted to investigate whether addition of these biomarkers to the current staging system could improve survival prediction, and hence support treatment decision making for patients with NSCLC.

Author Contributions: Conceptualization, U.C. and S.Y.P.; methodology, U.C.; software, U.C.; validation, U.C. and S.Y.P.; formal analysis, U.C.; investigation, U.C., S.Y.P., D.-G.C. and B.-Y.S.; resources, U.C.; data curation, U.C.; writing—original draft preparation, U.C.; writing—review and editing, S.Y.P., D.-G.C. and B.-Y.S.; visualization, U.C.; supervision, U.C.; project administration, U.C.; funding acquisition, U.C. All authors have read and agreed to the published version of the manuscript.

Funding: The authors wish to acknowledge the financial support of St. Vincent's Hospital, Research Institute of Medical Science (SVHR-2021-09).

Institutional Review Board Statement: The study was conducted according to the guidelines of the Declaration of Helsinki and approved by the Institutional Review Board of St. Vincent's Hospital (VC20SISI0017).

Informed Consent Statement: Patient consent was waived by the Institutional Review Board.

Data Availability Statement: Not applicable.

Conflicts of Interest: The authors declare no conflict of interest.

References

1. Sung, H.; Ferlay, J.; Siegel, R.L.; Laversanne, M.; Soerjomataram, I.; Jameal, A.; Bray, F. Global Cancer Statistics 2020: GLOBOCAN Estimates of Incidence and Mortality Worldwide for 36 Cancers in 185 Countries. *CA Cancer J. Clin.* **2021**, *71*, 209–249. [CrossRef] [PubMed]
2. Didkowska, J.; Wojciechowska, U.; Mańczuk, M.; Łobaszewski, J. Lung cancer epidemiology: Contemporary and future challenges worldwide. *Ann. Transl. Med.* **2016**, *4*, 150. [CrossRef] [PubMed]
3. Hanahan, D.; Weinberg, R.A. Hallmarks of Cancer: The Next Generation. *Cell* **2011**, *144*, 646–674. [CrossRef] [PubMed]
4. Pascale, R.M.; Calvisi, D.F.; Simile, M.M.; Feo, C.F.; Feo, F. The Warburg Effect 97 Years after Its Discovery. *Cancers* **2020**, *12*, 2819. [CrossRef]

5. Ancey, P.-B.; Contat, C.; Boivin, G.; Sabatino, S.; Pascual, J.; Zangger, N.; Perentes, J.Y.; Peters, S.; Abel, E.D.; Kirsch, D.G.; et al. GLUT1 Expression in Tumor-Associated Neutrophils Promotes Lung Cancer Growth and Resistance to Radiotherapy. *Cancer Res.* **2021**, *81*, 2345–2357. [CrossRef]
6. Shen, Y.M.; Arbman, G.; Olsson, B.; Sun, X.F. Overexpression of GLUT1 in colorectal cancer is independently associated with poor prognosis. *Int. J. Biol. Markers* **2011**, *26*, 166–172. [CrossRef]
7. Koh, Y.W.; Lee, S.J.; Park, S.Y. Differential expression and prognostic significance of GLUT1 according to histologic type of non-small-cell lung cancer and its association with volume-dependent parameters. *Lung Cancer* **2017**, *104*, 31–37. [CrossRef]
8. Zhang, B.; Xie, Z.; Li, B. The clinicopathologic impacts and prognostic significance of GLUT1 expression in patients with lung cancer: A meta-analysis. *Gene* **2019**, *689*, 76–83. [CrossRef]
9. Deng, Y.; Zou, J.; Deng, T.; Liu, J. Clinicopathological and prognostic significance of GLUT1 in breast cancer: A meta-analysis. *Medicine* **2018**, *97*, e12961. [CrossRef]
10. Creff, G.; Devillers, A.; Depeursinge, A.; Palard-Novello, X.; Acosta, O.; Jegoux, F.; Castelli, J. Evaluation of the Prognostic Value of FDG PET/CT Parameters for Patients With Surgically Treated Head and Neck Cancer: A Systematic Review. *JAMA Otolaryngol. Head Neck Surg.* **2020**, *146*, 471–479. [CrossRef]
11. Cacicedo, J.; Fernandez, I.; Del Hoyo, O.; Navarro, A.; Gomez-Iturriaga, A.; Pijoan, J.I.; Martinez-Indart, L.; Escudero, J.; Gomez-Suarez, J.; de Zarate, R.O.; et al. Prognostic value of maximum standardized uptake value measured by pretreatment 18F-FDG PET/CT in locally advanced head and neck squamous cell carcinoma. *Clin. Transl. Oncol.* **2017**, *19*, 1337–1349. [CrossRef]
12. Sokolović, E.; Cerić, T.; Cerić, Š.; Bešlija, S.; Vegar-Zubović, S.; Bešlić, N.; Sefić-Pašić, I.; Pašić, A. The Prognostic Value of SUVmax of 18F-FDG PET/CT in Patients with Metastatic Colorectal Cancer. *Acta Med. Acad.* **2020**, *49*, 1–8. [CrossRef]
13. Shim, J.R.; Lee, S.D.; Han, S.S.; Lee, S.J.; Lee, D.E.; Kim, S.K.; Kim, S.H.; Park, S.J.; Oh, J.H. Prognostic significance of 18F-FDG PET/CT in patients with colorectal cancer liver metastases after hepatectomy. *Eur. J. Surg. Oncol.* **2018**, *44*, 670–676. [CrossRef]
14. Wang, X.Y.; Zhao, Y.F.; Liu, Y.; Yang, Y.K.; Wu, N. Prognostic value of metabolic variables of [18F] FDG PET/CT in surgically resected stage I lung adenocarcinoma. *Medicine* **2017**, *96*, e7941. [CrossRef] [PubMed]
15. Zhao, K.; Wang, C.; Shi, F.; Huang, Y.; Ma, L.; Li, M.; Song, Y. Combined prognostic value of the SUVmax derived from FDG-PET and the lymphocyte-monocyte ratio in patients with stage IIIB-IV non-small cell lung cancer receiving chemotherapy. *BMC Cancer* **2021**, *21*, 66. [CrossRef] [PubMed]
16. Jhunjhunwala, S.; Hammer, C.; Delamarre, L. Antigen presentation in cancer: Insights into tumour immunogenicity and immune evasion. *Nat. Rev. Cancer* **2021**, *21*, 298–312. [CrossRef] [PubMed]
17. Park, H.S.; Cho, U.; Im, S.Y.; Yoo, C.Y.; Jung, J.H.; Suh, Y.J.; Choi, H.J. Loss of Human Leukocyte Antigen Class I Expression Is Associated with Poor Prognosis in Patients with Advanced Breast Cancer. *J. Pathol. Transl. Med.* **2018**, *53*, 75–85. [CrossRef]
18. Holub, K.; Conill, C. Unveiling the mechanisms of immune evasion in pancreatic cancer: May it be a systemic inflammation responsible for dismal survival? *Clin. Transl. Oncol.* **2020**, *22*, 81–90. [CrossRef]
19. Guo, G.; Yu, M.; Xiao, W.; Celis, E.; Cui, Y. Local Activation of p53 in the Tumor Microenvironment Overcomes Immune Suppression and Enhances Antitumor Immunity. *Cancer Res.* **2017**, *77*, 2292–2305. [CrossRef]
20. Nøst, T.H.; Alcala, K.; Urbarova, I.; Byrne, K.S.; Guida, F.; Sandanger, T.M.; Johansson, M. Systemic inflammation markers and cancer incidence in the UK Biobank. *Eur. J. Epidemiol.* **2021**, *36*, 841–848. [CrossRef]
21. Dupré, A.; Malik, H.Z. Inflammation and cancer: What a surgical oncologist should know. *Eur. J. Surg. Oncol.* **2018**, *44*, 566–570. [CrossRef] [PubMed]
22. Ethier, J.L.; Desautels, D.N.; Templeton, A.J.; Oza, A.; Amir, E.; Lheureux, S. Is the neutrophil-to-lymphocyte ratio prognostic of survival outcomes in gynecologic cancers? A systematic review and meta-analysis. *Gynecol. Oncol.* **2017**, *145*, 584–594. [CrossRef] [PubMed]
23. Templeton, A.J.; McNamara, M.G.; Šeruga, B.; Vera-Badillo, F.E.; Aneja, P.; Ocaña, A.; Leibowitz-Amit, R.; Sonpavde, G.; Knox, J.J.; Tran, B.; et al. Prognostic role of neutrophil-to-lymphocyte ratio in solid tumors: A systematic review and meta-analysis. *J. Natl. Cancer Inst.* **2014**, *106*, dju124. [CrossRef] [PubMed]
24. Cho, U.; Park, H.S.; Im, S.Y.; Yoo, C.Y.; Jung, J.H.; Suh, Y.J.; Choi, H.J. Prognostic value of systemic inflammatory markers and development of a nomogram in breast cancer. *PLoS ONE* **2018**, *13*, e0200936. [CrossRef]
25. Cho, U.; Sung, Y.E.; Kim, M.S.; Lee, Y.S. Prognostic Role of Systemic Inflammatory Markers in Patients Undergoing Surgical Resection for Oral Squamous Cell Carcinoma. *Biomedicines* **2022**, *10*, 1268. [CrossRef]
26. Li, B.; Zhou, P.; Liu, Y.; Wei, H.; Yang, X.; Chen, T.; Xiao, J. Platelet-to-lymphocyte ratio in advanced Cancer: Review and meta-analysis. *Clin. Chim. Acta* **2018**, *483*, 48–56. [CrossRef]
27. Jiang, S.; Liu, J.; Chen, X.; Zhen, X.; Ruan, J.; Ye, A.; Zhang, S.; Zhang, L.; Kuan, Z.; Liu, R. Platelet-lymphocyte ratio as a potential prognostic factor in gynecologic cancers: A meta-analysis. *Arch. Gynecol. Obstet.* **2019**, *300*, 829–839. [CrossRef] [PubMed]
28. Mandaliya, H.; Jones, M.; Oldmeadow, C.; Nordman, I.I. Prognostic biomarkers in stage IV non-small cell lung cancer (NSCLC): Neutrophil to lymphocyte ratio (NLR), lymphocyte to monocyte ratio (LMR), platelet to lymphocyte ratio (PLR) and advanced lung cancer inflammation index (ALI). *Transl. Lung Cancer Res.* **2019**, *8*, 886–894. [CrossRef]
29. Jin, J.; Yang, L.; Liu, D.; Li, W.M. Prognostic Value of Pretreatment Lymphocyte-to-Monocyte Ratio in Lung Cancer: A Systematic Review and Meta-Analysis. *Technol. Cancer Res. Treat.* **2021**, *20*, 1533033820983085. [CrossRef]
30. Dolan, R.D.; Lim, J.; McSorley, S.T.; Horgan, P.G.; McMillan, D.C. The role of the systemic inflammatory response in predicting outcomes in patients with operable cancer: Systematic review and meta-analysis. *Sci. Rep.* **2017**, *7*, 16717. [CrossRef]

31. Goldstraw, P.; Crowley, J.; Chansky, K.; Giroux, D.J.; Groome, P.A.; Rami-Porta, R.; Ostmus, P.E.; Rusch, V.; Sobin, L.; International Association for the Study of Lung Cancer International Staging Committee. The IASLC Lung Cancer Staging Project: Proposals for the revision of the TNM stage groupings in the forthcoming (seventh) edition of the TNM Classification of malignant tumours. *J. Thorac. Oncol.* **2007**, *2*, 706–714. [CrossRef] [PubMed]
32. Faubert, B.; DeBerardinis, R.J. Analyzing Tumor Metabolism In Vivo. *Annu. Rev. Cancer Biol.* **2017**, *1*, 99–117. [CrossRef]
33. Wahl, R.L.; Zasadny, K.; Helvie, M.; Hutchins, G.D.; Weber, B.; Cody, R. Metabolic monitoring of breast cancer chemohormonotherapy using positron emission tomography: Initial evaluation. *J. Clin. Oncol.* **1993**, *11*, 2101–2111. [CrossRef]
34. Christensen, T.N.; Andersen, P.K.; Langer, S.W.; Fischer, B.M. Prognostic Value of 18F-FDG-PET Parameters in Patients with Small Cell Lung Cancer: A Meta-Analysis and Review of Current Literature. *Diagnostics* **2021**, *11*, 174. [CrossRef]
35. Vansteenkiste, J.; Fischer, B.M.; Dooms, C.; Motersen, J. Positron-emission tomography in prognostic and therapeutic assessment of lung cancer: Systematic review. *Lancet Oncol.* **2004**, *5*, 531–540. [CrossRef] [PubMed]
36. Zhang, L.; Ren, Z.; Xu, C.; Li, Q.; Chen, J. Influencing Factors and Prognostic Value of ^{18}F-FDG PET/CT Metabolic and Volumetric Parameters in Non-Small Cell Lung Cancer. *Int. J. Gen. Med.* **2021**, *14*, 3699–3706. [CrossRef]
37. Liu, J.; Dong, M.; Sun, X.; Li, W.; Xing, L.; Yu, J. Prognostic Value of 18F-FDG PET/CT in Surgical Non-Small Cell Lung Cancer: A Meta-Analysis. *PLoS ONE* **2016**, *11*, e0146195. [CrossRef]
38. Goodwin, J.; Neugent, M.L.; Lee, S.Y.; Choe, J.H.; Choi, H.; Jenkins, D.M.R.; Ruthenborg, R.J.; Robinson, M.W.; Jeong, K.Y.; Wake, M.; et al. The distinct metabolic phenotype of lung squamous cell carcinoma defines selective vulnerability to glycolytic inhibition. *Nat. Commun.* **2017**, *8*, 15503. [CrossRef]
39. Werner, J.; Strobel, K.; Lehnick, D.; Rajan, G.P. Overall Neutrophil-to-Lymphocyte Ratio and SUVmax of Nodal Metastases Predict Outcome in Head and Neck Cancer Before Chemoradiation. *Front. Oncol.* **2021**, *11*, 679287. [CrossRef]
40. Ettinger, D.S.; Wood, D.E.; Aisner, D.L.; Akerley, W.; Bauman, J.R.; Bharat, A.; Bruno, D.S.; Chang, J.Y.; Chirieac, L.R.; D'Amico, T.A.; et al. Non–Small Cell Lung Cancer, Version 3.2022, NCCN Clinical Practice Guidelines in Oncology. *J. Natl. Compr. Cancer Netw.* **2022**, *20*, 497–530. [CrossRef]
41. Li, F.; He, C.; Yao, H.; Liang, W.; Ye, X.; Ruan, J.; Lin, L.; Zou, J.; Zhou, S.; Huang, Y.; et al. GLUT1 regulates the tumor immune microenvironment and promotes tumor metastasis in pancreatic adenocarcinoma via ncRNA-mediated network. *J. Cancer* **2022**, *13*, 2540–2558. [CrossRef] [PubMed]
42. McDonald, F.; De Waele, M.; Hendriks, L.; Faivre-Finn, C.; Dingemans, A.-M.C.; Van Schil, P.E. Management of stage I and II nonsmall cell lung cancer. *Eur. Respir. J.* **2017**, *49*, 1600764. [CrossRef] [PubMed]
43. Song, X.D.; Wang, Y.N.; Zhang, A.L.; Liu, B. Advances in research on the interaction between inflammation and cancer. *J. Int. Med. Res.* **2020**, *48*, 300060519895347. [CrossRef]
44. Karin, M.; Shalapour, S. Regulation of antitumor immunity by inflammation-induced epigenetic alterations. *Cell. Mol. Immunol.* **2022**, *19*, 59–66. [CrossRef] [PubMed]
45. Systemic Reprogramming of Monocytes in Cancer—PMC. 2022. Available online: https://www.ncbi.nlm.nih.gov/pmc/articles/PMC7528630/ (accessed on 10 November 2022).
46. Lin, S.; Fang, Y.; Mo, Z.; Lin, Y.; Ji, C.; Jian, Z. Prognostic value of lymphocyte to monocyte ratio in pancreatic cancer; a systemic review and metaanalysis including 3338 patient. *World J. Surg. Oncol.* **2020**, *18*, 186. [CrossRef]

Disclaimer/Publisher's Note: The statements, opinions and data contained in all publications are solely those of the individual author(s) and contributor(s) and not of MDPI and/or the editor(s). MDPI and/or the editor(s) disclaim responsibility for any injury to people or property resulting from any ideas, methods, instructions or products referred to in the content.

MDPI
St. Alban-Anlage 66
4052 Basel
Switzerland
www.mdpi.com

Diagnostics Editorial Office
E-mail: diagnostics@mdpi.com
www.mdpi.com/journal/diagnostics

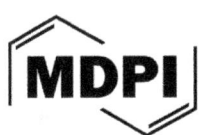

Disclaimer/Publisher's Note: The statements, opinions and data contained in all publications are solely those of the individual author(s) and contributor(s) and not of MDPI and/or the editor(s). MDPI and/or the editor(s) disclaim responsibility for any injury to people or property resulting from any ideas, methods, instructions or products referred to in the content.

www.ingramcontent.com/pod-product-compliance
Lightning Source LLC
LaVergne TN
LVHW070046120526
838202LV00101B/830